SMART MEDICINE
FOR YOUR EYES

Dr. Jeffrey Anshel

AVERY PUBLISHING GROUP

Garden City Park • New York

The therapeutic procedures in this book are based on the training, personal experiences, and research of the author. Because each person and situation are unique, the author and publisher urge the reader to check with a qualified health professional before using any procedure when there is any question regarding appropriateness.

The publisher does not advocate the use of any particular health program, but believes the information presented in this book should be available to the public.

Because there is always some risk involved, the author and publisher are not responsible for any adverse effects or consequences resulting from the use of any of the suggestions, preparations, or procedures described in this book. Please do not use this book if you are unwilling to assume the risk. Feel free to consult with a physician or other qualified health professional. It is a sign of wisdom, not cowardice, to seek a second or third opinion.

Cover designer: Doug Brooks
In-house editor: Elaine Will Sparber
Typesetter: Elaine V. McCaw and Gary A. Rosenberg
Printer: Paragon Press, Honesdale, PA

Avery Publishing Group
120 Old Broadway
Garden City Park, NY 11040
1–800–548–5757
www.averypublishing.com

The chart on page 227 is used by permission of You! Are Something Beautiful, La Hambra, CA.

Library of Congress Cataloging-in-Publishing Data

Anshel, Jeffrey.
    Smart medicine for your eyes : a guide to safe and effective
relief of common eye disorders / Jeffrey Anshel.
        p. cm.
        Includes bibliographical references and index.
        ISBN 0-89529-870-8 (pbk.)
        1. Eye—Care and hygiene—Popular works. 2. Eye—Diseases—
Popular works. I. Title.
    RE51.A633 1999
    617.7—dc21   98-51713
                                                          CIP

Contents

Part Three   Eye-Care Techniques and Procedures

Appendix

This book is dedicated to my son, Casey.
He continues to be my inspiration,
and a great example from whom I continue to learn.

Acknowledgments

No book can be written to this depth by one person alone.

I would like to thank Bill Parry, LAc, for his contribution on Chinese herbs; Pamela S. Nathan, BA, LAc, DHm (SA), and Harri Wolf, MA, for their contributions on homeopathy; and Carole Brown, herbalist, for her guidance on herb research. They were all very generous and giving of their time and knowledge.

And a special thank you to Kate Montgomery, who got the ball rolling on this project.

Preface

"The eye is the window to the soul." "An eye for an eye." "Seeing eye to eye." These are just a few of the sayings we use that indicate how important our eyes are to our everyday lives. Surveys have shown that of all our senses, the one we find the most frightening to lose is our sight. We live in a visual world. As the saying goes, "seeing is believing."

Over the past twenty years, I have been helping people to see better. It has been a very rewarding experience. However, what I have found is that most people (including me before I began to study optometry) know very little about their eyes. Parents don't know when they should have their children's eyes first examined. Parents and teachers don't realize that children's reading problems may be related to the eyes. And we all assume that getting cataracts is a normal part of the aging process. The fact is that most of us don't get eye examinations unless we have a problem.

Despite these misconceptions, however, many people are thirsty for knowledge about the eyes, but don't know where to find it. If you are like the average person, unless you have a specific eye concern, you don't go actively searching for eye-care information. And even if you go to an eye doctor, you may not get a complete picture of what your problem is and what alternatives are available in the way of treatment. Doctors in their office settings just don't have the time to explain all of the various conditions and remedies. But if you go to your doctor already possessing some general knowledge of what your problem may be and what might be available in the form of treatment, you and your doctor together can make an informed decision about what will work best for your visual well-being.

The eye-care industry, like the health-care industry in general, is going through significant changes in the face of managed care. Because of managed care, you have less access to the doctor of your choice, and you are treated more like a statistic than a patient. The bulk of your health care, including your eye care, is dependent upon your own education rather than the word of your doctor. My goal is to help you be as informed as possible.

I want this book to be a handy, yet comprehensive guide to all the vision problems that may crop up in your life. The information in this book is easily accessible, but thorough and up to date, offering the latest information on a large variety of eye problems and the possible treatments available for them. There are many things that you can do for yourself, not only to treat any eye problems that may arise, but also to prevent them. This book is not intended to undermine eye-care professionals, since they play an essential role in the care and treatment of vision problems, but to supplement their care. With the knowledge in this book and the care offered by your eye doctor, it is my hope that you will have clear vision and healthy eyes to last a lifetime.

How to Use This Book

This is an in-home guide that will help you care for your eyes through a unique approach that seeks to combine the best of conventional medicine, diet and nutritional supplementation, herbs, and homeopathy. Written by a practicing doctor of optometry, it offers advice and explanations of the full spectrum of options available to treat the many disorders related to the eyes.

This book is intended to help you make informed decisions regarding your eye care. The information and suggestions presented here are meant to be used in conjunction with the services of a trained eye doctor or other qualified health-care provider. This book is not meant to be used in place of such consultation. It is strongly suggested that if you have a problem with your eyes, you visit your eye doctor for a thorough examination, treatment, and personalized advice.

The subjects in this book have been divided into three parts. Part One, "The Elements of Eye Care," discusses the eyes and visual system, and offers suggestions on how to find eye-care providers. It also presents the basic history, theories, and practices of nutritional care, herbal therapy, and homeopathy.

Part Two, "Disorders of the Eye and Visual System," contains an alphabetic listing of the problems that commonly afflict the eyes, and outlines the different kinds of treatments appropriate for each. Every entry begins with a discussion of the problem, its causes, and how to identify the signs and symp-

toms. The treatment options follow, including recommendations for conventional treatment, nutritional supplementation, herbal treatment, and homeopathy. If emergency or first-aid treatment is appropriate, this is discussed in an inset in the margin adjacent to the entry. Many of the entries also have a section on self-treatment options including the most commonly helpful natural treatments, and general recommendations with tips for preventing the disorder or easing the symptoms. Part Two also contains a troubleshooting guide, consisting of a list of symptoms and the conditions that may be causing them; a first-aid section, providing care instructions for such eye emergencies as a black eye and corneal abrasion; and a list of common medications and their ocular side effects.

Part Three, "Eye-Care Techniques and Procedures," explains a number of the diagnostic and treatment procedures mentioned in Part Two. Eyeglasses and contact lenses, several surgical methods, vision therapy, and acupuncture and acupressure are explained and illustrated so that you will be able to discuss these options with your eye doctor.

Also included, in an appendix, are a glossary of some of the terms used in this book; a list of recommended suppliers of nutritional, herbal, and homeopathic products; and a roster of helpful resource organizations. A bibliography for further reading will guide you to books and periodicals for additional information on your particular area of concern.

Part One

The Elements of Eye Care

Introduction

You may never have thought about how easy it is for you to read the words on this page. That's because your eyes are probably doing the job pretty well. Consider the fact that over 80 percent of what you learn comes in through your eyes. That says a lot about the importance of vision in learning. You may be one of the 42 percent of Americans who don't wear corrective lenses. If so, congratulations! However, that doesn't mean you don't have a vision-related problem. More than likely, you're one of the 90 million Americans who are overdue for an eye examination. In 1997, a study showed that more people have their cars tuned than their eyes examined.

The act of seeing may seem automatic to you, so taking your eyes for granted is easy to do. We're born with two eyes that, for the most part, are fully functional at birth. However, the complex function of vision, which involves the processing and understanding of visual input, also requires learning. This learning takes place over the first decade of life, and if it doesn't occur, a child's development is impaired. Humans are visually-directed creatures; our eyes are our most important connection with the world.

Vision problems are often not painful and are usually slow to develop. Many of the problems are preventable, not just by reading letters on a chart once a year or eating a lot of carrots, but by taking a little extra time to learn about your eyes and how they work. A vision problem may start with occasional blurriness or a dull headache after reading for a short period of time. Or, you may have trouble seeing distant objects such as road signs. Your eyes may burn a bit or feel dry occasionally. Or, you may notice in the mirror that they look different. Fortunately, even if something does go wrong, you can usually correct the problem if you act quickly enough. There is such a thing as preventive eye care, and it's easier than you may think.

This book, by itself, will not give you the knowledge or the ability to cure all your eye problems or allow you to throw away your glasses. However, it will teach you about your eyes and how to interpret the messages they send, and may therefore help to keep you from being stuck behind glasses for the rest of your life—or at least from needing a stronger prescription every year. In addition, it will show you how to prevent serious eye damage or loss of vision. It's a lot easier to prevent eye problems than to reverse changes that have already taken place.

If you wear glasses, you should learn all you can about them. And, you might as well get glasses that enhance, rather than detract from, your appearance. Contact lenses are especially complicated and should be treated more like the medical devices they are than cosmetics. Whether you wear corrective lenses or not, you should have enough knowledge about vision to know when to see an eye doctor—and what kind of eye doctor to see. Studies continue to show that many people don't know if their eye-care professional is an optometrist, an optician, or an ophthalmologist.

The purpose of this book is to introduce you to the eyes and visual system, give you basic information on the fifty-six most common eye problems, provide an overview of what is available in traditional and alternative treatments for them, and guide you in finding more information. In Part One, we will discuss the various elements of eye care. Included are sections on the anatomy and physiology of the visual system, the development of vision, finding an eye-care professional, and the effects of nutrition on vision. Also offered are introductions to herbal therapy and homeopathy. Part One serves as the foundation for the subsequent information presented in the book.

The format of the book is simple, yet the facts presented are wide-ranging. The information is up to date and based on available research, my personal experiences, and common sense. My intention is for this book to be a comprehensive reference on eye care and eye health. It should answer your most common questions about your eyes and the way you see. I've tried to present the information in terms that are simple to understand, yet technical enough to accurately explain how your vision works. My hope is that this book will open your eyes to the world of vision and teach you about your eyes so that you can talk intelligently with your doctor about your vision problems. I also hope to dispel some myths about what's good for your eyes and what isn't. Should you have any questions about your condition or the appropriate treatment, contact an eye-care professional. In the meantime, here's looking at you!

The Eyes and Visual System

I'd like to introduce you to a part of your body that you don't see very much—your eyes. Since you're always seeing *with* your eyes, you don't often get a chance to look *at* them. You've got two fascinating organs of your own body that are available for you to observe, and I hope you'll get to know them well. So, get ready. You're about to start a fascinating trip into the world of vision. This book is not meant to be a technical medical synopsis of the anatomy and physiology of the human visual system. However, it is intended to give you at least a general understanding of how the eye is put together and how it works because you should have some background knowledge with which to make intelligent decisions regarding vision disorders and treatments. We'll start with some basic eye anatomy so that you will know what's what and where it is. Then we'll look at how the parts work together to create the fascinating sense of vision.

LOOK AT YOUR EYES

The eyeball is basically that—a ball. Its diameter is roughly one inch, and its circumference is about three inches. The part of the eye that is visible to the world—between the eyelids—is actually only one-sixth of the eye's total surface area. The remaining five-sixths of the eyeball is hidden behind the eyelids. The outer surface of the eye is divided into two parts—the *sclera* (SKLER-ah), the white part that is the outer covering of the eye, and the *cornea* (KOR-nee-ah), the transparent membrane in front of the eye. (For an illustration of the eye, see Figure 1.1, above right.) The cornea, which is steeper in curvature than the sclera, may be difficult to see because it is transparent and backed by the colored *iris* (EYE-ris). You can see the cornea easier if you look at a friend's eye from the side. The sclera is made of tough fibers, which allow

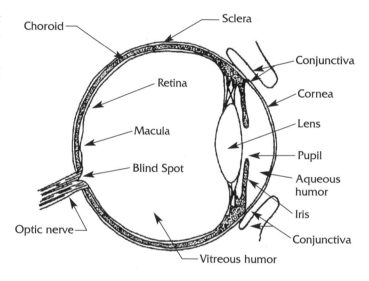

Figure 1.1. The eye.

it to perform its function of supporting the contents of the eyeball. It has a white appearance because the fibers are light in color and because it contains very few blood vessels.

Just inside the sclera and covering all of the same area is the *choroid* (KOH-royd), which is the main blood supply to the inner eyeball. Just inside the choroid is the *retina* (RET-in-ah), the nerve membrane that receives the light. A small but important area of the retina is the *fovea* (FOE-vee-ah). The fovea is the area used for sharp, detailed vision, needed for threading a needle or spotting a distant object, for example.

In addition to the blood vessels of the choroid, there are also blood vessels that enter the eye through the *optic nerve* and lie on the front surface of the retina. They supply nutrition to the retina and the other structures inside the eye. These parts all seem to be very basic when you think of what an eye must do.

The eye needs protection and support (provided by the sclera), a blood supply (provided by the vessels in the choroid and optic nerve), and a mechanism for seeing (provided by the retina).

When you look at an eye, the first thing you notice is the iris. If you look closely at the eye, you'll see that the iris is actually enclosed in what's known as a *chamber* (a closed space). The iris is also surrounded by a watery fluid called the *aqueous* (AY-kwee-us) *humor*, or *aqueous fluid*. The aqueous humor doesn't have anything to do with being funny; *humor* is just the Latin word for fluid. Just behind the iris is the *lens*, which facilitates focusing. The lens, also known as the crystalline lens, is transparent and can't really be seen from the outside unless special equipment is used. Behind the lens, and filling the main chamber within the eye, is the *vitreous* (VIT-ree-us) *humor*. The vitreous humor is more gel-like and less watery than the aqueous humor, and helps in the support of the retina and other structures.

HOW THE EYE WORKS

Let's look at the visual process by starting at the beginning. Light enters the eye by passing through the cornea, the aqueous humor, and the pupil; is focused by the lens; and then goes through the vitreous humor and on to the retina. The retina is actually an extension of the brain, since the nerve fibers from the retina go directly into the brain.

When light strikes the retina, it stimulates chemical changes in the light-sensitive cells of the retina, known as the *photoreceptors*. There are actually two kinds of photoreceptors—rods, which are long, slender cells that respond to light or dark stimuli and are important to night vision; and cones, which are cone-shaped, respond to color stimuli, and therefore are also called color receptors. There are about seventeen times as many rods as cones, or about 120 million rods and 7 million cones, in the retina of each eye. These rods and cones interconnect and converge to form networks of nerve fibers. About 1 million nerve fibers make up each optic nerve.

When the rods and cones are struck by light, they convert the light energy to nerve energy; we'll call this nerve energy a "visual impulse." This impulse travels out of the eye into the brain via the optic nerve at a speed of 423 miles per hour. It first reaches the middle of the brain, where a pair of "relay stations" combine the visual information the impulse is carrying with other sensory information. The impulse then travels to the very back part of the brain, the *visual cortex*. It is here that the brain interprets the shapes of objects and the spatial organization of scenes, and recognizes the visual patterns as belonging to known objects—for example, it recognizes that a flower is a flower. Further visual processing is done at the sides of the brain, known as the *temporal lobes*. Once the brain has interpreted this vital information about something the eyes have "seen," it instantaneously transfers the information to the different areas of the brain that must play a part in the response. For example, if the information is that a car is moving toward you, it is relayed to the motor cortex, which is the area that controls movement and enables you to get out of the car's way. The motor cortex is located in a band that goes over the top of your head from just above one ear to just above the other ear.

So, vision is really the combination of the eyeball receiving light and the brain interpreting the signals from the eye. We will discuss this process of vision in more detail in the next chapter.

REFRACTIVE ERRORS

The process I've just described is how the normal eye and visual system function when working perfectly well. This condition of the eye being optically normal is called *emmetropia* (em-e-TROH-pee-ah). (For an illustration of an emmetropic eye, see Figure 1.2 below.) Not all eyes, unfortunately, are emmetropic. Very often, there is something that goes wrong, and the visual process is disrupted. About 50 percent of the adults in the United States have difficulty seeing clearly at a distance, and about 60 percent have diffi-

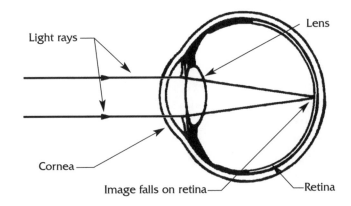

Figure 1.2. The emmetropic eye.

culty seeing up close with no corrective lenses. One of the more common problems is the misfocusing of light as it is directed onto the retina. Light can be focused too soon, it can be focused too late, or it can be distorted. Because the bending of light is technically called refraction, the misfocusing of light in the eye is called a *refractive error*.

First, let's define the necessary terms. *Nearsightedness*, also called myopia (my-OH-pee-ah), means having good near vision but poor distance vision. For the nearsighted person, a distant image (the image of something at least twenty feet away) falls in front of the retina and looks blurred. Nearsightedness results when an eye is too long, when the cornea is too steeply curved, when the eye's lens is unable to relax enough to provide accurate distance vision, or from some combination of these and other factors. (For an illustration of a nearsighted eye, see Figure 1.3, below.)

Farsightedness, also called hyperopia (hy-per-OH-pee-ah), is not exactly the opposite of nearsightedness. For the farsighted person, the image of an object that is twenty or more feet away is directed past the retina, so that it looks blurred because it hasn't yet been brought into focus. Farsightedness results when an eye is too short or a cornea too flat, or from some combination of these and other factors. (For an illustration of a farsighted eye, see Figure 1.4, above right.) The main difference between nearsightedness and farsightedness is that the eye can increase its focal power (to some degree) to compensate for farsightedness, but it cannot reduce its power to compensate for nearsightedness.

Theoretically, the surface of the cornea should be almost spherical in shape, like the surface of a ball, so that when light passes through it, it can be focused at a single point. However, nature isn't always perfect, and

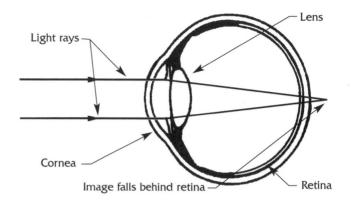

Figure 1.4. The farsighted eye.

the cornea is often "warped," resembling a barrel more than a ball. The lens, too, can be irregular in shape. These distortions can be significant enough so that light passing through the cornea and lens in the vertical orientation will focus at a different spot than light passing through in the horizontal orientation. Now you have two points of focus with a blur in between. This is known as *astigmatism* (a-STIG-ma-tism). (For an illustration of an astigmatic eye, see Figure 1.5, below.)

If the difference between these two points of focus is great enough, the eye will strain trying to decide which point of focus it should use. You might then develop occasional blurring of vision, tiring of the eyes, and headaches. Astigmatism in small amounts is very common and not of great concern. But, about 23 million Americans have significant amounts of astigmatism, requiring correction. Glasses correct astigmatism because the curvature of the eyeglass lens compensates for the curvature of the eye. This is a simple optical correction.

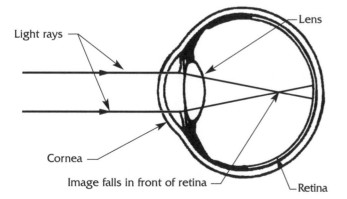

Figure 1.3. The nearsighted eye.

Figure 1.5. The astigmatic eye.

Glasses, however, will not change the amount of astigmatism—that is, they won't "cure" the problem.

SEEING CLEARLY NOW

Recall the last time you visited your eye doctor's office. You were probably given a full examination, had what seemed like a hundred different tests, and asked, "How are my eyes?" Your doctor may have said, "You have twenty-twenty vision!" You then walked out of the office satisfied that your eyes are in good shape. But are they? What does "twenty-twenty," written as "20/20" for short, refer to, and what does it mean?

The term "20/20" is a notation that relates to the resolving power of the eye. An eye's resolving power is its sharpness of sight, which we can define as the ability to distinguish two points from each other and not see them as just one point. This resolution occurs at its maximum in the fovea portion of the retina. If your vision is 20/20, it means that you can see at twenty feet what the "optically normal" eye can see at twenty feet—that is, your eyes can distinguish one point from another in a specific line of characters on a standard eye chart placed twenty feet away. The standard eye chart is called a Snellen chart. If your vision is, let's say, 20/40, it means that you can see at twenty feet what the normal eye can see at forty feet. You

have to be closer to the object than normal. And, if your vision is 20/100, you must be at twenty feet to see what the normal eye can see clearly at one hundred feet away. In short, the larger the bottom number is, the poorer is your resolving power, which is also known as your *visual acuity*. Visual acuity is measured for distance and near vision. So now you know that 20/20 is something like a grading, or scaling, of eyesight.

BLIND SPOTS

When you were in grade school, someone probably told you that everyone has blind spots in their eyes. I'm sure you looked and looked, but you could always see everything you looked at. This one is hard to believe if you haven't seen it for yourself. (To see it for yourself, take the blind-spot test, below.)

You know that the back of the inside of your eye is covered with the retina, which receives light and transmits nerve impulses to the brain. The cells in the retina are connected to nerve fibers that collectively make up the optic nerve, which leads to the brain. The area where the optic nerve leaves the retina heading for the brain is not covered with retinal cells, but serves solely as the exit for the nerve fibers. Since there are no cells to receive light, no perception occurs

Blind-Spot Test

The following test will help you locate the blind spots in your eyes. There is one blind spot in each eye.

1. Look at the illustration below. There is a plus sign on the left side of the page, and a large dot on the right side.

2. Hold the illustration six inches from your face. To test your right eye, cover your left eye and look at the plus sign.

3. Slowly move the illustration back to about twelve inches from your face. The dot on the right side of the page will disappear from the corner of your vision at about the twelve-inch point. You may have to move the illustration around a bit to get this effect because the blind spot is not very big. Keep the uncovered eye still and directed straight ahead.

To test your left eye, repeat the steps, but keep your right eye covered and look at the large dot.

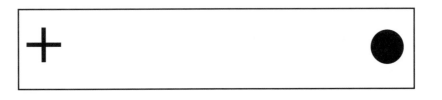

in this area; this area is actually blind. This blind area is called the *optic disk*.

Okay, you say skeptically, if your eyes have blind spots, why don't you see empty space in those areas? Well, if you remember, you have two eyes. Each of your eyes has a *visual field*, or area of visual perception. The fields of your two eyes overlap quite a bit, so there is a large area of *binocular* (two-eyed) *vision*. The blind spot in one eye is overlapped by a seeing portion of the other eye, so if both your eyes are open and functioning, you don't have any gaps in your visual field.

Blind spots are significant in the detection of eye diseases and other conditions, including brain tumors. For example, the eye disease glaucoma (glaw-KOH-mah), which involves an increase in the pressure in the eye, will cause the blind spot to enlarge. (For a discussion of glaucoma, see page 138.) Tracking the changes in the size of the blind spot can give a doctor information about the progression of a disease. If you ever perceive a blind area in your vision—other than the normal one just discussed—be sure to have it checked immediately.

PERIPHERAL VISION

Right now, you're reading the words on this page with (I hope) both your eyes. You have your eyes pointed at these words, and all you are really aware of is the page you see. But if someone were to sneak up behind you and then slowly come around to your side, you'd probably see the person move and know he or she was there (assuming the person didn't tip you off by knocking over a chair). But how could you see someone off to your side if your eyes are looking here? You'd be using your *peripheral (side) vision*, which accounts for a large percentage of your whole visual field. Your visual field is all you can see at one time without turning your head. A normal visual field extends about 170 degrees around, although certain conditions can narrow it. In fact, one definition of legal blindness is a visual field of less than 20 degrees. (For a discussion of legal blindness, also known as low vision, see page 162.)

About half of the inside of your eye is lined with the retina. When you look straight at an object, you line up that object with the *macula* (MAC-yoo-lah), a tiny, one-square-millimeter area of the retina that gives you the sharpest vision possible. So, there's a whole lot of retina that isn't completely "tuned in" to where you're looking. But, when people come up beside you, they move enough to alert the rest of your retina that something is there. Peripheral vision is very important when driving a car, for example, because you use it to catch glimpses of the cars on either side of you without actually turning your head or eyes completely to the side.

To test your peripheral vision, you'll need the help of a friend. You and your friend should sit facing each other, about two feet apart and at roughly the same eye level. (For an illustration of this positioning, see Figure 1.6, below.) You'll also need an object that you can hold at a slight distance from your hand, such as the eraser on a pencil. Have your friend cover one eye, and you cover the opposite eye. For example, your friend covers his or her right eye, and you cover your left eye. Look directly into each other's open eyes without moving. Now, with the pencil in your right hand, extend the eraser as far to your right as you can reach. Then, slowly bring the eraser in toward you and your friend, keeping it on an imaginary line midway between the two of you. You'll need to bend your elbow to do this. Both you and your friend should see the eraser come into view out of the corners of your eyes at about the same time. Be sure it's the eraser you see and not the pencil. If one person sees the eraser *much* sooner than the other, the one who sees it last might have decreased peripheral vision and should contact an eye doctor. A difference of four inches may be significant.

Now, do the technique again, but this time bring the eraser in from your left side. Then repeat the technique twice more, bringing the eraser down from over

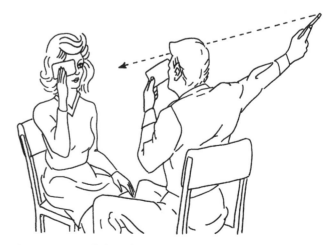

Figure 1.6. Peripheral Vision Test.

your head and up from your knees. Do the entire technique for the opposite eyes. Each time, both you and your friend should see the eraser at about the same time.

This home peripheral-vision test will pick up only very significant problems. For more accurate testing to find subtle defects in your visual field, see your eye doctor.

BINOCULAR VISION

Seeing a clear 20/20 is certainly a good indication that your eyes are doing their job well. However, sharp eyesight is just one of the functions that your eyes perform. Since there are two eyes, they must work in harmony with each other. One of the most fascinating abilities of the visual system is to take the images from the two eyes and put them together into one picture. This process is called *binocular vision*. You don't normally see two pictures, so the idea might sound strange, but double vision can occur and is one of the most dangerous manifestations of a vision problem. Imagine seeing two cars coming toward you as you drive down the road!

Here's how the brain keeps us from going off the road. Let's assume that you have two eyes that are working about equally well. As you look at an object, each eye receives an individual image of it. Both of these images are transmitted back to your brain, where they are "fused" together into one picture. In order for that to happen, however, both of your eyes must be pointed at the same object, at the same spot, with the images approximately equal in size and clarity.

Now, if one eye is not aimed at the same spot as the other, each eye will "see" a slightly different view of the object, and the two images won't match up. When these images are then transmitted back to the brain, they will stimulate two different groups of brain cells, and you will experience two pictures, otherwise known as "seeing double." After a short time, your brain will decide to turn off, or *suppress*, the image from the eye that is pointed in the wrong direction so that you can see one picture again. This suppression is necessary for our visual survival, but it is not the way we were meant to see.

Suppression of an image is the brain's way of making our daily tasks easy and comfortable in stressful situations. Thus, while you might think that suppression of an image is devastating, it actually works pretty well.

What is more serious, however, is *competition* between the eyes, when the eyes must struggle to work together. This problem is much more common than suppression. It is competition that causes a person to grapple with reading tasks, and that can lead to poor reading comprehension and job performance. Adequate binocular function is important for many common tasks. (For complete discussions of double vision and suppression, see pages 123 and 201, respectively.)

COLOR VISION

Color vision is actually nothing more than the perception of different wavelengths of light. This perception is accomplished by the cones in the retina. Color vision is a hereditary trait, as is color deficiency. (For a discussion of color deficiency, see "Colorblindness" on page 103.)

Before we can talk about color vision, we need to go over some of the basics of the nature of light. When light rays come from a source of light, they radiate from the light source like the waves formed in water when a rock hits its surface. These light waves travel in varying lengths, some shorter than others. The unit of length used to measure light waves is the nanometer (nan-AHM-iter), which is one millionth of a millimeter, or one billionth of a meter.

The range of light that humans can see is called visible light, and is the light with a wavelength of between 400 and 700 nanometers. (Ultraviolet light has a wavelength of less than 400 nanometers, and infrared light has a wavelength of more than 700 nanometers.) When white light bounces off a red apple, the apple absorbs all of the light rays except for those with a wavelength of about 650 nanometers. These light rays it reflects. Humans have learned to call this particular wavelength of reflected light "red." Each color that humans can see has its own wavelength—blue is about 460 nanometers, green is about 520 nanometers, and yellow is about 575 nanometers. When we perceive a colored object, what we see is that part of the light spectrum that is not absorbed by the object, but rather reflected back to our eyes.

As strange as it may seem, we still don't know for sure what happens in the retina and brain to enable us to have color vision. However, we do have some theories on the subject.

The trichromatic (try-kroh-MA-tik), meaning "three-color," theory says that there are three different types of cones in the retina. There are cones that respond to the color red, cones that respond to blue, and cones that respond to green. When these cones receive a light stimulus, they send a message to the brain via nerve fibers. Color mixing is accomplished by the cones firing in varying proportions, so that the color we perceive is a combination of the signals coming from the three types of cones. White, for example, is perceived when the red, blue, and green cones fire together.

This is a pretty good working model for color vision, but it's probably not the whole story. There are probably receptors that transmit light stimuli of particular wavelengths from the retina to the brain, and other receptors that inhibit light stimuli of particular wavelengths. The color we actually perceive is probably a result of some "yes" receptors and some "no" receptors sending messages to the brain. The eyes of humans can perceive about 7 million colors.

The quick little vision tests presented in this chapter are intended to help you become more familiar with your eyes and how they work. These tests will also tell you if your eyes are working properly. If you suspect that something may be amiss with your eyes, consult your eye doctor to confirm your suspicions. The more information you can take with you to your eye exam, the easier it will be for your doctor to detect any problems.

The Development of Vision

Since the vast majority of children are born with two eyes situated in the proper positions in their heads, it is easy to understand why we take seeing for granted. Children just assume that vision is "there," and that they see fine from the very beginning of life. Yet, as children grow, their eyes must develop along with the rest of their bodies or their maturation may be hindered. Young children with vision problems may think that everyone sees the way they do. They may not realize that they're supposed to be able to see the leaves on a tree from across the street or the letters on a blackboard from the rear of a classroom. These children may not know they have a problem. But the estimates are that one out of every twenty preschool children in the United States has a vision problem that will eventually lead to a needless loss of sight or a severe learning disability. Between 80 and 85 percent of our learning comes through vision. Vision is our most important sense. Most vision problems can be corrected if detected early. So, as a parent, it is your job to talk with your child and find out what is happening with his or her vision. Your child's vision is your responsibility.

This chapter will show you some techniques for testing your child's vision and for helping to improve his or her visual perception. If you have any doubts about whether your child's vision is developing on schedule, I advise you to consult your pediatrician or eye doctor. Developmental optometrists have a special interest in children's eyes and how they relate to the general maturation of children.

NORMAL VISION DEVELOPMENT

A child's eyeball closely resembles an adult's in structure and size by the age of three, with some growth and refinement continuing into adulthood. The macula is not refined at birth and must develop as the child grows. However, there is much more to vision than the physical structure of the eyeball—the "more" being the difference between "seeing" and "vision."

Visual perception develops in an individualized manner in every person, each person's way of seeing being just a little different from the next person's. This is due to the variety of stimuli that children receive (or don't receive) as they grow up. There is an ancient proverb that states, "We see things not as they are, but as we are." However, there are predictable stages of vision development, and they coincide with the *motor development*—the development of the large and small muscle movements—in a child's body.

At one time, people believed that the eyes were just two little balls that sat in the front of the face to catch light. But for many years now, we have known that the eyes are an integral part of the central nervous system and are very much influenced by the other parts of the body. As the body develops, so do the eyes. Vision is not a separate function, but is integrated with the total "action system" of the child, including posture, manual skills and coordination, intelligence, and even personality traits. This is the total vision process.

The development of the muscular system and the visual system together is known as *visual-motor development*. Although vision is one of our senses, the actions surrounding the visual process are motor, or muscle, driven. When we are awake, our eyes constantly respond to shifts in our body posture, or they initiate shifts. Thus, vision influences and is influenced by the sensitive patterns of movement of the total person. An excellent way to illustrate this point is to stand on one foot with your eyes looking straight ahead. Once you feel stable and secure, close your eyes. How quickly did you lose your balance?

And, just as it's possible to have poor coordination between two body parts, it is also possible to have poor coordination between the eyes and another body part, or even between the two eyes.

NORMAL VISUAL-MOTOR DEVELOPMENT

Motor development begins in infancy and continues throughout childhood. In the following description of normal motor and visual-motor development in children, any references to ages are approximations only. It is the sequence of development that is important. If you have any questions about your child's development, consult your pediatrician.

At birth, infants have only reflexes with which to work. However, these reflexes shape the patterns of their motor development.

The first basic motor patterns to develop are the *gross motor movements*. "Gross motor" refers to the movements of the large muscles, such as those in the arms and legs. The gross motor movements are crawling, standing, walking, moving the whole legs and arms, moving the head and neck, and other large-muscle actions. These movements are necessary for normal growth and development, enabling babies to move in space and use the perceptual tool that is the most developed during babyhood—touch.

Babies' explorations and touching experiments eventually lead to the second basic motor pattern—*fine motor movements*. Fine motor movements involve the small muscles and include finger bending, toe wiggling, wrist and ankle movements, and other subtle motor actions. These types of motor movements are necessary for fine manipulation and, in general, more detailed inspection of the environment by infants. Fine motor coordination is more difficult to achieve if the gross motor abilities did not develop on schedule.

The *oculomotor skills* develop simultaneously with the gross and fine motor skills. The eyes are controlled by the muscles that surround them and are directly connected to the brain. "Oculomotor development" refers to the development of the eye-related muscles and their coordination. Efficient eye movement is essential for good eyesight and good vision. The six *extraocular* (outside the eye) muscles have to be able to align each eye with a visual target, and the *intraocular* (inside the eye) muscles must be able to focus the light on the retina in order for the person to see the visual target. In addition, the movements of both eyes have to be coordinated in order to avoid excess strain or double vision. Once oculomotor development is underway, children can begin to "feel" with their eyes. The process starts slowly. At six to twelve months of age, touch is still children's main avenue of perception. But, once the eye muscles begin to coordinate with each other at about twelve to fifteen months, the majority of sensory input begins to be transferred to the eyes. Eventually, children don't have to crawl or walk across a room to identify an object by touch, but can merely look at it and see what it is.

The next phase of development is called *hand-eye coordination*. Hand-eye coordination is the ability of the brain to take in information through the eyes and speedily transfer it to the hands and back again. This ability takes off at around the age of two (although it is present to some degree well before that), but it really develops continually throughout life. Learning to play a sport at any age is a continuing process of developing hand-eye coordination.

As the visual system matures and oculomotor control increases, the first aspects of *form perception* begin to develop. Loosely defined, form perception is the perception of, first, the shapes of objects and, eventually, more abstract things, such as words on a page. Form perception starts as the perception of forms by oral investigation. Then, once fine motor development has been established, form perception is transferred to the fingers. Eventually, it is transferred to the eyes, with children recognizing forms from a distance based on previous experiences. *Advanced form perception* includes figure-ground discrimination (seeing the main form as different from the background), as well as perception of general shapes, size differentiation, differentiation of the details of configuration, and directional orientation. Research has shown that when experienced readers read, they don't perceive individual letters or even words, but rather "forms." Form perception is a complex process for the brain and the visual system to master, and it is crucial for good reading.

One aspect of advanced form perception is *laterality*. Laterality is the ability to perceive left and right in reference to your own body, and it begins to develop at about the age of five or six. After laterality comes *directionality*, which is the ability to make left-right distinctions for things other than yourself—say, for other people or objects in the room, or for letters on a piece of paper. This kind of perception usually develops at around the age of six or seven. If children can't tell their left from their right or can't make left-right distinctions for other objects, then words and letters don't have any meaning. The letter "p" may look the same as the letter "q," and "b" may look the same as "d," for example. These confusions, called *reversals*, are common and expected up to about the age of seven or eight. After that, children who still reverse letters need some help in figuring out which way is up! I'll describe some methods to help them later in this chapter.

The next step in the development of visual-motor skills is *visual memory*—the ability to recall visual images including everything from Mother's face to yesterday's dinner to a list of spelling words. Visual memory begins at about six months of age, but continues to develop as children mature. It is essential for the retention of written material, and is, in fact, one measure of intelligence.

A LOOK AT THE WHOLE CHILD

Children's eyes are closely influenced by their ever-changing muscle systems. Visual defects and deviations from the norm may not be apparent if all you look for is sharpness of vision such as can be measured using an eye chart. Vision problems in children may make themselves known as poor coordination, awkwardness, poor timing, hesitation, and sometimes lack of body movement. If you have any doubts about your child's visual-motor development, don't wait too long to have it checked out by a pediatrician or developmental optometrist.

Before Birth

The first rudiments of the eyes are evident in the fetus at the ripe age of twenty days after conception. The first trimester (first three months) of pregnancy is the most critical time for the eyes. Good nutrition, good prenatal care, and avoidance of medications and other chemicals (such as alcohol and tobacco) are all important for the development of the fetus's visual system.

There are some traits that are genetically determined, and eye color is one. All Caucasian babies are born with "blue" eyes because very little pigment has accumulated in their irises by birth. As children grow, more pigment is deposited in the iris, and it begins to look darker. The final eye color depends on how

much pigment has accumulated. A blue eye simply has less pigment than a brown eye does, and a green or hazel eye is somewhere in between.

Another hereditary trait is color deficiency. The gene for color deficiency is carried on the mother's X chromosome. Females have two X chromosomes, and males have an X and a Y. For a boy to develop color deficiency, he needs to have inherited only one defective X chromosome, from his mother. For a girl to develop color deficiency, she must have two defective X chromosomes—one from her mother and one from her father. This is the reason color deficiency is so much more common in boys than girls (8 percent of males are color deficient, compared to only .5 percent of females).

Nearsightedness, lazy eye, and strabismus (crossed eyes, wall eyes, or eyes turned upward or downward) do seem to "run in families," but I'm not convinced that genes are entirely to blame for these conditions. Children's genetic makeup may make them more or less likely to develop eye problems in any given environment, but it's my belief that the way children use their eyes in that environment can affect their vision. So, if you're nearsighted, don't throw up your hands and say, "I guess Johnny will be nearsighted, too." Start Johnny off right with regular eye examinations and good visual habits. Don't wait until it's too late.

Newborns

You might think that there is nothing that can be "tested" in newborn children. However, it is possible to do some eye testing on newborn babies. No, you can't hold an eye chart in front of your infant! However, there are certain visual reflexes that are present at birth, and you should know what they are and how to test for them, or ask your pediatrician to test for them.

The *pupil reflex* to light is present at birth and can easily be tested by shining a small light into either eye. When the light hits the pupil, *both* pupils should become smaller. The pupils should be approximately the same size and should stay small as long as the light is shined into the eye. (Adult eyes react the same way.)

To test for the *doll's-eye reflex*, gently nod your child's head back and forth as you look into his or her eyes. Notice whether the baby tries to compensate and keep looking at you. This is what the baby should do. This reflex was named after old-fashioned dolls of the more expensive type, which had eyes that swiveled as if to keep looking at you as you turned the doll's head.

The *blink reflex* is the fastest reflex in the body. This is a good indication of the importance of preserving our eyesight. Very carefully blow a tiny puff of air at your baby's eyes. (Do this very gently!) The eyes should blink immediately.

Our vision is dependent on these reflexes being present at birth, and visual development builds on these abilities. These reflexes are simple to test, so if you are unsure of the results, please contact your pediatrician immediately to confirm them.

Infants and Toddlers

During the first year of life, babies make the greatest leaps in development. They turn from helpless beings who sleep through most of the day into active toddlers interested in exploring all of the sights and sounds filling their worlds. Following are some rough guidelines you can use in evaluating your child's developing vision. If you have any doubts or questions about your child's eyes, contact your pediatrician or eye doctor.

At *one month old*, babies usually stare blankly around the room, although a bright light or window light should attract their attention. Occasionally, they will follow for a little bit an object brought in front of their face. Contrary to popular belief, babies are not born blind. However, the macula of the retina is not completely developed at birth, so babies' visual acuity is poor. (It gradually improves, until they ideally have a visual acuity of 20/20 at about the age of five or six years.)

At *two months old*, babies display a few additional eye movements, although these movements are still limited. At this age, children generally start to realize what their parents' faces look like and may be able to distinguish them from just any faces. This is the first indication of visual memory. Some authorities believe that babies are "programmed" to recognize faces better than other kinds of visual patterns. In terms of evolution and infant survival, this makes good sense.

At *three months old*, babies are able to follow a dangling object from one end of their visual gaze to the other, although their eye movements may be unsteady. If they get hold of a rattle, they may look at it occasionally. At this stage, babies prefer using the mouth over the eyes for investigational purposes. But,

since any kind of investigation that babies do is important to their developing vision, be sure to keep plenty of clean, harmless toys close by. Gross motor development at this point usually consists of lifting the head and chest when lying prone, as well as kicking the legs in random movements.

At *four months old*, babies stop occasionally to visually inspect things, such as their hands or a toy. Their head movements are more pronounced and should be more independent of their eye movements. This is the early stage of oculomotor development.

At *five months old*, babies may try to keep an object in sight as it is brought to their mouth. They release their fixation in an unsteady manner.

At *six months old*, babies are able to follow an object for a few seconds, although they may lose it to follow another object. Their eye movements are more fluid now, and any interest in an object across the room should be encouraged to help them learn about size and distance. Six-month-old children need plenty of room to crawl and explore. Their gross motor development is much more apparent now as their movement expands. They generally roll around and attempt to lift themselves upright now. As their fine motor development also progresses, they may attempt to manipulate toys, and their hands become more independent. Their movements are beginning to integrate all the parts of their body, matching sight with other kinds of perception, such as touch and hearing.

At *seven months old*, babies have noticeably improved eye movements, specifically convergence. They are now able to converge their eyes to inspect a toy at a close range, although they may momentarily lose this fixation and then regain it. Their hand-eye coordination begins to become refined, as they feel more comfortable with fine motor movements such as lifting a toy to inspect it. Their large muscles now allow them to sit up and start creeping.

At *eight months old*, babies begin to manipulate objects with more sophistication, turning the objects about in their hands to explore them visually. They may hold one toy while manipulating another. They become more aware of the space outside their reach and will watch other people across the room. They are well into crawling now. During the second six months of life, infants need plenty of crawling opportunities. Crawling is an important stage of development that allows children to fully integrate all of their major muscle groups with their perceptual abilities—at ground level. Unfortunately, many parents are too anxious for their little Johnny or Mary to walk and try to hurry their child through the crawling stage. Don't rush your child. I've seen many learning-disabled children with behavior problems who walked at an early age without the benefit of crawling.

At *ten months old*, babies are able to more easily move their head and trunk. Vertical surfaces become intriguing as they prepare to stand. Their eye muscles and large muscles work together in this process. Children now start to see the "whole" of objects, which is a rudimentary form of perception.

At *twelve months old*, babies have mastered their vertical orientation. Walking with assistance and standing alone temporarily indicate that gross motor development is proceeding on schedule. Visually, eye movements are more refined, and children may at times display unusual facial expressions as part of this process. Smooth, easy visual pursuit of objects and increased mobility of the eyes become apparent. Eye movements now are not necessarily associated with head movements.

Preschoolers

Between the ages of two and five years old, children make great strides toward adult visual capabilities. Their vision, as well as body and brain, get ready for the challenges of school and formal learning, including reading and writing. The guidelines presented here will help you to evaluate your preschooler's visual development. Again, the guidelines are rough. However, if your child's abilities deviate considerably from the norm, contact your pediatrician or eye doctor. Most problems are easier to correct before children enter school, when one problem can lead to another in a domino effect. (See "A Child's-Eye View," below.)

At *two years old*, children generally have good footing—good enough to be able to run without falling (well, at least some of the time). They use their eyes more responsively, watching what they do as they do it. The eyes and hands are less closely associated now than they were earlier, so children usually look, then act, instead of doing both simultaneously. Whirling disks and brightly colored objects are quite a source of

A Child's-Eye View

Let's say that right now you're sitting on a chair at a desk, reading. You are well aware of the distance from yourself to the desk, from the desk to the wall, from the room to the rest of the house. If you shift your attention from this book to the refrigerator in your kitchen, you remain aware of the book's location so you can return to it after eating without spending ten minutes looking for it around the house.

Now think of how preschool-aged children relate to these things. Each time they shift their attention from one object to another, they forget where the original object is. It's not really just poor memory; it's actually an inability to relate to spatial locations in their visual world until the age of about five or six years. If, for some reason, children are a little late at comprehending these spatial relationships and can't keep them straight in their heads, they can't progress in their development. Every new experience builds on the previous ones, and if a previous problem isn't conquered, a tool is missing for tackling the next.

What does all this have to do with children's vision and achievement? Just this: If children have a perceptual "lag" that persists into the school years, they may have trouble with arithmetic and spelling. They won't understand that two plus two equals four because this is a relationship among three different objects. They may have trouble remembering that the letters "g" and "o" spell "go" because these letters do this only if they are arranged in that particular order. A child who can't tell left from right (a spatial relationship) might come out with "og." This may be the basis of the reversals commonly seen in poor achievers and children with learning disabilities. As an adult, these problems may be difficult to understand unless you have experienced them yourself.

It's important to be aware of perception from a child's point of view. If you are, it will be easier to find ways to help your child catch on to what should be accomplished. This can easily be achieved by giving your child rich experiences with shapes, movements, and distances, and by scheduling regular eye examinations starting at the age of one year (earlier, if you suspect a problem). Then, all your child will need is love.

fascination at this age. Small objects might be studied with more intensity than before, a sure sign of increased visual discrimination. The attention span at this age is about seven minutes.

At *three years old*, children are definitely more organized in their actions than they were at two. Their hand-eye activities are more unified—they will color within the lines of pictures, and they can use their hands more freely without having their eyes riveted to them. Their eyes may take a more directive role, often not accompanied by head movements anymore, leading where they had previously been following. An increase in space orientation is evident; children know where they are and know more about where other objects are in relation to themselves. *Eye teaming*, in which the two eyes function as one unit, continues to develop. (To test one aspect of your child's ability to use both eyes together, see "Cover Test," below.) The attention span is about nine minutes now.

At *four years old*, children experience a definite leap in motor development. Enjoying bursts of racing, hopping, jumping, skipping, and climbing, they seem to be saying, "Look out, world! Here I come!" Motor patterns show a tendency for symmetry, with children using both hands and recognizing two halves as a whole picture. Eye teaming becomes more obvious. There is now a loose organization of the visual system that allows children's eyes to work together and to *accommodate* (adapt) better. The attention span is about twelve to fifteen minutes now.

At *five years old*, children reach a new maturity in terms of coordination, enjoying a greater ease and control of general body activity. Their movements are more refined, and so is their hand-eye coordination. Children move with more deliberation and a finer synchronization of movements. Their eyes can fix on things more easily, and their mechanical ability to focus is developed to the point where focusing is more accurate. The attention span is up to thirty minutes now.

School-Aged Children

School and vision—the two are practically synonymous. School is for learning, and at least 80 percent of learning is mediated by vision. All the skills and abilities that children develop during the preschool years come into play during the school years. And there is not a more demanding test of visual abilities than school.

Unfortunately, four out of ten grade-school children in the United States are visually handicapped for adequate school achievement. Visual handicaps include not only seeing a blur when looking at a blackboard, but poor oculomotor coordination, strabismus, lazy eye, focusing insufficiency, perceptual problems, and developmental lags.

Let's take a look at a few of the visual skills children need in school:

■ Near vision—the ability to see things fourteen to

Cover Test

As soon as your child is able to focus on objects for several seconds at a time (usually at about three years of age), you can try this test to see whether he or she can use both eyes together properly.

1. Have your child look at one particular object that will hold his or her attention. A good choice is a finger puppet with a small flashlight inserted inside.

2. While making sure your child stays focused on the object and not on your hand, cover one of his or her eyes while looking at the other eye. Did the uncovered eye move when the cover was put in place? Repeat this step a few times to be sure. If your child has both eyes focused on the object to

begin with, refocusing when one eye is covered should be unnecessary. In other words, your child shouldn't display any movement of the uncovered eye.

3. Remove the cover and let the child focus on the object with both eyes again.

4. Repeat step 2 with the other eye.

This test is to evaluate your child's ability to use both eyes together properly. If you saw any movement of the uncovered eye when the cover was put into position, consult your eye doctor. At this early age, any binocular dysfunction should be easy to rectify.

sixteen inches away (reading distance) clearly with both eyes.

■ Distance vision—the ability to see things at least twenty feet away with sharpness and very little effort.

■ Accommodation—the ability of the eyes to adjust for near-point tasks easily (with no effort). This process must be done with comfort and must be maintained for long periods of time.

■ Focusing flexibility—the ability to alternate between distance and near vision quickly and effortlessly.

■ Binocular coordination—the ability of both eyes to work together as a team using either distance or near vision. Tiring, double vision, poor reading ability, and headache are a few signs of inadequate binocular coordination.

■ Adequate field of vision—the ability to see up, down, left, and right while focusing on one spot. This saves unnecessary head and eye movements, and is crucial for reading.

These are only some of the visual abilities that are needed for good performance in school. Please keep in mind that a school vision "screening" does not substitute for a complete eye examination. Most schools do just the standard eye-chart test that is required by state law in many locations. By now, you should be aware that there are many other problems that can arise. Often, by the time a child's distance vision starts to decline enough to show up with the Snellen test, the problem is well on its way to becoming a permanent handicap. Distance vision is usually the last thing to go wrong, so a complete vision examination by an eye doctor is necessary to find any other problems first. (For a list of signs and symptoms of vision trouble, see "Know Your ABCs," below.) Make a complete vision examination a part of your child's back-to-school routine. And, if at any time your child has vision problems or is in the lower third of the class, take your child to the eye doctor for a complete vision examination.

HIGH-RISK AGES

Vision problems can develop at any age, but there do seem to be certain times during a child's school career when they are more likely to occur. Second grade, fourth grade, seventh grade, and ninth grade are key

---

Know Your ABC'S

Here are the ABC's of signs and symptoms that may signal vision trouble during the school years. Look for them in your child.

A. Appearance of Eyes
■ Crossed eyes or eyes pointing out, up, or down
■ Red eyes
■ Watery eyes
■ Encrusted lids
■ Frequent styes

B. Behavior
■ Squinting or closing one eye
■ Rigid body posture
■ Avoidance of close work
■ Rocking back and forth
■ Head turning
■ Excessive head movement

■ Sitting too close to the work
■ Using a finger to read
■ Blinking much and with effort
■ Rubbing the eyes during or after short periods of reading

C. Complaints
■ Blurred vision
■ Headaches
■ Nausea or dizziness
■ Burning or itching eyes
■ Double vision
■ Tiring quickly while reading

If your child has any of these signs or symptoms, contact your eye doctor for a complete eye examination.

years to pay special attention to your child's vision development.

In *second grade*, there is often a sudden increase in nearsightedness among students. This is understandable, since second grade is the time when children generally learn to read. In addition, the demand for close work is greatly increased over the previous school years.

In *fourth grade*, instead of learning to read, children begin reading to learn. This means that a possibly unmastered skill must now be used to investigate new areas of knowledge. It's as if you had just begun to learn French and suddenly had to study nuclear physics in the new language. The result of this kind of stress, and of the even more intense close work, is often nearsightedness.

In *seventh grade*, children are in the heart of middle school. The physical growth spurt that they experience combined with the tremendously increased demand for near-point work are a recipe for nearsightedness.

In *ninth grade*, the reading assignments pile up and the pressures to achieve increase. Teenagers may adapt to the stress by developing nearsightedness (if they haven't done so already). If vision problems go uncorrected, teenagers may give up on schoolwork and show declining achievement.

All of these periods of high stress require a good vision examination, which should be done every year anyway. So, when September rolls around and you buy new clothes and school supplies for your child and make appointments for medical examinations and dental checkups, don't forget about the one school supply that needs to be in the best working order—your child's vision.

SPECIAL PROBLEMS

There are a number of vision problems, as well as conditions that affect vision, that tend to occur in children. Among them is dyslexia. The term *dyslexia* (dis-LEX-ee-ah) was coined some years ago to describe a set of symptoms relating to the inability of some people to read and understand written language despite normal intelligence and educational opportunities. Early research in dyslexia looked for a single factor to explain the disorder. Some experts thought the problem had to do with visual acuity or binocular coordination, while others felt it was related to anything from an inner-ear condition to psychological difficul-

ties, faulty educational methods, or brain damage. As with most complex problems, it is now apparent that there is no simple answer to the puzzle of dyslexia. There are probably different causes for the symptoms in different children, although researchers have now uncovered some pretty hard evidence that certain areas of the brain develop more slowly in dyslexic children than they do in nondyslexic children.

Researchers continue to investigate the role of the visual system in dyslexia. The visual system is almost certainly involved in some way with the problem, although exactly how it is involved is not clear. Dyslexic children usually have good visual acuity, although they seem to have difficulty focusing their eyes. Interestingly, children with severe strabismus usually do not have difficulty reading because they manage to suppress the image from the severely affected eye and read with the good eye. Children with mild strabismus, on the other hand, may seem to be dyslexic because they struggle to fuse the two different images from their two eyes. This is not true dyslexia, but rather a binocular-vision problem that may mimic dyslexic symptoms. In the 1980s, psychologist Helen Irlen found another vision problem related to dyslexia. Her findings suggest that at least some dyslexics are extremely sensitive to light, a disorder that she named scotopic sensitivity syndrome (SSS). To assist persons with SSS, Dr. Irlen developed a treatment using special light-filtering lenses, now called Irlen lenses. (For a discussion of this treatment, see "Irlen Lenses" on page 21.)

Instead of dyslexia, underachieving children often have a similar affliction called attention deficit disorder (ADD). Because "ADD" has become a buzzword in learning today, vision problems are often masked and labeled as ADD. If children cannot pay visual attention to close work, they will look far away (daydream) or try to stir up other children in the immediate area. Paying attention to near-point work requires a sophisticated visual system that must be controlled carefully and for long periods of time.

If you suspect that your child may have dyslexia, it's best to get a thorough vision examination, as well as educational and perceptual testing, including an assessment of the child's visual-motor development. Contact your pediatrician or school nurse for a referral to the appropriate specialist. Many optometrists who specialize in vision development can also perform appropriate tests to rule out any visual compo-

Irlen Lenses

In the 1980s, Dr. Helen Irlen, a psychologist, developed a theory that at least some dyslexic people have an unusual sensitivity to light that interferes with their reading ability. According to Dr. Irlen's theory, these people use their night vision all the time, which creates some visual distortion when they try to read black letters on a white background. Irlen named this problem scotopic sensitivity syndrome (SSS).

In an effort to find a way to help people with SSS, Dr. Irlen experimented with colored light-filtering lenses to use while reading. These lenses are now called Irlen lenses. The approach used by the Irlen Institute is to first give the patient a complete vision examination to rule out any refractive problems—that is, make sure the patient can see clearly. Next, an evaluation is made to determine the exact visual dis-

tortions experienced relating to light sensitivity, visual resolution (blurring), span of focus, and sustained focus during the reading process. Lastly, lenses are designed to minimize or eliminate the distortions using the appropriate tint from among 150 different color possibilities. Dr. Irlen's process has created some controversy in the medical community, but my sense is that there may be some reading disabilities that the Irlen colored lenses can benefit.

For more information on the Irlen method and Irlen lenses, see *Reading by the Colors: Overcoming Dyslexia and Other Reading Disabilities Through the Irlen Method* by Helen Irlen or write to the Irlen Institite. (For the current address and phone number of the Irlen Institute, see "Resource Organizations" on page 255.)

nents that may be contributing to the problem. To find such an optometrist, contact the College of Optometrists in Vision Development. (For the address and telephone number, see "Resource Organizations" on page 255.)

Several recent studies have shown that using blue filters for reading has brought about improved reading abilities in previously diagnosed "dyslexic" children. This lends additional support to the work done by Dr. Irlen and suggests a visual-processing component to this condition. Some doctors also use the therapeutic technique of syntonics to treat these types of problems. For a discussion of syntonics, see page 234.

You may need to take your child to a number of professionals before you find one who is able to tie all of the various components together for a comprehensive program. Many school systems have educational psychologists who have resources for helping children with dyslexia and SSS symptoms.

WHAT TO LOOK FOR WHEN CHILDREN READ

To evaluate your child for dyslexia and other vision problems that may affect reading, look for the following signs while watching and listening to him or her read. Remember that many vision problems are normal at certain stages, and that children develop at their own pace. Some things to look for are:

■ Poor reading comprehension.

■ Loss of place often during reading.

■ Short attention span for reading.

■ Frequent omission of words.

■ Writing uphill or downhill on paper.

■ Rereading or skipping lines unknowingly.

■ Failure to recognize the same word in the next sentence.

■ Confusing two or more words with the same or similar beginnings.

■ Failure to visualize what is read.

■ Repeated confusion over left-right directions.

■ Poor orientation of drawings on the page.

■ Quick loss of interest.

Be sure to take your child to the eye doctor for a thorough vision examination to ensure that he or she gets off to a good start in reading.

YOUR CHILD'S EYE EXAMINATION

When you take your child for an eye examination, the doctor should be able to explain any visual difficulties that your child may have in a way that you can understand. If you don't understand something, don't hesitate to ask questions. This chapter may have helped you to decide which questions to ask. In any case, be sure you understand the following aspects of the examination:

■ *Visual acuity.* Although 20/20 is only an arbitrary figure, it will still give you an idea of how close to "normal" your child's vision is.

■ *Refractive errors.* You should understand your child's nearsightedness, farsightedness, or astigmatism, if any of these is present, and how the condition can be corrected.

■ *Health of the eyes.* The external and internal health of the eyes is a very basic and necessary finding, since the eyes must be healthy to see well.

■ *Eye-brain coordination.* You should know about any special eye-brain coordination problems, such as strabismus or lazy eye, and the possible treatment plans.

■ *Focusing ability and flexibility.* It should be determined if your child can maintain his or her focus for near and for distance vision, and can switch easily from near to far and back again.

■ *Binocular efficiency.* This is a critical area in children's vision. It is extremely important to determine if your child can maintain binocular fixation on a certain point for a sustained period of time, and the quality of his or her depth perception.

■ *Color vision.* If your child is a boy, his color vision should be tested and particular color deficiencies, if any, determined.

■ *Perception and development.* If your child is having some difficulty in school, a series of tests may be recommended to determine if the problems are due to perceptual difficulties or a developmental lag. Make sure you understand the purpose and results of each test. If vision therapy is prescribed, it, too, should be thoroughly explained to you.

In addition to understanding the different aspects of the examination, make sure you understand all of the instructions the doctor gives you if glasses or contact lenses are prescribed. If glasses are prescribed, be sure you and your child know exactly for which activities to wear the glasses and how to care for them. If contacts are prescribed, be sure you and your child know how to insert them, remove them, and take care of them.

GROWING UP WITH TELEVISION AND COMPUTERS

It's no surprise to anyone that some children want to spend as much time watching television as they spend at school. Television has been a powerful influence on kids (and adults) for several generations. Now, computers have taken over as the video-of-choice for most children. Since watching a television or computer screen involves intensive use of the eyes, many people have become concerned about the visual effects of extended viewing. A few studies have been done in this area, and some interesting conclusions have been reached. Here are answers to some of the more frequently asked questions about television, computers, and vision.

How does watching television affect the eyes? The eyes suffer less focus strain from viewing television than from doing close work such as reading or operating a computer. However, close concentration and staring at the television screen over an excessive period of time may result in general fatigue and tired eyes.

Can a room be too bright for comfortable television viewing or computer use? Yes. Excessively bright room lighting tends to reduce the contrast on the screen and to wash out the picture. Lamps and other lights should be positioned so that no glare or reflections will be seen on or near the screen.

What is the best way to adjust the lighting when watching television or working on a computer? It is better to first turn on the desired room light and to then adjust the brightness and contrast of the television picture or computer screen. Adapt the television set or computer screen to the room lighting, not vice versa.

Should television be watched in a totally darkened room? No! The contrast between the screen and the surrounding area is too great for comfortable and efficient vision. When the room is softly illuminated, this undesirable high contrast is kept to a minimum.

What's the best distance to sit from the screen? A television picture appears much sharper and better defined if viewed from a distance that is at least five times the diagonal dimension of the screen. For example, if you have a nineteen-inch screen—measured from the lower-left to the upper-right corner of the screen—you should sit at least eight feet away from it. Nearsighted children are the ones most likely to persist in sitting two or three feet from the screen. (There is really no such thing as sitting too far from the television.) When working at a computer, you should sit about twenty or more inches from the screen.

Is radiation emitted by televisions or computers? Some radiation is emitted by both black-and-white and color television sets, with more emitted from a color screen. At this time, however, it does not seem to pose a health hazard, although many experts still think you should not sit too close to a color screen. Stick with the distance recommended—five times the diagonal dimension of the screen—for safety as well as comfort. No studies to date have shown any negative radiation effects from sitting in front of a computer.

Does body posture affect viewing comfort? Yes. Watching television in a twisted or leaning position will cause one eye to see much more than the other eye. This will lead to eyestrain because the vision is not balanced equally between the eyes. An erect, straight-ahead position is the best for television watching. A computer screen, which is usually situated closer than a television set, should be in a lowered position, enabling you to look straight ahead and see over its top. This is obviously more difficult to set up for children, who are usually much shorter when sitting in a chair. Special considerations for comfort should be addressed when children use computers.

With a little common sense and these few facts, you and your child can learn to live with televisions and computers, and make the most of the experiences. Junk-food commercials aside, television has much to offer children. See page 104 for more information on computer vision syndrome and some recommendations.

GOOD VISION—HOW PARENTS CAN HELP

If you've read this chapter, you know that children's vision is an integral part of their whole development, and goes hand-in-hand with the maturation of the large and small muscles, and the brain. Most of the time, vision, like the rest of the body, develops properly and on schedule. Once in a while, it seems delayed or deficient, which usually means you'll need to seek help from your pediatrician, eye doctor, or school-associated professional. Even when vision does seem to be developing properly, there are things that you, as a parent, can do to ensure that it stays on track. With young children, try some of the following activities for good fun and good vision.

■ *Coordination* is the ability to move your body in a controlled manner. To assist your child's development of coordination, do the following:

● Let your child crawl over, under, and around chairs and tables. (Watch for sharp corners.)

● Play "Mother, May I?" with your child. Use running, hopping, crawling, and jumping skills in the game.

● Ask your child to walk backwards or sideways when you go for walks together.

● Have your child hop first on one foot and then on the other. Have your child hop on both feet or run in place to music while you count to ten.

● Have your child jump forward or backward over a line or a crack.

● Have your child run on tiptoes, and then stand on tiptoes for ten seconds.

● Play "Simon Says" with your child. Use directions that include the terms "right" and "left," and encourage any activity that requires and reinforces the concepts of left and right.

● Practice naming parts of the body while touching them.

● Bounce a ball to your child, and have your child catch and bounce the ball back.

● Have your child hop forward on the right foot, and then walk the left foot up to the right.

● If you have a two- by four-inch balance beam available, have your child walk along it with arms outstretched or clasped behind the body. Also, have your child try different techniques and games on the beam, including walking back and forth with the eyes closed. (Do *not* allow your child to do these things without a spotter.)

■ *Visual-motor control* is the ability to control the movements of the small-muscle groups in conjunction with the eye muscles. To assist your child's development of visual-motor control, do the following:

● Have your child make pictures using scrap materials such as string, buttons, beads, and shells.

● Draw a line pattern on a piece of paper, and have your child trace the pattern with a finger.

● Have your child practice turning the pages of a book or magazine.

• Have your child string pieces of macaroni like beads.

• Fold a piece of paper into many parts. Open the paper up, and have your child draw along the crease lines.

• Help your child practice tying knots and bows in shoelaces and pieces of string.

• Put some cornmeal or sand in a tray, and have your child draw shapes and letters in it.

• Make dotted letters, and have your child trace over them with a pencil, pen, or crayon.

• Have your child color in the "O's" in a newspaper article.

■ *Visual perception* is the ability to perceive such things as colors, shapes, sizes, letter forms, and words. To assist your child's development of visual perception, do the following:

• Place some objects on the floor, and have your child arrange them according to size or color.

• Play "smaller-larger." For example, ask your child to "find something smaller than your head, but larger than your hand."

• Talk about colors.

• Have your child separate teaspoons and tablespoons into two stacks.

• Have your child measure the sizes of things such as furniture, paper, and rooms.

• Have your child take a piece of string and find five things longer and five things shorter than it.

• Draw arrows in different directions on one index card, and one arrow on a second index card. Hold the second card so that the single arrow faces in different directions, and have your child match the arrow to the correct arrow on the first index card.

■ *Visual memory* is the ability to reproduce letters and other objects and images from memory. To assist your child's development of visual memory, do the following:

• Have your child circle all the words in a newspaper article that begin with a certain letter.

• Play "What's Missing?" For example, set out a few articles of clothing, and have your child look at them. Then, have the child close his or her eyes while you remove one article, then open the eyes and tell you which article is missing.

• Touch several objects on a table. Have your child try to touch the same objects in the same order.

• Arrange three shapes in a certain sequence. Then mix them up, and have your child put them back in the same sequence.

• Open a storybook to a certain page. Let your child look at the page for a moment, then close the book and have your child find the page again.

• Write three numbers, then quickly cover them and have your child write the numbers from memory.

For older children who have begun to read, here are some activities that will encourage the continued development of their abilities:

• Correct the mistakes your child makes when reading to you (but have him or her continue reading to avoid loss of concentration).

• When your child reads a page, ask him or her questions about it.

• Have your child look for words on a page that start or end with a certain letter.

• Have your child look at the picture in a storybook, then guess what the story is about before reading it.

• Encourage your child to write stories.

• Let your child see you reading often. Imitation is a strong teacher.

For most children, vision, like other skills, develops on schedule with few problems. But for some children, it does not. When a child has vision problems, it falls to the child's parents and teachers to pick up the clues that vision or visual-motor skills may be lacking, and to get the child the help that he or she needs.

Finding Eye Care

Okay, it's time for your eye examination. Now, how do you find an eye doctor? Which type of eye doctor should you see? (Are there really different *types* of eye doctors?) How do you know you're making the right choice? There seems to be an endless series of questions surrounding eye doctors and their services. Let's take a look at the different types of eye-care professionals, and see if we can figure out who does what and which one is appropriate for you.

THE THREE O'S

There are three different kinds of professionals involved with the care of the eyes, so it may not come as a surprise to you that there is some confusion on the part of the general public over who does what. What's the difference between an ophthalmologist, an optometrist, and an optician? Time and again, studies show that most people don't know the differences and probably never will. Let's see if we can explain them here.

Ophthalmologists

An ophthalmologist (of-thal-MAHL-oh-jist) is a medical doctor (MD) who specializes in eye health and disease. After graduating from college and medical school, an ophthalmologist spent three more years learning about the diseases and surgeries of the eye. (All ophthalmologists are surgeons.) In order to become what is known as a board-certified ophthalmologist, the MD passed a written, oral, and practical certifying examination in the specialty of ophthalmology.

As you can see, an ophthalmologist has a lot of training. However, that doesn't mean an ophthalmologist is the correct professional for every eye problem.

Ophthalmologists are the people to see when you have a serious eye injury or an eye disease requiring surgery. Most ophthalmologists also prescribe glasses or contact lenses for healthy eyes, but many refer all or part of this work to someone else. For example, in a recent survey of about 600 ophthalmologists, 75 percent indicated that someone in their practice fitted contact lenses, but only 60 percent said that they did fittings themselves.

Ophthalmologists sometimes specialize within the specialty of ophthalmology. Some are retinal specialists, while others specialize in the problems of the cornea or lens. Some are pediatric ophthalmologists, specializing in children's eye problems. Some confine themselves to surgery or even specific kinds of surgery, such as cataract surgery. There are also refractive surgeons, who perform only prescription-changing procedures.

In telephone directories, ophthalmologists are listed under the general heading of "Physicians."

Optometrists

An optometrist (op-TAHM-e-trist) is a doctor of optometry (OD). Optometrists are defined as health-care professionals trained and state licensed to provide primary eye-care services. These services include comprehensive eye-health and vision examinations; diagnosis and treatment of eye diseases and vision disorders; detection of general health problems; prescribing of glasses, contact lenses, low-vision rehabilitation, vision therapy, and medication; performing of certain surgical procedures; and counseling of patients regarding their surgical alternatives and vision needs as related to their occupations, avocations, and lifestyles. Optometrists also have their areas of specialization. Some of these are contact lenses, low vision, vision therapy, sports vision, and occupational vision.

Optometrists completed pre-professional undergraduate education at a college or university, and four years of professional education at a college of optometry. Some optometrists also completed residencies. There is a national board examination for licensing in optometry, and most states accept passage of this examination along with passage of an additional practical or oral examination of their own.

To find an optometrist or optometric specialist, contact your local or county chapter of the Optometric Society, listed in telephone directories under the general heading of "Optometrists."

OPTICIANS

An optician (op-TISH-an) is a technician trained to fill prescriptions for lenses written by optometrists and ophthalmologists. Opticians are trained to make glasses, fit eyeglass lenses into frames, and adjust eyeglass frames to people's faces. In some states, they are also allowed to do fittings of contact lenses.

Opticians generally have an associate college degree, which is normally awarded for completing a two-year undergraduate program. Most states license opticians and require continuing education. There is also an American Board of Opticianry, which certifies opticians. However, not all states accept this certification as qualifying an optician to practice. At this time, the requirements vary a great deal from state to state.

CHOOSING THE CORRECT PROFESSIONAL FOR YOUR NEEDS

You've got an eye problem and decide you need some professional help. But whom do you see? Are all three types of eye-care professionals trained to treat your condition?

There are no hard-and-fast rules to help you make the decision of which eye-care specialist to see because, if you are like most people, you are unsure of exactly what your problem is and what treatment it requires. We can, however, make some generalizations that should make the decision easier. If you are just having trouble seeing clearly, either at a distance or up close, or have some eyestrain, you probably need the services of an optometrist. If your child is having difficulty reading in school (or is a "problem" student), then a

developmental optometrist is appropriate. If all you want to do is trade in your glasses for contact lenses, an optometrist who fits contacts is your answer. But if you have a family history of glaucoma and have been noticing some halos around light at night, an optometrist who treats eye diseases is the correct choice. If you believe you might have a condition that could require surgery, then start with an ophthalmologist for an opinion. If you just broke your glasses and need them repaired, but your last examination was very recent, visit an optician.

You might be reading this and saying, "Well, he's an optometrist, so of course he'll say that they do everything!" Well, yes and no. I am an optometrist, and we do have an expanded range of services to offer the public, but we don't do it all. It is acknowledged, though, that the optometrist is the "general practitioner" of eye care who can determine if a problem needs further attention from another specialist. And since optometrists have started treating diseases and prescribing medications, this is now even more true than ever.

Occasionally, you may need to work with a variety of professionals for one particular problem. If, for example, you visit an optometrist for a routine examination and a cataract is diagnosed, the optometrist may want to follow you for some time before recommending a surgical procedure. The optometrist may make nutritional recommendations or other environmental suggestions first, thus delaying surgery. However, if it is determined that surgery is the best route for you, an ophthalmologist will take charge of your care. Following the surgery, you will probably be referred back to your optometrist for continued follow-up care.

SELECTING THE INDIVIDUAL DOCTOR

You've decided which kind of professional you should see, but now you've got to pick the individual doctor. How do you know whether you've got the right person? This is a tough one! There are as many different types of individual doctors as there are types of people. One of the best sources of good doctors is word of mouth. If you have a friend who wears glasses or contacts, and has been with a good doctor for several years, there's a good chance that this doctor will be good for you, too.

When looking for a doctor, don't bypass an experienced practitioner for a young professional fresh out of school. Although recent graduates may possess the latest technical knowledge, there's something to be said for experience in any field. And, some new doctors are so cautious that they may keep you in the chair for hours doing every test in the book instead of just the ones related to your problem.

To avoid the high costs of setting up offices of their own, new graduates of optometry school sometimes begin their practices in chain-store operations, which are usually located in shopping malls. In these kinds of stores, you may find young doctors with good technical knowledge but little time to apply it because of the large numbers of patients the stores book into each time slot. These young doctors often don't stay around for very long—usually just long enough to get on their feet financially—so if you frequent these stores for your eye care, there is little chance that you'll see one doctor more than one time.

On the other hand, you should also be cautious of older doctors who have been in the same location since prehistoric times. If they have been keeping up with the advancements in eye-care technology and knowledge, they are perfectly fine doctors to see, but things change fast and not everyone keeps up. Since all states require continuing education as part of the re-licensing process for optometrists, checking to make sure that your doctor has a valid license should give you some comfort that he or she has kept abreast of at least the most important developments in the field.

I don't advise browsing through the telephone directory for a doctor. It still amazes me how many people choose an eye doctor based simply on the size of the display ad or the cost of the examination. I often wonder if these people would shop around for a bargain-priced brain surgeon as well!

QUESTIONS TO ASK

To become familiar with the doctors on your list of possibilities and to make an intelligent choice from among them, you should inquire about their educational and professional backgrounds. You could ask each doctor for a résumé and any office promotional materials. Here are a few questions to ask their receptionists when telephoning their offices for the first time:

■ How long has the doctor been in practice?

■ How long does the examination take?

■ Will your eyes be dilated for the examination?

■ How much does the examination cost?

■ Does the doctor specialize in (or have experience with) the particular condition or service you are interested in?

Here are some questions to ask the doctor before the examination:

■ Will a case history be taken? (Be sure the doctor sits down and talks about your problems, medical history, medications, and lifestyle.)

■ How extensive is the examination form? (Although the form will probably look mysterious, see how big it is and how much of it should be filled out by the end of the examination. Be suspicious of an examination form that's the size of an index card.)

■ Is a full range of distance- and near-vision tests included in the examination?

■ Is a glaucoma test a regular part of the examination?

■ Does the doctor work with a number of different contact-lens companies? (If you want contact lenses, it's important to have a doctor who is not tied to one manufacturer. There are many different kinds of contacts available now.)

■ Will the doctor describe the different tests while performing them?

■ Does the doctor offer treatment alternatives (for example, contact lenses, glasses, or vision therapy) according to the patient's preferences?

■ Does the doctor regularly refer patients to other doctors when appropriate or necessary?

Much of what you determine about a doctor will be based on just plain old gut feelings about the office in general. If you feel you aren't getting high-quality, personalized service from your eye doctor, you may want to go elsewhere. Sometimes it takes a little faith and trust to find a good eye-care professional. A good doc is hard to find, but once you find one, stay with him or her, and appreciate the good vision care.

THE COMPONENTS OF AN EYE EXAMINATION

A complete eye examination should be so thorough that it tires you out. There are some basic procedures that are included in every complete examination. The additional procedures will vary depending upon your doctor and your complaints.

Every examination should begin with a *case history*. Your doctor should ask you questions about your health and lifestyle, starting with, "Why are you here?" You should also be questioned about the date of your last examination, your history with glasses and contact lenses, the quality of your distance and near vision, any headaches you may be having, any medications you may be taking, your job-related visual tasks, and your family history of eye diseases. Beware of a doctor who doesn't ask you any questions before beginning the testing.

Every examination should also include *visual-acuity testing*. This is a test of the sharpness of your vision using the Snellen chart. Each eye should be tested individually for distance and then again for near. This will give the doctor an idea of how well you see the world.

Also included in every examination should be a check of your *external eye health*. This involves checking the outer area of each eye, including the pupil, iris, cornea, sclera, conjunctiva (the mucous membrane covering the front of the eye and lining the inside of the eyelids), lids, eyelashes, eyebrows, and surrounding skin area. This is usually done with a flashlight, although occasionally more sophisticated instruments are used to magnify the eye.

Your *internal eye health* is also important. Using an ophthalmoscope (of-THAL-moh-scope), the doctor should look into the back of each eye to see the retina, optic nerve, blood vessels, and surrounding tissue to rule out any diseases in those areas. This examination will often be done after your eyes have been dilated so that the doctor can see the entire retina more easily. (For a discussion of dilated examinations, see below.)

Refraction, used in connection with an eye examination, is the determination of refractive errors in vision. Refraction is done using a machine called a refractor, which contains all the different lens combinations. Using the refractor, the doctor can determine your distance prescription and near prescription. The refractor will also provide information about your eye-muscle balance, focusing strength, and focusing flexibility. This portion of the examination usually takes the most time.

Glaucoma testing is a normal part of the eye examination. The pressure of each eye is measured with an instrument called a tonometer. Many of today's tonometers blow a puff of air at the eye. Although glaucoma testing, because of this puff of air, can be the most irritating part of the complete eye examination, it is also the most crucial.

Many doctors also perform *visual-field testing* to determine whether your peripheral vision is intact. Visual-field testing is most often performed if glaucoma or another disorder is suspected, but it can be done at any time, and some doctors do it routinely. The old-fashioned way to test the visual field utilized a black-felt board and white-tipped pointer. The patient would tell the doctor when the pointer appeared in his or her peripheral vision. Modern visual-field testing is done using a computerized system. The patient's head is positioned in a shell-like machine, and lights are flashed all around. The patient indicates when the flashes appear in the peripheral vision.

Every complete eye examination should end with a *consultation*. The doctor should spend some time

Dilated Examinations

Many patients wonder whether eye drops that dilate (widen) the pupil will be used during their eye examination, and how long it will take the drops to wear off. Drops are used for two purposes—to enable the doctor to get a better view of the inner eye for the detection of eye diseases and retinal problems, and to paralyze the focusing muscle of the eye. Some doctors dilate the eyes routinely, and in fact, the practice is becoming the "standard of care." It may be especially necessary to use drops in older patients with very small pupils, especially if eye disease is suspected, and in children, who often have trouble focusing at the required distances for the examination. Doctors may also use the drops if they suspect an unusual refractive problem.

If your eyes are dilated as part of your eye examination, they will most likely return to normal by the next morning. In the meantime, they will be extremely sensitive to light, and you will be unable to read or to focus for any near-point activities. Your doctor will probably offer you disposable sunglasses to help with any excessive glare.

explaining the results of all the tests and the recommendations for your eyes. Be certain that you understand the test results and all the options that you are given. Be cautious of a doctor who pushes one option, especially one with which you may not be comfortable.

THE COST OF AN EYE EXAMINATION

It's difficult to put a price tag on eye care, but you should have some idea of what to expect when you walk into a doctor's office for an examination. The prices of examinations, contact lenses, and other services vary around the country.

A survey of optometrists around the nation in 1998 found that the average cost of a complete eye examination was $69. A similar survey of ophthalmologists in 1997 found that the average cost of a comprehensive examination was $120. The cost of a contact-lens examination is always additional.

Sometimes you'll see "specials" offered for eye examinations. These are popular in shopping malls, and are designed to entice you into the store, where you will hopefully purchase other services, such as contact lenses or glasses. In other words, the examination is a "loss leader" technique used by some large chain operations. The emphasis in these stores is usually on eye*wear* rather than eye *care*.

My personal belief is that you shouldn't do *much* shopping around when it comes to your vision. Find a professional whom you can trust, and stick with him or her. Quality usually doesn't come cheap.

You may not be able to judge the quality of an eye examination or your doctor's expertise, but hopefully, you will feel that the doctor you choose does a thorough job, and offers you alternatives for your eye-care needs. By asking a lot of questions and reading this book, you'll at least be familiar with the process of vision and what can go wrong. It is hoped that together, you and your doctor can deal effectively with any problems that may arise.

Nutrition and Vision

By now you should be getting the idea that the eyes and visual system are an integral part of the body. It makes sense, therefore, that they require proper nutrition to maintain their optimal function. You might be surprised to find out that the brain and visual system, while composing only about 2 percent of your body weight, use up about 25 percent of your nutritional intake. So let's take a look at what your eyes—and your body—need for optimal performance.

This chapter is designed to give you an overview of nutrition, explaining how it works and how it generally affects the body. In addition, the macronutrients (water, carbohydrates, protein, and fats) are discussed, as are selected micronutrients (vitamins and minerals) that are important to vision.

DIGESTION, ABSORPTION, AND METABOLISM

Nutrition is the process by which the body digests food to obtain the nutrients it needs for growth and repair purposes. Proper nutrition involves consuming foods and supplements that supply the correct nutrients in adequate amounts for optimal health. In this section, we will examine how the body processes these nutrients.

The foods eaten by humans are chemically complex. They must be broken down by the body into simpler chemical forms so that they can be taken in through the intestinal walls and transported by the blood to the cells. In the cells, they provide energy and building materials to maintain human life. The processes that work together to complete this job are digestion, absorption, and metabolism.

Digestion

Digestion is a series of physical and chemical processes that break down food in preparation for the absorption of its nutrients from the intestinal tract into the bloodstream. These processes take place in the digestive tract, which includes the mouth, pharynx, esophagus, stomach, small intestine, and large intestine.

The active materials in the digestive juices that cause the chemical breakdown of food are called enzymes. Enzymes are complex proteins that are capable of inducing chemical changes in other substances without being changed themselves. Each enzyme is capable of breaking down only a single specific substance. For example, an enzyme capable of breaking down fats cannot also break down proteins or carbohydrates.

Digestion actually begins in the mouth, where the large pieces of food are broken down into smaller pieces via chewing. The salivary glands in the mouth produce saliva, a fluid that moistens the food for swallowing and contains an enzyme necessary for carbohydrate breakdown. Active chemical digestion begins in the middle portion of the stomach, where the food is mixed with gastric juices containing hydrochloric acid, water, and enzymes that break up protein and other substances. After one to four hours, muscle action pushes the food, now in a liquid form, out of the stomach and into the small intestine.

When the liquid food enters the small intestine, the pancreas secretes digestive juices that are added to the mixture. If fats are present in the food, bile, an enzyme produced by the liver and stored in the gallbladder, is secreted. The pancreas also secretes a substance that neutralizes the digestive acids in the food, as well as additional enzymes that continue the breakdown of the proteins and carbohydrates. Finally, the undigested portions of the food enter the large intestine for eventual excretion. No digestive enzymes are secreted in the large intestine, and little occurs there aside from the absorption of water.

Absorption

Absorption is the process by which nutrients—in the form of glucose from carbohydrates, amino acids from protein, and fatty acids and glycerol from fats—are taken up by the intestines and passed into the bloodstream to function in cell metabolism. Absorption takes place primarily in the small intestine. The lining of the small intestine is covered with minute fingerlike projections called villi. These villi contain lymph channels called lacteals and tiny blood vessels called capillaries, which are the principal channels of absorption. About 60 to 70 percent of fats and fat-soluble vitamins are absorbed by the lacteals into the lymphatic system and transported to the liver. The remaining nutrients are absorbed by the capillaries into the bloodstream and transported to the liver.

In the liver, many different enzymes help to change the nutrient molecules into new forms for specific purposes. Unlike the earlier changes, which prepared the nutrients for absorption and transport, the reactions in the liver produce the actual products needed by the cells. Some of these products are used by the liver itself, but the rest are held in storage by the liver, to be released as needed into the bloodstream. From the blood, they are picked up by the individual cells and put to work.

Metabolism

Metabolism is the final stage of food handling. It includes all the chemical changes that nutrients undergo from the time they are absorbed until they either become a part of the body or are excreted from the body. Metabolism is the conversion of digested nutrients into building materials for living tissues or energy to meet the body's needs.

Metabolism occurs in two general phases, anabolism and catabolism, which take place simultaneously. Anabolism involves all the chemical reactions that nutrients undergo in the construction or building up of body chemicals and tissues such as blood, enzymes, hormones, and glycogen. Catabolism involves all the reactions that break down various compounds and tissues to supply energy. Energy for the cells is derived primarily from the metabolism of glucose, which combines with oxygen in a series of chemical reactions to form carbon dioxide, water, and cellular energy. The carbon dioxide and water are waste products, carried away from the cells by the bloodstream. Energy is also derived from the metabolism of essential fatty acids and amino acids, although the major purpose of amino-acid metabolism is to provide material for the growth, maintenance, and repair of tissues. The waste products of essential-fatty-acid and amino-acid metabolism are also carried away from the cells by the bloodstream.

The process of metabolism requires that the body maintain extensive systems of enzymes to facilitate the thousands of different chemical reactions that take place and to regulate the rate at which these reactions occur. These enzymes often require the presence of specific vitamins and minerals to perform their functions. For proper growth, the body needs the the four basic nutrients of water, carbohydrates, protein, and fat—called macronutrients—as well as vitamins and minerals—called micronutrients. In the remainder of this chapter, we will describe these various nutrients and how they interact to supply the eyes with the materials they need to perform the amazing function of vision.

THE MACRONUTRIENTS

The macronutrients are the essential ingredients among the building blocks of nutrition. They are water, carbohydrates, protein, and fat, all of which are required for the process of metabolism—the conversion of food to useable nutrients. Although the macronutrients are critical for life itself, there are no Federal guidelines regarding their intake, such as there are for the vitamins and minerals. All of the macronutrients are required to some degree, and are available from the foods we eat. Let's review the macronutrients, and see how they interact with our bodies to supply the fuel for life.

Water

Water is an essential nutrient, involved in every function of the body. It helps to transport other nutrients and waste products in and out of the cells. It is necessary for all of the digestive, absorptive, circulatory, and excretory functions of the body, as well as for the body's utilization of the water-soluble vitamins. It is also needed for the maintenance of proper body temperature. The human body is two-thirds water.

Replenishing your body's supply of water, which is continually drained through sweating and elimination, is very important. To keep your body functioning properly, you must drink at least eight 8-ounce glasses of quality water each day. While the body can survive without food for about five weeks, it cannot survive without water for more than five days.

Carbohydrates

Carbohydrates supply the body with the energy it needs to function. They are found almost exclusively in plant foods, such as fruits, vegetables, and legumes. Milk and milk products are the only animal foods that contain a significant amount of carbohydrates.

Carbohydrates are divided into two groups—simple and complex. The simple carbohydrates, sometimes called simple sugars, include fructose (fruit sugar), sucrose (table sugar), and lactose (milk sugar). Fruits are among the richest natural sources of simple carbohydrates. Complex carbohydrates are also made of sugars, but the sugar molecules are strung together into longer, more complex chains. The complex carbohydrates include fiber and starches. Foods rich in complex carbohydrates are vegetables, whole grains, and legumes.

Carbohydrates are the main source of blood glucose, which is a major fuel for all of the body's cells and the only source of energy for the brain and red blood cells. Except for fiber, which cannot be digested, both simple and complex carbohydrates are converted into glucose. The glucose is then either used directly to provide energy for the body or stored in the liver for future use. When a person consumes more calories than the body needs, a portion of the carbohydrates consumed may also be stored in the body as fat.

Protein

Protein is essential for growth and development. It provides the body with energy, and is needed for the manufacture of hormones, antibodies, enzymes, and tissues. It also helps to maintain the proper acid-alkaline balance in the body. When protein is consumed, it is broken down in the body into amino acids, which are called the building blocks of protein. Some amino acids are considered nonessential. This does not mean that they are unnecessary, but rather that they do not have to come from the diet because they are manufactured by the body from other amino acids. The remaining amino acids are considered essential, mean-

ing that they are not synthesized by the body and must be obtained from the diet.

Because of the importance of consuming proteins that provide all of the essential amino acids, dietary proteins are divided into two groups according to the amino acids they contain. Complete proteins, which constitute the first group, contain ample amounts of all of the essential amino acids. These proteins are found in meat, fish, poultry, cheese, eggs, and milk. Incomplete proteins, which constitute the second group, contain only some of the essential amino acids. These proteins are found in foods such as grains, legumes, and leafy green vegetables.

Although it is important to consume the full range of amino acids, both essential and nonessential, it is not necessary to get them from meat, fish, poultry, and the other complete-protein foods. In fact, because of their high fat content, most of those foods should be eaten in moderation. It is possible to create complete proteins by combining various incomplete-protein foods. This is called food combining. For instance, although beans and brown rice are both quite rich in protein, each lacks one or more of the essential amino acids. However, when you combine beans and brown rice with each other, or when you combine either one with any of a number of other protein-rich foods, you form a complete protein that is a high-quality substitute for meat.

Fats

Although much attention has been focused on the need to reduce the amount of fat in the diet, the body does need some fat. During infancy and childhood, fat is necessary for normal brain development. Throughout life, it provides energy and supports growth. Fat is, in fact, the most concentrated source of energy available to the body. However, after the age of two, the body requires only small amounts of fat—much less than what is provided by the average American diet.

Fats are composed of building blocks called fatty acids. There are three major categories of fatty acids—saturated, polyunsaturated, and monounsaturated. Saturated fatty acids are found primarily in animal products, including dairy items such as whole milk, cream, and cheese and fatty meats such as beef, veal, lamb, pork, and ham. The fat marbling that you see in beef and pork is composed of saturated fat. Some vegetable products—including coconut oil, palm kernel, oil, and vegetable shortening—are also high in saturates. The liver uses saturated fats to manufacture cholesterol. Therefore, excessive dietary intake of saturated fats can significantly raise the blood-cholesterol level, especially the level of low-density lipoproteins (LDLs), or "bad" cholesterol.

Polyunsaturated fatty acids are found in the greatest abundance in corn, soybean, safflower, and sunflower oils. Certain fish oils are also high in the polyunsaturates. Unlike the saturated fats, the polyunsaturates may actually lower your total blood-cholesterol level. In doing so, however, they also have a tendency, when present in large amounts, to reduce your high-density lipoproteins (HDLs), or "good" cholesterol. For this reason, the guidelines state that the intake of polyunsaturated fats should not exceed 10 percent of the total caloric intake.

Monounsaturated fatty acids are found mostly in vegetable and nut oils such as olive, peanut, and canola. These fats appear to reduce the LDL blood level without affecting the HDL level in any way. However, this positive impact upon LDL cholesterol is relatively modest. The guidelines recommend that the intake of monounsaturated fats be kept between 10 and 15 percent of the total caloric intake.

Although most foods contain a combination of all three types of fatty acids, one of the types is usually predominant. Thus, a fat or oil is considered saturated or high in saturates when it is composed primarily of saturated fatty acids. Saturated fats are usually solid at room temperature. A fat or oil composed mostly of polyunsaturated fatty acids is called polyunsaturated, while a fat or oil composed mostly of monounsaturated fatty acids is called monounsaturated.

THE MICRONUTRIENTS

The same as the macronutrients, vitamins and minerals are essential to life. They are therefore also considered nutrients. However, they are needed in such small amounts compared to the macronutrients that they are called micronutrients.

Because vitamins and minerals are so necessary for health, the U.S. Food and Nutrition Board of the National Research Council (NRC) has formulated recommended consumption levels, called the Recommended Daily Allowances (RDAs). But the amounts cited in these recommendations usually are

adequate for maintaining a minimal level of health—that is, freedom from disease—rather than optimal health. Therefore, any adult not suffering from a specific disorder should obtain more than the RDAs of the vitamins and minerals from food and/or supplement sources. People who are active or exercise, are under great stress, are on restricted diets, are mentally or physically ill, take medication, are recovering from surgery, or smoke or consume alcoholic beverages all need higher than the normal amounts. Women who take oral contraceptives also need increased amounts. The RDAs and intake recommendations for each substance are provided in the following listings.

Vitamins

Vitamins are essential to life. They contribute to good health by regulating the metabolism and assisting the biochemical processes that release energy from digested food. Some vitamins are water-soluble, while others are fat-soluble. The water-soluble vitamins must be taken into the body daily, as they cannot be stored and are excreted within one to four days. These include the B vitamins and vitamin C. The fat-soluble vitamins can be stored for longer periods of time in the body, in fatty tissues and the liver. These include vitamins A, D, E, and K. Both the water-soluble and fat-soluble vitamins are needed by the body for proper functioning.

Vitamin A and Beta-Carotene

Of all the micronutrients that are important to visual function, vitamin A is probably the most well known. Vitamin A is a fat-soluble vitamin that occurs in nature in a variety of chemical forms. It is found as retinol in animal tissues. It is found as beta-carotene in plants, with the highest amounts present in fruits such as apricots and cantaloupes, and in vegetables such as carrots, pumpkins, sweet potatoes, spinach, squash, and broccoli. While retinol is readily absorbed as is by the body, beta-carotene must be broken down before it can function as a vitamin.

Beta-carotene is a carotenoid, a class of compounds related to vitamin A. Some carotenoids, such as beta-carotene, can act as precursors of vitamin A. When a food or supplement containing beta-carotene is consumed, the beta-carotene is converted into vitamin A in the liver. According to recent reports, beta-carotene appears to aid in cancer prevention by scavenging, or neutralizing, free radicals.

Vitamin A is the molecule in the retina that is responsible for the transformation of light energy into nerve impulses. It is therefore critical in the function of the eye. A lack of vitamin A can cause some forms of night blindness. Since vitamin A is also necessary for the maintenance of the mucous lining of various tissues including the eye, it is important to the support of a proper tear level and prevention of dry-eye syndrome.

Vitamin A additionally enhances immunity, may heal gastrointestinal ulcers, protects against pollution and cancer formation, and assists in the maintenance and repair of mucous tissue. It is important in the formation of bones and teeth, aids in fat storage, and protects against colds, influenza, and infections of the kidneys, bladder, lungs, and mucous membranes. Vitamin A also acts as an antioxidant. (For a discussion of antioxidants, see page 45.)

The upper intestinal tract is the primary area of absorption of vitamin A, since it's here that fat-splitting enzymes and bile salts convert carotene into a usable nutrient. This conversion is stimulated by thyroxine, an amino acid obtained from the thyroid gland. Once converted into vitamin A, carotene is absorbed the same way as preformed vitamin A. The conversion of carotene into vitamin A is never 100-percent complete. Approximately one-third of the carotene in food is converted into vitamin A. Less than one-fourth of the carotene in carrots and root vegetables undergoes conversion, and about one-half of the carotene in leafy green vegetables does. Some unchanged carotene is absorbed into the circulatory system and stored in the fat tissues rather than in the liver. Unabsorbed carotene is excreted.

The degree to which carotene is utilized by the body varies with the food source and the way the food is prepared. Cooking, puréeing, and mashing of a vegetable rupture the cell membranes and therefore make the carotene more available for absorption. Factors interfering with the absorption of vitamin A and carotene include strenuous physical activity performed within four hours of consumption of the nutrient, intake of mineral oil, excessive consumption of alcohol, excessive consumption of iron, and the use of cortisone and other medications. The intake of polyunsaturated fatty acids with carotene results in rapid destruction of the carotene unless antioxidants also are present. Even cold weather can hinder the

transport and metabolism of vitamin A and carotene. Diabetics cannot convert carotene to vitamin A.

Approximately 90 percent of the body's vitamin A is stored in the liver, with small amounts deposited in the fat tissues, lungs, kidneys, and retinas of the eyes. Under stressful conditions, the body uses this reserve supply if it doesn't receive enough vitamin A from the diet. Gastrointestinal and liver disorders, infections of any kind, or any condition in which the bile duct is obstructed can limit the body's capacity to retain and use vitamin A. Factors affecting the absorption of vitamin A include the amount of the nutrient consumed, the influence of other substances present in the intestines, and the amount of the vitamin stored in the body. For these reasons, the recommended dietary amounts vary for each individual.

A deficiency of vitamin A may be apparent if night blindness, dry hair or skin, dry eyes, or poor growth is present. Other possible results of a vitamin A-deficiency are abscesses in the ears; insomnia; fatigue; reproductive difficulties; sinusitis; pneumonia, frequent colds, and other respiratory infections; skin disorders including acne; and weight loss.

Precautions and Recommendations. Taking large amounts of vitamin A over long periods of time can be toxic to the body, mainly the liver. The RDAs for vitamin A are 1,500 international units (IU) for infants and children up to four years old, 3,000 IU for children from four to twelve years old, and 5,000 IU for children over twelve years old and adults. These amounts increase during disease, trauma, pregnancy, and lactation. The requirements vary for people who smoke, who live in highly polluted areas, who easily absorb vitamin A, and who have pneumonia or nephritis (inflammation of the kidney). Increased intakes of vitamins C and E will help to prevent excessive oxidation (free-radical damage) of stored vitamin A.

Research indicates that no more than 50,000 IU per day of vitamin A can be utilized by the body except in therapeutic cases, where up to 100,000 IU is recommended. It has been suggested that the best level is somewhere between 25,000 and 50,000 IU per day. However, do not take an excess of vitamin A without first consulting your physician or health-care practitioner. Toxic levels of vitamin A are associated with abdominal pain, amenorrhea (halt of menstruation), enlargement of the liver and/or spleen, gastrointestinal disturbances, hair loss, itching, joint pain, nausea and vomiting, water on the brain, and small cracks and scales on the lips. Vitamin C can help prevent the harmful effects of vitamin-A toxicity. Overdose is impossible with beta-carotene, although if you take too much, your skin may turn slightly yellow-orange in color. It is important to take only natural beta-carotene or a natural carotenoid complex.

Vitamin A has been successfully used in treating several eye disorders, including Bitot's spots (white, elevated, sharply outlined patches on the sclera), blurred vision, night blindness, cataracts, strabismus, and nearsightedness. Therapeutic dosages of vitamin A are necessary for the treatment of glaucoma, dry-eye syndrome, and pinkeye.

Vitamin-B Complex

All the B vitamins are water-soluble substances that can be cultivated from bacteria, yeasts, fungi, or molds. The known B-complex vitamins are B_1 (thiamine), B_2 (riboflavin), B_3 (niacin), B_5 (pantothenic acid), B_6 (pyridoxine), B_{12} (cyanocobalamin), biotin, choline, folic acid, inositol, and para-aminobenzoic acid (PABA). The grouping of these water-soluble compounds under the term "B complex" is based upon their common sources, their close relationship in vegetable and animal tissues, and their functional relationships.

The B-complex vitamins are active in providing the body with energy, basically by converting carbohydrates into glucose, which the body burns to produce energy. They are vital in the metabolism of fats and protein. In addition, the B vitamins are necessary for the normal functioning of the nervous system, and may be the single most important factor in the health of the nerves. They are essential for the maintenance of muscle tone in the gastrointestinal tract, and for the health of the skin, hair, eyes, mouth, and liver.

All of the B vitamins are natural constituents of brewer's yeast, liver, and whole-grain cereals. Brewer's yeast is the richest natural source of the B-complex group. Another important source of the B vitamins is intestinal bacteria. These bacteria grow best on milk sugar and small amounts of fat in the diet.

Precautions and Recommendations. Because of the water-solubility of the B-complex vitamins, any excess vitamin is excreted rather than stored. Therefore, the B vitamins must be continually replaced. All of the B vitamins, when mixed with saliva, are readily absorbed. Sulfa drugs, barbiturates (sleeping pills), insecticides, and estrogen can create a condition in the digestive tract that can destroy the B vitamins. Certain B vitamins are lost through perspiration.

The most important thing to remember is that all of the B vitamins should be taken together. They are so interrelated in function that a large dose of any one of them may be therapeutically valueless or may cause a deficiency of other B vitamins. For example, if you take extra B_6, you must take a complete B complex along with it. In nature, we find the B-complex vitamins in yeast and green vegetables, but nowhere do we find a single B vitamin isolated from the rest. The need for the B-complex vitamins increases during infection and stress. Alcoholics and individuals who consume excessive amounts of carbohydrates require higher intakes of the B vitamins for proper metabolism. Coffee uses up the B vitamins. Children and pregnant women need extra B vitamins for normal growth.

The B vitamins are so meagerly supplied in the American diet that almost every person in this country lacks some of them. If you are tired, irritable, nervous, depressed, or even suicidal, suspect a vitamin-B deficiency. Gray hair, baldness, acne and other skin problems, poor appetite, insomnia, neuritis (disease of the peripheral nerves), anemia, constipation, and a high cholesterol level also are indicators of a vitamin-B deficiency. One reason there is such a great vitamin-B deficiency in the American population is that we eat so much processed food from which the B vitamins have been removed. Another reason for the widespread deficiency is the high amount of sugar we consume. Sugar and alcohol destroy the B-complex vitamins.

The B vitamins have been used in the treatment of barbiturate overdose, alcoholic psychosis, and drug-induced delirium. An adequate dose has been found to control migraine headaches and attacks of Meniere's syndrome (a disease of the inner ear). Some heart abnormalities have responded to the use of the B complex because the nerves affecting the heart need the B-complex vitamins for smooth, quiet functioning. Massive dosages of the B-complex vitamins have been used to cure polio, to improve the condition of hypersensitive children who fail to respond favorably to medications such as Ritalin, and to improve cases of shingles. Nervous individuals and persons working under tension can greatly benefit from taking larger than normal doses of the B vitamins. The B vitamins may also help beriberi (caused by a vitamin-B_1 deficiency), pellagra (caused by a deficency of vitamin B_3, specifically nicotinic acid), constipation, burning feet, tender gums, eyelid twitching, double vision, fatigue, lack of appetite, skin disorders, cracks at the corners of the mouth, anemia, and dry, burning eyes.

Vitamin B_1 (Thiamine)

Vitamin B_1, also known as thiamine, is a water-soluble vitamin that combines with pyruvic acid to form a coenzyme necessary for the breakdown of carbohydrates into glucose, which is then oxidized by the body to produce energy. Thiamine is vulnerable to heat, air, and water in cooking. It is a component of the germ and bran of wheat, the husk of rice, and that portion of all grains which is commercially milled away to give the grain a lighter color and finer texture.

Thiamine enhances circulation, assists in the formation of blood, and aids in the production of hydrochloric acid, which is important for proper digestion. Thiamine also optimizes cognitive activity and brain function. It has a positive effect on energy, growth, appetite, and learning capacity, and is needed for muscle tone in the intestines, stomach, and heart. It also acts as an antioxidant, protecting the body from the degenerative effects of aging, alcohol consumption, and smoking.

Precautions and Recommendations. Thiamine deficiency can lead to inflammation of the optic nerve, called optic neuritis, as well as to impairment of the central nervous system. (For a discussion of optic neuritis, see page 179.) The first signs of thiamine deficiency include easy fatigue, loss of appetite, irritability, and emotional instability. If the deficiency is not addressed, confusion and loss of memory appear, followed closely by gastric distress, abdominal pain, and constipation.

The RDA for thiamine is 1.1 to 1.4 milligrams per day. A thiamine intake of 1.4 milligrams daily is recommended during pregnancy and lactation. The need for thiamine increases during severe diarrhea, fever, stress, and surgery. Thiamine has no known toxic side effects.

The richest food sources of thiamine include brown rice, egg yolks, fish, legumes, liver, pork, poultry, rice bran, wheat germ, and whole grains. Other sources are asparagus, brewer's yeast, broccoli, Brussels sprouts, dulse, kelp, most nuts, oatmeal, plums, dried prunes, raisins, spirulina, and watercress. Herbs that contain thiamine include alfalfa, bladderwrack, burdock, catnip, cayenne, chamomile, chickweed, eyebright, fennel, fenugreek, hops, nettle, oat straw, parsley, peppermint, raspberry, red clover, rose hips, sage, yarrow, and yellow dock.

Vitamin B_2 (Riboflavin)

Vitamin B_2, also known as riboflavin, is a water-soluble vitamin that occurs naturally in the same foods containing the other B vitamins. Riboflavin is stable to heat, oxidation, and acid, but disintegrates in the presence of alkalis or light, especially ultraviolet (UV) light.

Riboflavin functions as part of a group of enzymes involved in the breakdown and utilization of carbohydrates, fats, and protein. Riboflavin is necessary for cell respiration because it works with enzymes in the utilization of cell oxygen. It is also necessary for the maintenance of good vision, skin, nails, and hair.

Riboflavin deficiency is the most common vitamin deficiency in the United States. This deficiency can result from long-established faulty dietary habits, food idiosyncrasies, alcoholism, arbitrarily selected diets used for the relief of digestive problems, and/or prolonged dietary restriction. The most common symptoms of a lack of B_2 are cracks and sores in the corners of the mouth; a red, sore tongue; a feeling of grit and sand on the insides of the eyelids; burning eyes; eye fatigue; dilated pupils; corneal changes; light sensitivity; lesions on the lips; scaling around the nose, mouth, or forehead; trembling; sluggishness; dizziness; and vaginal itching.

Riboflavin plays an important role in the prevention of some visual disturbances, especially cataracts. Under-nourished women at the end of pregnancy often suffer from conditions such as visual disturbances, burning eyes, excessive tearing, and failing vision. These conditions can be helped by supplementing the diet with large doses of B_2.

Precautions and Recommendations. The RDA for riboflavin is 1.6 milligrams for adult males and 1.2 milligrams for adult females. During pregnancy and lactation, the requirement goes up to 1.5 milligrams and 1.7 milligrams, respectively. There are no known toxic side effects to the use of riboflavin. However, prolonged ingestion of large doses of any one of the B-complex vitamins, including riboflavin, may result in high urinary losses of the other B vitamins. Therefore, it is important to take a complete B complex along with any single B vitamin.

Vitamin B_3 (Niacin)

Niacin is another member of the B-complex family of vitamins, and is also water soluble. It is more stable than either thiamine or riboflavin, and is remarkably resistant to heat, light, air, acids, and alkalis. As a coenzyme, niacin assists enzymes in the breakdown and utilization of protein, fats, and carbohydrates. Niacin is effective at improving circulation and reducing the blood-cholesterol level. It is vital to the proper function of the nervous system, and for the formation and maintenance of healthy tongue and digestive-system tissues, and skin.

Relatively small amounts of pure niacin are present in most foods. The niacin "equivalent" listed in dietary tables refers either to pure niacin or to tryptophan, an amino acid that can be converted into niacin by the body. Lean meats, poultry, fish, and peanuts are rich sources of both niacin and tryptophan, as are such dietary supplements as brewer's yeast, wheat germ, and desiccated liver. Niacin is difficult to obtain except from these foods.

Precautions and Recommendations. The RDAs suggest that the daily allowance of niacin be based on caloric intake, with 6.6 milligrams of niacin recommended for every 1,000 calories. There have been no toxic side effects reported for niacin, but taking extremely large doses can cause tingling and itching sensations, intense flushing of the skin, and throbbing in the head.

Excessive consumption of sugar and starches depletes the body's supply of niacin, as does taking certain antibiotics. The symptoms of niacin deficiency are many. In the early stages, they include muscular weakness, general fatigue, loss of appetite, indigestion, and various skin eruptions. Niacin deficiency may also cause bad breath, small ulcers, canker sores, insomnia, irritability, nausea, vomiting, recurring headaches, tender gums, strain, tension, and deep depression.

Vitamin B_6 (Pyridoxine)

Vitamin B_6 is a water-soluble vitamin consisting of three related compounds—pyridoxine, pyrdoxinal, and pyridoxamine. It is required for the proper absorption of vitamin B_{12}, and for the production of hydrochloric acid and magnesium. Pyridoxine plays an important role as a coenzyme in the breakdown and utilization of carbohydrates, fats, and protein. It is required for the production of antibodies and red blood cells. In addition, it facilitates the release of glycogen for energy from the liver and muscles.

Vitamin B_6 helps to maintain the balance between sodium and potassium, which regulate the body fluids and promote the normal functioning of the nervous and musculoskeletal systems. The best sources of vitamin B_6 are meats and whole grains, specifically desiccated liver and brewer's yeast.

Precautions and Recommendations. According to the RDAs, the daily allowance of vitamin B_6 is based on protein intake. Adults need 2.0 milligrams of pyridoxine for every 100 grams of protein they consume per day. Children need 0.6 to 1.2 milligrams for every 100 grams of protein they consume. The need for vitamin B_6 doubles during pregnancy, lactation, exposure to radiation, cardiac failure, aging, and use of oral contraceptives.

In cases of vitamin-B_6 deficiency, there is low blood sugar and low glucose tolerance, resulting in a sensitivity to insulin. Deficiency may also cause loss of hair, water retention during pregnancy, cracks around the mouth and eyes, numbness and cramps in the arms and legs, slow learning, visual disturbances, neuritis, arthritis, heart disorders, and increased urination.

Vitamin B_{12} (Cyanocobalamin)

B-complex member vitamin B_{12} is unique in that it is the first cobalt-containing substance found to be essential for longevity. In addition, it is the only vitamin that contains essential mineral elements. Vitamin B_{12} cannot be made synthetically, but must be grown, like penicillin, in bacteria or molds. One of the only foods in which B_{12} occurs naturally in substantial amounts is animal protein. Therefore, vegetarians frequently are low in vitamin B_{12}. At the same time, high blood levels of folic acid, also common in vegetarians, can mask a vitamin-B_{12} deficiency. Liver is the best source of B_{12}, and kidney, muscle meats, fish, and dairy products are other good sources.

Vitamin B_{12} is necessary for the normal metabolism of nerve tissue, and is involved in protein, fat, and carbohydrate metabolism. The actions of B_{12} are closely related to those of four amino acids, vitamin B_5, and vitamin C. Vitamin B_{12} also helps iron to function better in the body, and aids folic acid in the synthesis of choline.

Precautions and Recommendations. The human requirement for vitamin B_{12} is minute, but the vitamin is essential to health. The RDA for vitamin B_{12} is 3 micrograms for adults and 4 micrograms for pregnant and lactating women. Infants require a daily intake of 3 micrograms, and growing children need 1 to 2 micrograms. No cases of vitamin-B_{12} toxicity have ever been reported.

The symptoms of a vitamin-B_{12} deficiency may take five or six years to appear. Deficiency of the vitamin is usually due to a lack of the intrinsic factor, a glycoprotein necessary for the absorption of B_{12}. Deficiency begins with changes in the nervous system such as soreness and weakness in the legs and arms, diminished reflex response and sensory perception, difficulty walking and speaking, and jerking of the limbs. The condition known as tobacco amblyopia, a loss of vision due to tobacco poisoning, has been improved with injections of vitamin B_{12}, whether or not the patient stopped smoking. The symptoms of tobacco amblyopia are blackouts, headaches, and far-sightedness.

Choline

Choline is considered one of the B-complex vitamins. It functions with inositol, also considered a B-complex vitamin, as a basic constituent of lecithin. It is present in the bodies of all living cells, and is widely distributed in animal and plant tissues. Lecithin is the richest source of choline, but other rich dietary sources are egg yolks, liver, brewer's yeast, and wheat germ.

Choline appears to be associated primarily with the utilization of fats and cholesterol in the body. It prevents fats from accumulating in the liver, and facilitates their movement into the the cells. In the liver, choline combines with fatty acids and phosphoric acid to form lecithin. It is essential for the health of the liver and kidneys.

Choline is also essential for the health of the myelin sheaths of the nerves. The myelin sheaths are the principal components of the nerve fibers. Choline plays an important role in the transmission of the nerve impulses. Choline also helps to regulate and improve liver and gallbladder functioning, and aids in the prevention of gallstones.

Precautions and Recommendations. The daily requirements for choline are not known. The average American adult diet has been estimated to contain 500 to 900 milligrams of choline per day.

Vitamin C

Vitamin C, also known as ascorbic acid, is a water-soluble nutrient. Although fairly stable in acid solutions, it is normally the least stable of the vitamins, and is very sensitive to oxygen. Its potency can be lost through exposure to light, heat, or air, all of which stimulate the activity of the oxidative enzymes.

The primary function of vitamin C is to maintain the body's collagen, a protein necessary for the formation of the connective tissue in the skin, ligaments, bones, and, most importantly for our purposes, sclera of the eye. Vitamin C plays a role in the healing of wounds and burns because it facilitates the formation of connective tissue in scars. Vitamin C also aids in the formation of red blood cells and the prevention of hemorrhaging. In addition, vitamin C fights bacterial infections and reduces the effects on the body of some allergens. For these reasons, vitamin C is frequently used in the prevention and treatment of the common cold.

Vitamin C is present in most fresh fruits and vegetables. Natural-vitamin-C dietary supplements are prepared from rose hips, acerola cherries, green peppers, and citrus fruits.

The level of ascorbic acid in the blood reaches a maximum about two or three hours after the ingestion of a moderate quantity of the nutrient, then decreases as the vitamin is eliminated in the urine and through perspiration. Most vitamin C is out of the body in three to four hours. Because vitamin C is a "stress vitamin," it is used up even more rapidly under stressful conditions. Humans, apes, and guinea pigs are the only animals that must obtain vitamin C from their food because they are unable to meet the body's needs by synthesis alone. Ascorbic acid is readily absorbed from the gastrointestinal tract into the bloodstream. Two factors that influence its absorption are the manner in which the vitamin is administered and the presence of other substances in the intestinal tract. The normal human body, when fully saturated, contains about 5,000 milligrams of vitamin C, of which 30 milligrams are found in the adrenal glands, 200 milligrams in the extracellular fluids, and the rest in varying concentrations throughout the cells of the entire body.

Vitamin C promotes bone and tooth formation while protecting the dentine and pulp of teeth. Some types of viral and bacterial infections are prevented or cured by vitamin C. One school of thought regarding the effects of vitamin C on the development of nearsightedness is that the sclera of the eye, being connective tissue, is fortified by the vitamin. If there is a lack of vitamin C for an extended period of time, especially during the high growth years, the eye structure will weaken, allowing the pressure inside the eye to expand the length of the eye, which leads to nearsightedness. In addition, it is a fact that the fluid filling the anterior chamber of the eye—between the cornea and the lens—maintains a vitamin-C level approximately twenty times higher than that of the blood plasma. This is considered significant in the nutrition of the lens, which has no blood supply and depends on the aqueous fluid for its nourishment. It only stands to reason that the level of vitamin C should be upheld or increased as we age to maintain a clear and healthy lens within the eye.

Precautions and Recommendations. The RDA for vitamin C is 45 milligrams for adults. However, the now-famous Dr. Linus Pauling suggested that the optimal daily intake of vitamin C for most human adults is from 2,300 to 9,000 milligrams. This wide range takes into account differences in weight, activity level, metabolism, ailments, and age.

Toxicity symptoms usually do not occur with high intakes of vitamin C because the body simply discharges whatever it cannot use. However, a daily intake of 5,000 to 15,000 milligrams may cause side effects in some people. The toxicity symptoms of vitamin C include a slight burning sensation during urination, loose bowels, and skin rashes.

The body's ability to absorb vitamin C is reduced by smoking, stress, high fever, prolonged intake of antibiotics or cortisone, inhalation of petroleum fumes, and ingestion of aspirin or other painkillers. Baking soda destroys vitamin C, as does cooking with copper utensils. The signs of deficiency include shortness of breath, impaired digestion, poor lactation, bleeding gums, weakened tooth enamel or dentine, tendency to bruising, swollen or painful joints, nosebleeds, anemia, lowered resistance to infections, and slow healing of wounds. Severe deficiency results in scurvy.

Vitamin D

Vitamin D is a fat-soluble vitamin that can be acquired both from food and through exposure to sunlight. It is known as the "sunshine vitamin" because the sun's UV rays activate a form of cholesterol present in the skin, converting the substance to vitamin D.

Vitamin D aids in the absorption of calcium from the intestinal tract, and in the breakdown and assimilation of phosphorus, which is required for bone formation. In the mucous membranes, it helps to synthesize enzymes that are involved in the active transport of available calcium. Vitamin D is necessary for normal growth in children, for without it, the bones and teeth do not calcify properly.

Adults also benefit from vitamin D. It is valuable for maintaining a stable nervous system, normal heart action, and normal blood clotting because all these functions are related to the body's supply and utilization of calcium and phosphorus. Vitamin D is best utilized by the body when taken with vitamin A. Fish-liver oils are the best natural sources of vitamins A and D.

Precautions and Recommendations. Most of the body's need for vitamin D can be met by sufficient exposure to sunlight and ingestion of small amounts of food. However, the sun's action on the skin can be inhibited by such factors as air pollution, clouds, window glass, and clothing. The RDA for vitamin D is set at 400 IU per day, which should meet the requirements of most healthy individuals who are not regularly exposed to UV light.

Being a fat-soluble vitamin means that vitamin D can be stored in the body. Excessive blood levels of the vitamin often cause a rise in the blood levels of calcium and phosphorus, and excessive excretion of calcium in the urine. This leads to calcification of the soft tissues and of the walls of the blood vessels and kidney tubules, a condition known as hypercalcemia. The symptoms of acute overdosage are increased frequency of urination, loss of appetite, nausea, vomiting, diarrhea, muscular weakness, dizziness, weariness, and calcification of the soft tissues of the heart, blood vessels, and lungs. These symptoms disappear within a few days of discontinuation of the overdosing.

A deficiency of vitamin D leads to inadequate absorption of calcium from the intestinal tract and retention of phosphorus in the kidneys. The inability of the soft bones to withstand the stress of the body's weight results in skeletal malformations. Rickets, a bone disorder in children, is a direct result of vitamin-D deficiency. Adult rickets, called osteomalacia, can also occur. One study showed that a vitamin-D deficiency may cause nearsightedness. An imbalance of the vitamin with calcium is at the root of this disorder. Other possible effects are keratoconus (cone-shaped cornea), pinkeye, cataracts, and arteriosclerosis.

Vitamin E

Vitamin E, a fat-soluble vitamin, is composed of a group of compounds called tocopherols. Seven forms of tocopherol—alpha, beta, delta, epsilon, eta, gamma, and zeta—exist in nature. Of these, alpha tocopherol is the most potent and has the greatest nutritional and biological values. The tocopherols occur in the highest concentrations in cold-pressed vegetable oils, whole raw seeds and nuts, and soybeans. Wheat germ oil is the source from which vitamin E was first obtained.

Vitamin E is an antioxidant, which means it opposes the oxidation of substances in the body. It plays an essential role in the cellular respiration of the muscles, especially the cardiac and skeletal muscles. It makes it possible for these muscles and their nerves to function with less oxygen, thereby increasing their endurance and stamina. It also causes dilation of the blood vessels, permitting a fuller flow of blood to the heart, as well as to the other organs.

Vitamin E is effective against the formation of elevated scar tissue on the surface of the body and within the body. In ointment form, it is used on burns to promote healing and to lessen the formation of scars. As a diuretic, vitamin E helps to lower elevated blood pressure. It protects against the damaging effects of many environmental poisons in the air, water, and food.

There are several substances that interfere with, or even cause a depletion of, vitamin E in the body. For example, when iron, especially the inorganic form, and vitamin E are administered together, the absorption of both is impaired. Chlorine in drinking water, ferric chloride, rancid oil or fat, and inorganic-iron compounds destroy vitamin E in the body. Mineral oil used as a laxative depletes vitamin E. Large amounts of polyunsaturated fats or oils in the diet increase the oxidation rate of vitamin E. The more unsaturated fats or oils that are consumed, the more vitamin E is necessary.

Vitamin E has many beneficial effects. It works to treat and prevent heart diseases, such as coronary thrombosis, a heart attack caused by vessels being blocked by blood clots. Vitamin E causes arterial blood clots to disintegrate. Angina, a condition in which chest pain results from an insufficient supply of blood to the heart tissues, is successfully treated with alpha tocopherol. Vitamin E is beneficial to persons with atherosclerosis if used as a therapy before irreparable damage occurs. It relieves pain in the extremities, speeds up blood flow, and reduces clotting tendencies.

Vitamin E can aid in the healing of burned tissue, skin ulcers, and abrasions. It prevents or dissolves scars. It is also helpful in counteracting premature aging of the skin. It is useful to apply vitamin E to the skin in ointment form while also taking it orally, because it affects cell formation by replacing the cells on the outer layer of the skin. Vitamin E also helps to counter the gradual decline in metabolic processes during aging.

Vitamin-E therapy has been suggested as beneficial in a number of other conditions, including bursitis (inflammation of a bursa resulting in joint pain), gout (defective uric-acid metabolism), arthritis, nearsightedness, strabismus, varicose veins, thrombosis (thickening of the blood resulting in blood clots), phlebitis (inflammation of the wall of a vein), nephritis, and even headaches.

Precautions and Recommendations. The RDA for vitamin E is based upon metabolic body size and level of polyunsaturated fatty acids in the diet, rather than upon weight or caloric intake. The requirements increase along with any increases in the amount of polyunsaturated fatty acids consumed. The RDA is 4 to 5 IU daily for infants, 7 to 12 IU for children and adolescents; 15 IU for adult males, 12 IU for adult females, and 15 IU for pregnant or lactating females. However, many nutritionists consider these allowances exceedingly low.

The first sign of a vitamin-E deficiency is the rupture of red blood cells, resulting from the cells' increased fragility. A deficiency could result in a reduction of membrane stability and shrinkage of collagen. Also, a tendency toward muscular wasting or abnormal fat deposits in the muscles, and an increased demand for oxygen can occur in a deficiency state. The essential fatty acids are altered so that blood cells break down and hemoglobin formation is impaired. In addition, the body's ability to utilize several amino acids is impaired, and the level of functioning of the pituitary and adrenal glands is reduced. Iron absorption and hemoglobin formation also are impaired. A severe deficiency can cause damage to the kidneys and liver.

A prolonged deficiency of vitamin E can cause faulty absorption of fat and the fat-soluble vitamins. Poor utilization of vitamin E or an increased demand for it can cause anemia.

The Bioflavonoids

The bioflavonoids, sometimes known as vitamin P, are water soluble and composed of a group of brightly colored substances that often appear in fruits and vegetables as companions to vitamin C. The members of the group are citrin, hesperidin, rutin, the flavones, and the flavonals.

The bioflavonoids were first discovered as substances in the white part, not the juice, of citrus fruits. The edible part of citrus fruits contains ten times more bioflavonoids than the strained juice. The sources of the bioflavonoids include lemons, grapes, plums, black currants, grapefruits, apricots, buckwheat, cherries, blackberries, and rose hips.

The bioflavonoids are essential for the proper absorption and use of vitamin C. They assist vitamin C in keeping the collagen in healthy condition. They also have the ability to increase the strength of the capillaries and to regulate the capillaries' permeability. These actions help to prevent hemorrhages and ruptures in the capillaries and connective tissue, and to build a protective barrier against infections. The blood-vessel leakage that occurs within the retina of the eye may be reduced to some degree by the use of a vitamin C-bioflavonoid combination.

Precautions and Recommendations. The absorption and storage properties, daily requirements, deficiency symptoms, and body utilization of the bioflavonoids are all similar to those of vitamin C.

Minerals

Minerals are nutrients that exist in the body and in food, in organic and inorganic combinations. Approximately seventeen minerals are essential in human nutrition. Although minerals make up only 4 or 5 percent of the human body's weight, they are vital to overall mental and physical well-being. All of the tissues and internal fluids of living things contain varying quantities of minerals. Minerals are constituents of the bones, teeth, soft tissue, muscle, blood, and nerve cells. They are important in maintaining the physiological processes, strengthening the skeletal structure, and preserving the vigor of the heart, the brain, and all of the muscle and nerve systems.

Although we will discuss a number of minerals separately in the following pages, it is important to note that the actions of all the minerals within the body are interrelated; no one mineral functions without affecting the others. Physical and emotional stress can cause a strain on the body's supply of minerals. A mineral deficiency often results in illness, which may be corrected by adding the missing mineral to the diet.

Calcium

Calcium is the most abundant mineral in the body. About 99 percent of the calcium in the body is deposited in the bones and teeth, with the remainder found in the soft tissues. To function properly, calcium must be accompanied by magnesium, phosphorus, and vitamins A, C, and D.

The major function of calcium is to act in cooperation with phosphorus to build and maintain the bones and teeth. Calcium is essential for healthy blood, eases insomnia, and helps to regulate the heartbeat. An important calcium partner in cardiovascular health is magnesium. Calcium assists in the process of blood clotting and helps to prevent the accumulation of too much acid or alkali in the blood. It also plays a part in muscle growth, muscle contraction, and nerve transmission. Calcium aids in the body's utilization of iron, helps to activate several enzymes, and helps to regulate the passage of nutrients in and out of cell walls.

Calcium absorption is very inefficient, with usually only 20 to 30 percent of ingested calcium absorbed. When it needs calcium, however, the body can absorb it more effectively. Therefore, the greater the need for calcium and the smaller the dietary supply are, the more efficient is the absorption. Absorption is also increased during periods of rapid growth. Calcium absorption depends upon the presence of adequate amounts of vitamin D, which works with the parathyroid hormone to regulate the amount of calcium in the blood. Phosphorus is needed in at least the same amount as calcium. Vitamins A and C are also necessary for calcium absorption. Fat consumed in moderate amounts and moving slowly through the digestive tract facilitates absorption. A high intake of protein also aids in the absorption of calcium.

Precautions and Recommendations. Certain substances inhibit calcium absorption. When excessive amounts of fat combine with calcium, the result is an insoluble compound that cannot be absorbed. Calcium combined with oxalic acid, found in chocolate, spinach, and rhubarb, makes another insoluble compound and may form into stones in the kidney or gallbladder. Other interfering factors are lack of exercise, excessive stress, and too rapid a flow of food through the intestinal tract.

One of the first signs of a calcium deficiency is a nervous affliction called tetany, which is characterized by muscle cramps, and numbness and tingling in the arms and hands. A calcium deficiency can result in bone malformation, causing rickets in children and osteomalacia in adults. Another ailment that results from calcium deficiency is osteoporosis, in which the bones become porous and fragile because calcium is withdrawn from them, as well as from other body areas, faster than it is deposited. Moderate cases of calcium deficiency may lead to cramps, joint pains, heart palpitations, eyelid twitching, slow pulse rate, tooth decay, insomnia, impaired growth, and excessive irritability of the nerves and muscles.

Chromium

Chromium is an essential mineral found in concentrations of twenty parts of chromium to one billion parts of blood. It stimulates the activity of enzymes involved in the metabolism of glucose for energy and the synthesis of fatty acids and cholesterol. Chromium also appears to increase the effectiveness of insulin, thereby facilitating the transport of glucose into the cells. In the blood, it competes with iron in the transport of protein. Chromium may also be involved in the synthesis of protein through its binding action with ribonucleic-acid (RNA) molecules.

The sources of chromium include corn oil, clams, whole-grain cereals, and meats. Fruits and vegetables contain trace amounts. Brewer's yeast provides a dependable supply without the problems of high carbohydrate intake and high cholesterol levels. Chromium is difficult to absorb. Only about 3 percent of dietary chromium is retained in the body, and the amount of chromium stored in the body decreases with age.

Precautions and Recommendations. A chromium deficiency may upset the function of insulin, and result in depressed growth rates and severe glucose intolerance in diabetics. It is also believed that the interaction of chromium and insulin is not limited to glucose metabolism, but also affects amino-acid metabolism. Chromium may inhibit the formation of aortic plaques, and a deficiency may contribute to atherosclerosis. Chromium deficiency has also been shown to be a factor in the development of nearsightedness.

Magnesium

Magnesium is an essential mineral that accounts for about .05 percent of the body's total weight. Nearly 70 percent of the body's supply is located in the bones together with calcium and phosphorus, while 30 percent is found in the soft tissues and body fluids.

Magnesium is involved in many essential metabolic processes. Most of the body's magnesium is found inside the cells, where it activates enzymes necessary for the metabolism of carbohydrates and amino acids. By countering the stimulative effect of calcium, magnesium plays an important role in neuromuscular contraction. It also helps to regulate the acid-alkaline balance in the body.

Magnesium helps to promote the absorption and metabolism of other minerals, as well as the utilization of the B vitamins and vitamins C and E. It aids during bone growth and is necessary for the proper functioning of the nerves and muscles.

Magnesium is widely distributed in food sources, but is found chiefly in fresh green vegetables, where it is an essential element of chlorophyll. Other excellent sources are unmilled raw wheat germ, soybeans, figs, corn, apples, and oil-rich seeds and nuts, especially almonds. Dolomite, a natural dietary supplement, is also rich in magnesium.

Precautions and Recommendations. The RDA for magnesium is 350 milligrams for adult males and 300 milligrams for adult females. The amount for females increases to 450 milligrams during pregnancy and lactation. It is estimated that the typical American diet provides only about 120 milligrams.

Evidence suggests that the balance between calcium and magnesium is especially important. If calcium consumption is high, magnesium intake must also be high. The magnesium requirement is further influenced by the amounts of protein, phosphorus, and vitamin D in the diet. The need is also increased when the blood-cholesterol level is high or the consumption of protein is high. Magnesium oxide is preferred over dolomite. When dolomite is taken, additional supplementation with hydrochloric acid is needed to ensure that the dolomite is dissolved properly. Because magnesium acts as an alkali, it should not be taken after meals.

Large amounts of magnesium can be toxic, especially if the calcium intake is low and the phosphorus intake is high. Excessive magnesium is usually excreted adequately, but in the event of kidney failure, there is a greater danger of toxicity because the rate of excretion is much lower.

Magnesium deficiency can occur in patients who have diabetes, pancreatitis, or kidney malfunction; are alcoholic; or consume a high-carbohydrate diet. A deficiency is thought to be related to coronary heart disease, since it results in the formation of clots in the heart and brain, and may contribute to calcium deposits. The symptoms include apprehensiveness, muscle twitching, tremors, confusion, and disorientation.

Selenium

Selenium is an essential mineral found in minute amounts in the body. It works closely with vitamin E in some of its metabolic actions, and in the promotion of normal body growth and fertility. Selenium is a natural antioxidant and appears to preserve the elasticity of tissue by delaying the oxidation of polyunsaturated fatty acids, which can cause solidification of tissue proteins.

Selenium is found in the bran and germ of cereals; in vegetables such as broccoli, onion, and tomatoes; and in tuna. The liver and kidneys contain four to five times as much selenium as do the muscles and other tissues. Selenium is normally excreted in the urine. Its presence in the feces is an indication of improper absorption.

Precautions and Recommendations. The RDA for selenium for adults is extremely minute—five to ten parts of selenium per one million parts of food or other minerals is considered toxic. This is due to the tendency of selenium to replace sulfur in biological compounds and to inhibit the action of some enzymes. Selenium can be toxic in its pure form, so supple-

ments should be taken with care. Reported instances of toxicity have occurred in areas where the selenium content of the soil is high.

A deficiency of selenium may encourage premature aging. This is because selenium preserves tissue elasticity. This is of major significance for the lens within the eye, which becomes less flexible with age. (For a discussion of this, see "Presbyopia" on page 187.)

Sodium

Sodium is an essential mineral found predominantly in the extracellular fluids such as the vascular fluids within the blood vessels and the interstitial fluids surrounding the cells. The remaining sodium in the body is found within the bones.

Sodium functions with potassium to equalize the acid-alkaline balance in the blood. Along with potassium, it helps to regulate the water balance within the body—that is, it helps to control the distribution of fluids on either side of the cell walls. Sodium and potassium are also involved in muscle contraction and expansion, and in nerve stimulation. Another important function of sodium is keeping the other blood minerals soluble so that they will not build up into deposits in the bloodstream. It helps to purge carbon dioxide from the body, aids digestion, and functions in the production of hydrochloric acid in the stomach. In addition, it acts with chlorine to improve blood and lymph health.

Sodium is found in virtually all foods, especially in sodium chloride (table salt). High concentrations are found in seafood, carrots, beets, poultry, and meat. Kelp is an excellent supplemental source of sodium.

Precautions and Recommendations. There is no established dietary requirement for sodium, but it is generally observed that the usual intake far exceeds the need. The average American ingests 3 to 7 grams of sodium and 6 to 18 grams of sodium chloride each day. The NRC recommends a daily sodium-chloride intake of 1 gram for every 1 kilogram (35 ounces) of water consumed.

An excess of sodium in the diet may cause potassium to be lost in the urine. Abnormal fluid retention accompanied by dizziness and swelling of the legs or face can also occur. A daily intake of 14 to 28 grams of sodium chloride is considered excessive. Diets containing excessive amounts of sodium contribute to an increase in blood pressure. The simplest way to reduce sodium intake is to eliminate table salt from the diet.

Zinc

Zinc is an essential trace mineral that occurs in the body in a larger amount than any other trace element except iron. The human body contains approximately 1.8 grams of zinc, compared to nearly 5.0 grams of iron.

Zinc has a variety of functions. It is related to the normal absorption and action of the vitamins, especially vitamin A and the B complex. It is a constituent of at least twenty-five of the enzymes involved in digestion and metabolism. It is a component of insulin, and part of the enzyme that is needed to break down alcohol. It also functions in carbohydrate digestion and phosphorus metabolism. It has an important role in general growth and development, the function of the prostate gland, the healing of wounds and burns, and the synthesis of deoxyribonucleic acid (DNA).

The best sources of all the trace elements in proper balance are natural unprocessed foods, especially those grown in organically enriched soil. Diets high in protein, whole-grain products, brewer's yeast, wheat bran, wheat germ, and pumpkin seeds are usually high in zinc.

Precautions and Recommendations. The RDA for zinc is 15 milligrams a day for adults. An additional 15 milligrams is recommended during pregnancy, and an additional 25 milligrams is recommended during lactation. Zinc is relatively nontoxic, although poisoning may result from eating a food that has been stored in a galvanized container. High intakes of zinc interfere with copper utilization, causing incomplete iron metabolism. When zinc is added to the diet, vitamin A is also needed in larger amounts.

ANTIOXIDANTS

All the vitamins and minerals that are antioxidants operate in a similar manner in the body. They play an important role in the body's basic defense system against disease, infection, premature aging, and, possibly, the adverse effects of strenuous athletic performance. Here is some background on how the antioxidants work.

At the root of many diseases and the aging process are a group of highly reactive substances called free radicals or oxidants. These chemical compounds consist of two or more elements bound together by a chemical bond, with an unpaired, or "extra," electron. The unpaired electron makes the free radical very reactive and unstable. To stabilize itself, a free radical seeks out and grabs an electron from a stable compound. This, in turn, creates a new free radical. A chain reaction is begun, thus extending the damage of even a small number of these reactive compounds.

Once in the body, free radicals attack cell components and cause damage to cells and tissues in the body. Common sites of attack are the polyunsaturated fatty acids in cell membranes. This free-radical-induced damage alters the cell-membrane structure and function. The membrane is no longer able to transport nutrients, oxygen, or water into the cell, or to regulate the removal of waste products. Continued free-radical attack ruptures the cell membrane, causing the loss of the cellular components and rendering the cell useless. The intracellular chemicals leak into and damage the surrounding tissues. This process is associated with the initiation of numerous disorders from arthritis to cardiovascular disease.

Free-radical damage to tissues or molecules might be an initiating factor of atherosclerosis. Oxidative damage to the arteries attracts platelets, while the damaged artery becomes a place for cholesterol to accumulate. Oxidized LDLs might contribute to the process and increase adhesion at the site of the injury. Free radicals also damage the cells' mitochondria (energy factories), which results in limited or halted production of energy for all the cell processes. Free-radical damage to enzymes and other proteins limits the building of body tissues and causes the accumulation of protein fragments. Both of these conditions are noted in the premature aging of tissues. Finally, a cell cannot reproduce normally when its genetic code has been altered by free radicals. At best, the cell dies. At worst, the cell mutates into a cancerous cell.

Free radicals are unavoidable. They are formed during the normal metabolic process. They also are obtained from some foods, inhaled with polluted air and tobacco smoke, and generated in the environment by radiation and herbicides. Fortunately, the body has an anti-free-radical system composed of antioxidant enzymes such as superoxide dismutase (SOD) and glutathione peroxidase; vitamins such as C, E, and beta-carotene; minerals such as zinc and selenium;

herbs such as bilberry and ginkgo; and other nutrients such as cysteine, pine bark extract, coenzyme Q_{10}, and the bioflavonoids. These antioxidants intercede, deactivating the free radicals and rendering them harmless before they can cause irreversible damage to the body's tissues. They are currently being thoroughly investigated for their role in the prevention of many major diseases, including eye diseases such as cataracts and age-related macular degeneration.

Two recently discovered, powerful antioxidants are the carotenes lutein and zeaxanthin. Lutein and zeaxanthin are similar to beta-carotene in that they are found in spinach, kale, and other vegetables and fruits. They are not converted to vitamin A, but they do serve as potent antioxidants. They make up the yellow pigment in the retina, and appear to protect the macula in particular. Research shows that higher dietary levels of lutein and zeaxanthin are associated with greater protection of the macula, which can help to prevent macular degeneration. Lutein and zeaxanthin have also been shown to lead to a lower level of cataract formation.

Nutrition is the relationship of foods to the health of the human body. Proper nutrition implies receiving adequate foods and supplements to convey the nutrients required for optimal health. Without proper nutrition, optimal health and well-being cannot be obtained.

This statement is also true for the visual system. Our eyes are very complex organs and require an extremely high proportion of nutrients to maintain their proper function. With a little attention paid to general nutritional guidelines, you should be able to "feed your eyes" optimally and see well for years to come.

Herbal Therapy

Herbs, by definition, are plants that lack the woody characteristics of shrubs and trees. Over the years, many substances have been extracted from numerous herbs, as well as from other plants, and used successfully to heal the human body. Herbs are food for the body. They contain natural medicines, vitamins, and minerals, and have remarkable histories of curative effects when used in the proper way. Herbs have been used for centuries, and many of today's modern medicines have their foundations in herbal therapy.

The exact reasons for the positive effects that herbs exert on the human body are not always known. It is evident, however, that the nutrients stored within the plants' cellular structures are in forms that are easily metabolized by the body. The therapeutic actions of herbs come from alkaloids, organic compounds that cause certain chemical reactions within the body. Alkaloids also help the body to resist disease, strengthen tissues, and improve the nervous system. It is an often overlooked fact that the organic chemical structures of hemoglobin (the substance within red blood cells that carries oxygen and gives blood its red color) and chlorophyll (the substance within green plants that absorbs light and gives plants their green color) are very similar.

In this chapter, we will discuss herbs and herbal therapy. We will describe the twenty-eight most popular herbs used for the eyes, as well as the most common Western herbal combinations and the traditional Chinese herbal combinations used for eye problems.

WESTERN HERBS VERSUS CHINESE HERBS

Herbs are grown all over the world. Some of the more popular herbs are Chinese herbs. In China, unlike in other parts of the world, herbalists have sought out special tonic herbs that can be taken daily to improve the physical condition, enhance the energy, increase the resistance to disease, and prolong life. These herbs in particular help to distinguish Chinese herbalism from other forms of the art, such as Western herbalism. The term "Western" as used in herbalism really applies to the methods of using herbs rather than to the origins of herbs. This is why Western herb books often list substances from places such as Asia, Africa, South America, and Egypt. Individual herbs are used for their reputed health benefits, not because of the way they may act against a complex health syndrome or interact with other herbs in a combination formula.

Chinese herbalism, also known as traditional Chinese medicine, arranges physical signs and symptoms into patterns of organ disharmony, which can then be treated with acupuncture and herbal combinations to restore harmony and balance in the human body. The treatment of disease by traditional Chinese medicine is generally a complicated procedure and should be performed by an experienced practitioner. The herbal formulas are often adjusted as the symptoms change during recovery. Some of these formulas are meant for short-term therapy only. There are several patented medicines made in China and the United States that can be used to treat vision problems and benefit overall health. Their use, too, however, should be overseen by a health-care professional.

FORMS OF HERBAL PREPARATIONS

Herbal preparations can be applied in many different forms. The best are the tincture and the extract, which remain potent longer than any other form. A tincture is an herb mixed in an alcohol solution. It is made by adding a powdered herb to alcohol, then adding enough water to make a 50-percent alcohol solution. Let the mixture stand for two weeks, shaking the bottle once or twice a day, then strain it before using it. An extract is made by hydraulically pressing an herb, then soaking it in alcohol or water. The excess liquid is allowed to evaporate, and the result is a concentrated liquid. Before using an extract, dilute it in a small amount of water. *Warning: Never use an alcohol-based extract, no matter how diluted it is, directly in the eye. A tincture also should not be used in the eye.* No alcohol preparation should come in contact with this delicate structure.

Capsules are a pleasant way to take herbs, especially when the herbs are bitter-tasting or mucous-forming. Capsules generally consist of gelatin capsules filled with powdered herb. If prepared capsules are purchased from a first-class herb company or health-food store, the herbs generally are clean and combined in the correct proportions. To comfortably wash down and properly dissolve a capsule, take it with eight ounces of pure water or herb tea.

An herbal compress will achieve an effect similar to that of an ointment, but has the advantage of the therapeutic action of heat. To make a compress, bring one or two heaping tablespoons of the herb to a boil in one cup of water. Dip a cotton pad or piece of gauze in the strained liquid, let the excess liquid drain off, and place the pad or gauze over the *closed* eyelid while still warm. Keep the compress in place until it has cooled off.

An infusion is made by pouring hot water over dry or powdered herb, and steeping the herb for several minutes to extract its active ingredients. This method of preparation minimizes the loss of the herb's volatile elements. The usual amounts are about one-half to one ounce of herb to one pint of water. Use an enamel, stainless steel, porcelain, or glass pot with a tight-fitting lid to prevent evaporation and loss of the essential oils (the main medicinal part of some herbs). Steep the herb for about ten to twenty minutes. To drink an infusion, strain it into a cup, and drink it lukewarm or cool. For directions on how to prepare and use an infusion as an eyewash, see below.

A decoction is similar to an infusion. Instead of steeping the dry herb, however, simmer it for about twenty to thirty minutes. Be careful not to boil the herb.

A poultice is a warm, mashed, moist mass of fresh or ground herb tied in a piece of muslin or other loosely woven cloth. It is applied directly to the skin to relieve inflammations, boils, and abscesses, and to promote proper cleansing and healing of the affected area. Oil the skin before applying a poultice. Because

Eyewashes

Having herb tea as a late-afternoon pick-me-up or just before bed to help release the tensions of the day has become as common in the United States today as tea time has been in England for centuries. But herb tea can be used as more than a drink. Used as an eyewash, an herb tea, infusion, or decoction can bring relief to a stressed eye through the direct application of the properties that make the herb so beneficial.

To prepare an herb tea or other mixture for external application to the eye, use a piece of cheesecloth or filter paper, and strain the mixture repeatedly until it runs clear. In addition to being free of any debris that could scratch or irritate the eye, the mixture must also be allowed to cool to room temperature before being used. Any leftover liquid can be kept in the refrigerator for future use. However, never use a mixture that is more than two weeks old.

To apply an herb mixture as an eyewash, use an eyedropper and simply instill two drops of liquid in each eye. To do this, lean your head back, gently pull the lower lid down from the eye, and instill the drops in the pocket that is created. Another method is to instill the drops in the corner of the eye. Do not attempt to drop the liquid directly on the eye. The blink reflex, as already mentioned, is the quickest reflex in the body.

Apply the eyewash to one eye at a time. Put the drops in the first eye, then close the eye for about thirty seconds to keep the drops in contact with the eye tissue. Instead of an eyedropper, you can use an eye cup. Place a small amount of the herb mixture in the cup (be careful to not overfill the cup), place the cup up against your eye socket, tilt your head back, and look up, blinking a few times. Remove the cup, and keep the eye closed for another thirty seconds. Repeat with the other eye.

the skin around the eyes is very thin, make sure that the poultice is not too hot. A warm poultice is fine, but one that is too hot can easily cause a burn. Once a poultice has cooled, discard it. A cooled poultice should never be reheated and reused.

THE BEST HERBS FOR THE EYES

There are twenty-eight herbs that are commonly used to treat eye conditions. In the following list, they are presented according to their most popular common names, with their Latin names following. Also included are general information on each herb, what the herbs contain nutritionally, what conditions they are used to treat, and how they affect the eyes.

Most herbs can be purchased in bulk from local health-food stores or by mail order. (For a listing of mail-order companies, see "Recommended Suppliers" on page 253.) When buying an herb, make sure that you have selected the correct variety, since quite a few herbs are known by more than one name. If you are unsure of the specific herb to buy, or of the action of an herb, consult an herbalist. It is best to store bulk herbs in airtight containers in a dark, cool place.

Alfalfa

Alfalfa (*Medicago sativa*) contains health-building properties. Because of its vitality and nutrient content, it is beneficial for all ailments. Alfalfa helps the body to assimilate protein, calcium, and other nutrients. In addition, it contains high levels of chlorophyll, and therefore is a good body cleanser, infection fighter, and natural deodorizer. It also breaks down poisonous carbon dioxide. Alfalfa's components are properly balanced to allow for complete absorption.

Alfalfa has very rich supplies of vitamins A, D, and K. It is also high in calcium, and contains iron, phosphorus, potassium, and eight essential enzymes. It is the richest land source of trace minerals.

Bayberry

Bayberry (*Myrica cerifera*) can be useful in warding off colds at the first sign, especially when taken along with the herb capsicum (*Capsicum frutescens*). It is also helpful when used as a gargle for tonsillitis and sore throats. It is beneficial in the rejuvenation of the adrenal glands, cleansing the bloodstream, washing out wastes from the

veins and arteries, and ridding the system of toxins. In India, the powdered root bark of bayberry is combined with ginger (*Zingiber officinale*) to successfully combat cholera. Bayberry has long been used as a tonic, stimulating the system to help raise vitality and resistance to disease; as an aid to digestion and nutrition; and to build the blood.

Bayberry contains a high amount of vitamin C. It kills germs, and is stimulating to the mucous membranes around the eye.

Bilberry

The bilberry plant is a small shrubby perennial that grows in the woods and meadows of northern Europe. Its berries have been used for centuries to make jams and jellies, but it wasn't until after World War II that its therapeutic benefits became known.

Bilberry (*Vaccinium myrtillus*) acts as a potent antioxidant, enhances blood circulation, has anti-inflammatory properties, and enhances the regeneration of rhodopsin (visual purple) in the retina. It has been shown to be completely nontoxic, with no side effects and no contraindications. Some of the uses of bilberry for the eye include improving night vision, cataracts, nearsightedness, diabetic retinopathy, eyestrain, macular degeneration, and glaucoma. Bilberry contains anthocyanin, which is a type of antioxidant, as well as vitamins A and C, the bioflavonoids, and mineral salts.

Blackberry

Blackberry (*Rubus villosus*), when used as a tea, can dry up sinus drainage. An infusion made from unripe berries is highly esteemed for curing vomiting and loose bowels. The root contains astringent properties. The Chinese believe that the fruit increases the yin principle, in addition to giving vigor to the whole body.

Blackberry contains vitamins A and C. It also has calcium, iron, vitamins B_2 and B_3, and some vitamin B_1. It can be used as an eyewash when infused and strained as a tea.

Black Walnut

Black walnut (*Juglans nigra*) oxygenates the blood to kill parasites. It is used to help balance the blood-sugar level. It also is able to burn up excessive toxins and fatty materials. The extract is very useful against poison oak, ringworm, and skin problems.

Black walnut is rich in pangamic acid, occasionally referred to as vitamin B_{15}, and manganese. It contains protein, calcium, iron, magnesium, phosphorus, potassium, and silica.

Borage

Borage (*Borago officinalis*) is especially soothing in cases of bronchitis and digestive upset. It promotes the activity of the kidneys and adrenal glands. It is soothing to the mucous membranes, such as the covering of the eye. Borage tea can be used as an eyewash for sore eyes. Borage contains calcium and potassium.

Catnip

Catnip (*Nepeta cataria*) has a sedative effect on the nervous system. As a warm infusion, it has been known to help prevent a cold when taken at the first symptom. It helps to fight fatigue and improves circulation, and it has been used to ease infant colic. It also helps to reduce swelling under the eyes.

Catnip is high in vitamins A, B-complex, and C. It contains magnesium, manganese, phosphorus, and sodium, and a trace amount of sulfur.

Chamomile

Chamomile (*Anthemis nobilis*) is one of the best herbs to keep handy for emergencies. It is excellent as a tea for the nerves and for cramps, including menstrual cramps. Chamomile helps to promote a natural hormone similar to thyroxine that helps to rejuvenate the texture of the hair and skin. It helps with mental alertness, and is excellent for soothing an upset stomach and colic in babies. In addition, chamomile is effective against insomnia.

Chamomile is high in calcium and magnesium. It also has iron, manganese, potassium, zinc, and some vitamin A.

Chaparral

Chaparral (*Larrea divaricata*) has the ability to cleanse deep inside the muscles and tissue walls. It is a potent healer in the urethral tract and lymphatics, tones up the system, and rebuilds the tissues. It is a strong antioxidant, anti-tumor agent, painkiller, and antiseptic. It is one of the best herbal antibiotics. It has been recommended for cataracts.

Chaparral is high in protein, potassium, and sodium. It also contains aluminum, barium, chlorine, silicon, sulfur, and tin.

Chickweed

Chickweed (*Stellaria media*) is valuable for treating blood toxicity, fevers, and inflammations. It has antiseptic properties in the blood, and also helps to dissolve plaque out of the blood vessels and fatty substances out of the system. It is used as a poultice for boils, burns, skin diseases, sore or inflamed eyes, and swollen testes. Chickweed is mild, and has been used as a food as well as a medicine.

Chickweed is rich in vitamin C, copper, and iron. It contains calcium and sodium, and has a high amount of the B-complex vitamins. It also contains phosphorous and zinc, and some vitamin D and manganese.

Comfrey

Comfrey (*Symphytum officinale*) is one of the most valuable herbs known to botanical medicine. It has been used successfully for centuries as a wound healer and bone knitter. It feeds the pituitary with a natural hormone, and helps to strengthen the body skeleton. It helps to maintain the calcium-phosphorus balance by promoting strong bones and healthy skin. It encourages the secretion of the digestive enzyme pepsin, and is a general aid to digestion. It has a beneficial effect on all the parts of the body, and is therefore used as an overall tonic.

Comfrey is rich in vitamins A and C. It is high in protein, calcium, phosphorus, and potassium. It contains copper, iron, magnesium, sulfur, and zinc, as well as eighteen amino acids.

Eyebright

Eyebright (*Euphrasia officinalis*) aids in stimulating the liver to cleanse the blood and relieve the conditions that affect the clarity of vision. It is useful against inflammations because of its cooling and detoxifying properties. It has antiseptic properties that fight infections of the eyes. Eyebright has traditionally been used as a remedy for eye problems such as failing vision, pinkeye, ulcers, and even eye strain. It strengthens all the parts of the eye.

Eyebright is extremely rich in vitamins A and C. It contains the vitamin-B complex, vitamin D, and some vitamin E. It also has copper, iron, silicon, zinc, and a trace of iodine.

Ginkgo

Ginkgo (*Ginkgo biloba*) improves brain functioning by increasing the cerebral and peripheral blood flow, circulation, and oxygenation. Because it improves circulation, it may also relieve leg cramps. Ginkgo is good against depression, headache, memory loss, and tinnitus (ringing in the ears). In addition, it has been shown to be beneficial in cases of asthma, eczema, macular degeneration, and heart and kidney disorders. Ginkgo contains the bioflavonoids, which function as antioxidants.

Goldenseal

Goldenseal (*Hydrastis canadensis*) has been used to boost a sluggish glandular system, and to promote youthful hormone harmony. The active ingredient of the herb goes directly into the bloodstream and helps to regulate the liver's functioning. Goldenseal has a natural antibiotic ability to stop infection and to kill poisons in the body. It is now considered an endangered species, so is used rarely by responsible herbalists. It is also very expensive.

Goldenseal is valuable against all of the mucous-forming conditions in the nasal, bronchial, throat, intestinal, stomach, and bladder areas. It has the ability to heal mucous membranes anywhere in the body. When taken with other herbs, its tonic properties are increased for whatever ailment is being treated.

Goldenseal contains vitamins A and C. It also has the B-complex vitamins and vitamin E; the minerals calcium, copper, iron, manganese, phosphorus, potassium, sodium, and zinc; and unsaturated fatty acids.

Hawthorn

Hawthorn (*Crataegus oxycantha*) is a vasodilator that opens the blood vessels of the heart and also lowers the cholesterol level. It increases the intracellular vitamin-C level, and is useful against anemia, cardiovas-

cular and circulatory disorders, high cholesterol, and lowered immunity.

Hawthorn contains vitamins B_1, B_2, B_3, B_6, B_{12}, and C, as well as citric acid, choline, the flavonoids, folic acid, PABA, and selenium.

Marigold

Marigold (*Calendula officinalis*) is very useful as a first-aid remedy. It has been used as a tea for acute ailments, especially fevers, and is effective as a tincture when applied to bruises, sprains, muscle spasms, and ulcers. It relieves earache, boosts the heart and circulation, and cleanses the lymphatic system. Recently, it was discovered that the petals of the marigold flower have a significant amount of lutein, a yellow pigment found in the retina that can protect the retina against damage from the sun.

Marigold is high in phosphorus, and contains vitamins A and C.

Marshmallow

Marshmallow (*Althaea officinalis*) contains a mild expectorant that helps to soothe and heal the bronchial tubes. It is valuable against all lung ailments. It is especially good for asthma, and helps to remove mucous from the lungs. Marshmallow heals inflammations. Applied externally as a poultice with cayenne, it can be used to treat blood poisoning, gangrene, burns, bruises, and wounds.

Marshmallow contains 286,000 IU of vitamin A per pound. It is very high in calcium and extremely rich in zinc. It also contains the B-complex vitamins, iodine, iron, and sodium.

Oat Straw

Oat straw (*Avena sativa*) is used for stress-related conditions. It is rich in body-building materials, and is used to rebuild nerve tissue. It has been used in the treatment of arthritis, rheumatism, paralysis, liver infections, and skin diseases. Hot oat-straw poultices applied to areas in pain from kidney-stone attacks have brought relief. Oat straw has many elements that have antiseptic properties, and it is said to be a natural preventive against contagious diseases when taken frequently as a food.

Oat straw is high in silicon and rich in calcium. It contains vitamins A, B_1, B_2, and E, and phosphorus.

Parsley

Parsley (*Petroselinum sativum*) should be used as a preventive herb. It is so nutritious that it boosts resistance to infections and diseases, and has been used as a cancer preventive. It increases the iron content of the blood. Parsley has a tonic effect on the entire urinary system. The roots and leaves are very good for all liver and spleen problems when jaundice or venereal disease is present. The fresh juice has helped in cases of pinkeye and eyelid inflammation.

Parsley is high in the vitamin-B complex and potassium. It is said to contain a substance in which cancerous cells cannot multiply. It is rich in vitamins A and C, chlorophyll, and iron. It also contains some calcium, cobalt, copper, silicon, sodium, and sulfur.

Passion Flower

Passion flower (*Passiflora incarnata*) is used to treat insomnia and hysteria, as well as hyperactivity and convulsions in children. It is an herb that is quieting and soothing to the nervous system, and should be recommended to patients who wish to wean themselves from synthetic sleeping pills or tranquilizers. Passion flower helps to reduce high blood pressure and tachycardia, and is an effective antispasmotic. It is good for inflamed eyes and eyestrain. Passion flower contains the flavonoids, a subgroup of the antioxidants called the bioflavonoids.

Red Clover

Red clover (*Trifolium pratense*) is useful as a tonic for the nerves and as a sedative for nervous exhaustion. Native Americans used the plant for sore eyes and, as a salve, for burns. It is useful mixed with honey and water as a cough syrup. It is also good as an aid for strengthening the systems of delicate children. Red clover is effective against coughs, a weak chest, wheezing, bronchitis, lack of vitality, and nervous energy. It has also been included in some well-known cancer mixtures.

Red clover is a good source of vitamin A. It is high in iron, and contains the B-complex vitamins, vitamin C, the bioflavonoids, and unsaturated fatty acids. It is valued for its high mineral content. For example, it is rich in calcium, copper, and magnesium, and contains some cobalt, manganese, nickel, selenium, sodium, and tin.

Rose Hips

Rose hips (*Rosa canina*) play an important role in treatments where vitamins A, C, and E are needed. They are very nourishing to the skin. Rose hips contain a natural fruit sugar. They help to prevent infections, and also help when an infection has already developed.

Rose hips are very high in the vitamin-B complex, and are very rich in vitamins A, C, and E. They also contain vitamin D and the bioflavonoids. Rose hips are high in calcium and iron. They also have some potassium, silica, sodium, and sulfur.

Rosemary

Rosemary (*Rosmarinus officinalis*) is a stimulant, especially of the circulatory system and pelvic region. It is considered a proven heart tonic, and is a treatment for high blood pressure. Rosemary is used externally on bites and stings. In cases of colds or flu, it can be taken in the early stages as a warm infusion, and may be used as a cooling tea when the symptoms include restlessness, nervousness, and insomnia. It has been considered one of the most powerful remedies to strengthen the nervous system. Rosemary is a good tonic for the reproductive organs. It has also been effective against diarrhea, especially in children.

Rosemary contains vitamins A and C. It is high in calcium, and also contains iron, magnesium, phosphorus, potassium, sodium, and zinc.

Rue

Rue (*Ruta graveolens*) has the ability to expel poisons from the system, and therefore has been used for snake, scorpion, spider, and jellyfish bites. It has been found to be very effective at preserving sight by strengthening the eye muscles. It helps to remove deposits that tend to form in the tendons and joints, especially in the wrist joints, with age. It has also been found to be effective at treating high blood pressure, and helps to harden the bones and teeth.

Rue contains a large amount of rutin. Rutin is a bioflavonoid that is known for its ability to strengthen the capillaries and veins.

Sarsaparilla

Sarsaparilla (*Smilax officinalis*) is a valuable herb used

in glandular-balancing formulas. Its stimulating properties are noted for increasing the metabolic rate. Sarsaparilla also contains precursors of both the male and female hormones. It has been used to relieve sore eyes.

Sarsaparilla contains vitamins A, B-complex, C, and D. It also has copper, iodine, iron, manganese, silicon, sodium, sulfur, and zinc.

Siberian Ginseng

Siberian ginseng (*Eleutherococcus*) is very effective at increasing the circulation, especially around the heart; normalizing the blood pressure; and combating stress and fatigue. It increases brain and physical efficiency, improves the concentration span, and increases speed and accuracy in work. It also strengthens the adrenal and reproductive glands. Siberian ginseng contains the B-complex vitamins, vitamin E, and eleutherosides, a type of complex sugar molecule with beneficial effects.

Taheebo

Taheebo (*Tabebuia*) also goes by the names pau d'arco, lapacho, and ipe roxo. It is found in South America, and is a very powerful antibiotic with virus-killing properties. Taheebo is said to contain compounds that seem to attack the causes of diseases. One of its main actions purportedly is to put the body into a defensive posture, to give it the energy needed for defense against and resistance to disease.

Taheebo contains a high amount of iron, which aids in the proper assimilation of nutrients and the elimination of wastes.

Wild Cherry

Wild cherry (*Prunus serotina*) is considered to be a very useful expectorant. It is a valuable remedy for all mucous-forming conditions, and is beneficial against bronchial disorders caused by hardened accumulations of mucous. Wild cherry contains a volatile oil that acts as a local stimulant in the alimentary canal and aids digestion. It is a useful tonic for persons convalescing from diseases. Wild cherry contains cyanogenic glycoside, a type of complex sugar molecule with beneficial effects.

HERBS TO AVOID

As much as we can reap positive effects from herbal remedies, we also need to take some precautions in their use. For example, the following herbs have the same anti-inflammatory effect as steroids—and can cause the same ocular problems, such as cataracts, glaucoma, herpes simplex keratitis (corneal inflammation), light sensitivity, and retinal-blood-vessel problems:

■ Bethroot	■ Damiana
■ Fenugreek	■ Ginseng
■ Licorice	■ Saw palmetto
■ Blue cohosh	■ False unicorn root
■ Figwort	■ Goldenrod
■ Red sage	■ Wild yam

There are also some herbs that have the same effects as aspirin (salicylates), as well as the same ocular effects of blurred vision, disturbed accommodation, optic atrophy, retinal edema (swelling), and visual-field constriction. These herbs are:

■ Birch	■ Sweet violet
■ Chickweed	■ Black willow
■ Pansy	■ Meadowsweet
■ Black cohosh	■ Wintergreen
■ Crampbark	■ Blue flag

Diuretics are substances that affect the fluid and electrolyte balances in the body. They can cause blurred vision, disturbed accommodation, dry eyes, light sensitivity, xanthopsia (yellow vision), and nearsightedness. Herbs that act as diuretics are:

■ Bearberry	■ Shepherd's purse
■ Couch grass	■ Buchu
■ Parsley	■ Juniper
■ Birch	■ Stone root
■ Dandelion	■ Bugleweed
■ Pelletory of the wall	■ Licorice
■ Blue flag	■ Sweet violet
■ Fumitory	■ Carline thistle
■ Saw palmetto	■ Night blooming cereus
■ Boldo	■ Wild carrot
■ Gravelroot	■ Cleavers

■ Sea holly   ■ Pansy

■ Broom tops   ■ Yarrow

■ Hydrangea   ■ Corn silk

Some herbs contain volatile or aromatic oils that can cause ocular effects such as excessive tearing, irritation, contamination of contact lenses, and disorders of the central nervous system. These herbs are:

■ Cinnamon   ■ Fennel

■ Peppermint   ■ Rosemary

■ Tansy   ■ Wild carrot

■ Clove   ■ Garlic

■ Prickly ash   ■ Selfheal

■ Thuja   ■ Willow

■ Cudweed   ■ Ginger

■ Queen's delight   ■ Skunk cabbage

■ Thyme   ■ Wintergreen

■ Echinacea   ■ Pennyroyal

■ Red sage   ■ Southernwood

■ Valerian

Some herbs have a drying effect on the eye tissue. This can, in some cases, be detrimental, especially if you have a dry-eye condition or are wearing contact lenses. Some of these drying herbs are:

■ Bistort   ■ Cudweed

■ Eyebright   ■ Golden seed

■ Mouse ear   ■ Pokeroot

■ Coltsfoot   ■ Daisy

■ Golden root   ■ Ground ivy

■ Myrrh   ■ Scots pine

Other herbs and their possible side effects are:

■ Arnica—eye irritation.

■ Bittersweet—blurred vision, dilated pupils, loss of accommodation, glaucoma, light sensitivity.

■ Bladderwrack—metabolic changes due to altered thyroid activity.

■ California poppy—constricted pupils.

■ Ephedra—dilated pupils, dry eyes, increased eye pressure.

■ Shepherd's purse—blurred vision, red eyes, constricted pupils.

■ Squill, figwort, hawthorne, lily of the valley, night blooming cereus—lazy eye, blurred vision, central blind spot, double vision, disturbed color vision, disturbed accommodation, light sensitivity.

Herbs are naturally occurring substances in nature that have medicinal-type actions on our bodies. We can use herbs to treat disease, avoiding many of the negative side effects of medications. But like medications, herbs can also be harmful if taken inappropriately. Therefore, you should take care when choosing an herbal therapy. I strongly recommend consulting a qualified herbalist to discuss your options before taking any herb for any reason.

HERBAL COMBINATIONS FOR EYE PROBLEMS

Herbal combinations have more than one function in the fight against eye problems, since they consist of several substances that each have their own benefits and that work together in natural harmony. When taken over a period of time, an herbal combination will condition the body to react in a way that is comparable to the effects produced by certain medications, but in a less drastic manner and without the unwanted side effects. This is because the herbs trigger neuro-chemical reflexes in the body that over time become automatic and continue even after the person stops taking the herbs. One advantage of using an herbal combination instead of a medication is that the herbs help the body to bring about its own recovery and make it unlikely to be susceptible to the same complaint during or after convalescence. Unlike medications, which treat symptoms, herbal combinations go right to the root of the disorder and treat its cause.

Two herbal combinations that work especially well for the eyes are Herbal Combination Number One and Herbal Combination Number Two. Herbal Combination Number One consists of the following herbs:

■ Bayberry—high in vitamin C; kills germs; stimulates the mucous membranes.

■ Eyebright—boosts the body's immunity to eye problems.

■ Goldenseal—acts as a natural antibiotic against eye infections; kills poisons in the body.

Bayberry, eyebright, and goldenseal are three of the more common herbs used for external eye conditions.

Although each one used separately is effective, the combination benefits several types of eye conditions, which make this combination a good choice if you are not sure of exactly what is wrong with your eyes. Specifically, Herbal Combination Number One has been shown to be good for cataracts, iritis, pinkeye, weak eyes, and night blindness.

Herbal Combination Number Two consists of the three herbs from Herbal Combination Number One plus the following herbs:

■ Raspberry—effective against styes; astringent action helps to stop discharge.

■ Capsicum—acts as a stimulant and a relaxant; high in vitamin A and a number of minerals.

Use caution with Herbal Combination Number Two. Capsicum is a very powerful herb and can cause severe damage to delicate tissues if not used properly. If the eye is very inflamed and has a discharge, use a very small amount of capsicum in the mixture. Herbal Combination Number Two will help to increase the circulation in the eye area to rid the tissue of toxins. Consult an herbalist if you have any concerns or questions about the proper combination of herbs to use.

When using an herbal combination, follow the same precautions outlined for single herbs at the beginning of this chapter. A number of pre-mixed herbal combinations are available from health food stores and by mail order, but you can also mix a combination yourself if you are careful to keep your ingredients, tools, and work area clean. The usual recipe calls for approximately equal amounts of the different herbs. To prepare a tea, infusion, or other desired mixture, follow the procedures described for single herbs in "Forms of Herbal Preparations" on page 47.

TRADITIONAL CHINESE HERBAL COMBINATIONS FOR EYE PROBLEMS

Chinese medicine is a science and art form that is well over 5,000 years old. The procedures and symptomology of Chinese medicine differ significantly from those of Western medicine. For example, a Chinese medical practitioner generally asks different types of questions and performs different diagnostic tests than does a Western medical practitioner. The emotional aspects of illness are often of more concern to Chinese practitioners than to Western practitioners, and Chinese and Western practitioners often find different patterns in the health of the patient to be of interest.

Oftentimes, there is no correlation between our Western medical terminology and diagnoses, and those of traditional Chinese medicine.

Some of the traditional Chinese herbal combinations contain herbs chosen because of the way they interact with one another. It is rare for Chinese practitioners to use one herb alone. Some combinations include as many as twenty-five different herbs. A number of combinations also include nonherbal ingredients, such as minerals, plants, and animal organs. Therefore, many of the combinations in the following list are not used strictly for eye conditions. Since Chinese medicine strives to treat the whole person—the body, mind, and spirit—the treatment oftentimes is also directed toward a whole other set of symptoms, which may or may not be apparent.

The Chinese use their observations of nature to describe the workings of the inner body. For example, if a practitioner talks about "heat from the liver," he or she may be describing a series of conditions caused by an emotional constraint or blockage of energy in the liver. This "heat from the liver" may manifest as an inflammation (a Western medical term) in the head area—for example, a sore throat, earache, red eyes, or irritability. A person's condition is a very individualized expression of a disorder, and different people may display completely different combinations of symptoms. The different combinations of symptoms that are possible are what have given rise to the various herbal combinations used in traditional Chinese medicine.

Some of the more common traditional Chinese herbal combinations that may have beneficial effects on eye conditions are the following:

■ *An mian pian.* This combination cools liver "heat." The symptoms it helps to relieve include anxiety, red eyes, and eye irritation.

■ *Er ming zuo ci wan.* This combination is used to treat a liver deficiency that is causing symptoms such as headaches, high blood pressure, pressure behind the eyes, insomnia, thirst, and eye irritation.

■ *Long dan xie gan wan.* This is the classic combination for purging liver and gallbladder "heat." Use it for headaches; red, burning eyes; ringing in the ears; sore throat; fever blisters on the mouth; scanty urination; and constipation.

■ *Ming mu di huang wan.* This combination replenishes the energy in the liver and kidneys. The symptoms it can be used for include dry eyes; red, itchy eyes; poor eyesight; light sensitivity; excessive tearing; and eye diseases such as glaucoma and cataracts.

■ *Ming mu shang qing pian.* This combination dispels "heat," clears the vision, and sedates the liver. Use it for liver "heat" that is affecting the eyes, causing redness, itching, tearing, and swelling (pinkeye).

■ *Nei zhang ming yan wan.* This combination benefits the clarity of vision, nourishes the liver and kidneys, reduces "heat," and helps the circulation. Use it when your vision is impaired due to a liver deficiency, to aid recovery from eye surgery, and for cataracts, glaucoma, disturbed day or night vision, and itchy, painful eyes.

■ *Niu huang shang qing wan.* Use this combination for systemic "heat" rising from the liver, causing headaches, eye pain or red eyes, sore throat, toothache, or a fever with thirst.

■ *Qi ju di huang wan.* This combination nourishes the kidneys, boosting their energy. The symptoms it helps include blurred vision; dry, painful eyes; pressure behind the eyes; and disturbed night vision. It can also be used for dizziness, headaches, pain behind the eyes, and restlessness.

■ *Shi hu ye guang wan.* This combination improves vision, especially eyesight that is beginning to become blurry or is affected by dizziness. It is valuable in the early stages of cataract formation. It is also suitable for

use with tearing eyes, red or itchy eyes, dry eyes, or hypertensive changes within the eyes.

■ *Xiao yao wan.* This is a basic combination for stagnation of the liver due to a blood deficiency. The symptoms it relieves are diverse and include digestive dysfunction, menstrual and premenstrual disorders, vertigo, headaches, fatigue, blurred vision, and red, painful eyes. It is also useful for treating food allergies, chronic hay fever, and hypoglycemia.

■ *Zhong guo shou wu zhi.* This combination is an excellent tonic for the blood. It nourishes the liver and kidneys, and benefits the eyes and tendons.

Since herbal preparations are not "pure" substances, you need to use caution when taking them. The problem is that different parts of the herbs—the roots, leaves, pods, bark, seeds, flowers—are often used, giving different batches varying degrees of potency, or strength. In some cases, the potency of the active ingredient in an herb matches or exceeds that of the medication manufactured using that ingredient. Furthermore, some companies package and market their products in a way that fosters misuse of natural products by consumers who believe that natural equals weak and safe. And, of course, some products do have undesirable side effects, which can lead to dire consequences. I highly recommend consultation with an experienced herbalist before taking any herb or herbal combination.

Homeopathy

Homeopathy (ho-me-OP-a-thee) is a system of medicine whose principles are even older than Hippocrates. It seeks to cure in accordance with the natural laws of healing, and uses medicines made from natural animal, vegetable, and mineral substances. These remedies are prepared in such a way that they are nontoxic and do not cause side effects. They are available at a fraction of the cost of most prescription and nonprescription medications.

Homeopathic medicines are prescribed according to an age-old principle that recognizes the body's ability to heal itself. This is not a new approach to healing. This approach was "discovered" in the early 1800s by a German physician named Samuel Hahnemann. It was extremely popular in the United States in the nineteenth century, then declined because of the new "wonder drugs" and other political and economic changes in the practice of medicine. The holistic movement that surfaced in the early 1970s has been advocating a return to the natural laws of healing and has sparked a revival of interest in this scientific system of medicine.

Because you may not be familiar with the process used to produce homeopathic remedies and the system of diagnosis and treatment, we will describe the laws of homeopathy in this chapter. We also will discuss the specific remedies that can be used to help the eyes and the visual system.

THE LAWS OF HOMEOPATHY

Like any science, the system of homeopathy is governed by certain "laws" that dictate how the process works. These laws must be followed in order for the process to be considered homeopathic. These laws are called the law of similars, the law of proving, and the law of potentization.

The Law of Similars

The term "homeopathy" comes from the Greek *homoios* ("similar") and *pathos* ("suffering" or "sickness"). The fundamental law upon which homeopathy is based is called the law of similars, which states that "like is cured by like." According to the law of similars, a remedy can cure a disease if it produces, in a healthy person, symptoms that are similar to those of the illness.

The basic concept of the law of similars is attributed to Hindu sages from the tenth century B.C., who described the law as, "Through the like, disease is produced, and through the application of the like, it is cured." The following is an example of how the law works: A man develops a fever, with a flushed face, dilated pupils, rapid heartbeat, and feeling of restlessness. His homeopathic physician studies all these symptoms, then searches for a remedy that, under scientifically controlled conditions, has produced all these symptoms in a healthy person. Within a short time after taking the remedy, the man's fever drops to normal, and he begins to feel well again. In other words, using the law of similars, a doctor selects the one medicine needed by the patient by matching the symptoms of the patient's disorder to the symptoms the remedy is known to induce.

The Law of Proving

The second law of homeopathy, the law of proving, refers to the method used to test a substance to determine its medicinal effect. To prove a remedy, half of a group of healthy people is given a dose of the test substance, and the remaining half is given a placebo (an inactive substance). Conforming to the standard double-blind method used in pharmacological experiments, neither the subjects nor the researchers know which substance a particular person is taking. Every day, all the subjects carefully record the symptoms they experience. When the proving is complete, it is determined who took what, and all the symptoms experienced by the persons taking the substance are listed as a characteristic remedy picture in the reference book. To treat a patient, a physician looks up the remedy picture in the reference book, and, when the symptoms fit, applies the law of similars.

The Law of Potentization

The third law of homeopathy, the law of potentization, refers to the method of preparation of a homeopathic remedy. All homeopathic remedies are prepared using a controlled process consisting of dilution followed by succussion (shaking), which may be repeated until the resulting medicine contains few or no molecules of the original substance. These dilutions are called potencies. Lesser dilutions are known as low potencies, and greater dilutions are known as high potencies. As strange as it may seem, the more a remedy is diluted, the greater is its potency. The potencies are designated by a number followed by an "x" or "c." The "x" represents 10, and signifies that the mother tincture has been diluted to 1 part in 10. The "c" represents 100, and signifies that the mother tincture has been diluted to 1 part in 100. The mother tincture is an alcohol-based extract of the substance as it comes directly from the plant, animal, or mineral. The number preceding the "x" or "c" indicates the number of times the remedy has been diluted. Thus, a 3x-potency remedy has been diluted three times, and a 6c-potency remedy has been diluted six times. For purposes of consistency, the recommended homeopathic remedies in this book are all 6c and should be used three to four times daily.

When the process of potentization was devised roughly 200 years ago, the idea that medicine containing an infinitesimal amount of matter could be curative was inconceivable. In this nuclear age, however, the power of minute quantities is all too well established. The dose of vitamin B_{12} that is used to treat certain anemias contains one-millionth of a gram of cobalt. Trace elements, essential for physical development and functioning, are present in the body in barely measurable amounts. The human body manufactures only fifty- to one-hundred-millionth of a gram of thyroid hormone each day, yet a small devia-

tion in the amount can seriously affect the health of an individual.

The power of the infinitesimal dose is not clearly understood, but neither are the actions of many modern medications. The process of potentization makes it possible to use as medicines substances such as certain metals, charcoal, and sand, which are inert in their natural states. Potentized remedies do not contain sufficient matter to act directly on the tissues, which means that homeopathic medicines are nontoxic and cannot cause side effects.

SINGLE REMEDIES

Contrary to the current medical practice of prescribing two or more medicines for use at the same time, most homeopaths usually recommend only one remedy at a time. It is unknown what the effect of using two remedies would be, but the effects of using a single remedy are well known. Single remedies have been proved, or tested, on healthy subjects.

Many homeopathic remedies are sold today in health food stores under the description of the symptoms, for example, "Colds," "Flu," or "Teething." These are combination remedies and may be as effective as single remedies, but probably are not.

HOMEOPATHY VERSUS HERBALISM

Many people are confused about the differences between homeopathy and herbalism because both systems use herbs as medicines. The methods of preparing the remedies are very different, however. An herbalist may use an age-old formula for making an herb tea or a poultice, but can also improvise like a cook, personalizing the recipe. In addition, using intuition and experience, herbalists often combine a number of herbs to increase the effect desired. Homeopathy is somewhat more scientific, its remedies prepared, tested, and prescribed according to specific laws and procedures.

Some herbs, by themselves, are toxic, particularly when they are ingested in large amounts. Herbalists cannot use these herbs. Although many homeopathic remedies are made from poisonous herbs or plants, the potentized remedies contain only minute amounts of the original substances and are nontoxic. It cannot be overemphasized that caution should be taken with any self-remedy. Although a homeopathic remedy may be harmless because of its low potency, it can

COMMON HOMEOPATHIC REMEDIES

Remedy	Indications
Aconite	For any kind of pain or injury.
Agaricus	For dimmed vision.
Allium cepa	For headaches, mostly in the forehead area.
Anacardium	For swollen eyes.
Antimonium crudum	For eyelid inflammation.
Apis mellifica	For bee stings; puffy swelling around the eyes.
Argentum nitricum	For sticky eyelids.
Arnica montana	For eye injuries; black eyes; any kind of bruising.
Arsenicum album	For the late stages of head colds; red eyes; foggy vision.
Aurum	For any kind of pain; double vision.
Belladonna	For dilated pupils; red eyes; light sensitivity.
Bryonia	For headaches; dry, hard coughs.
Calcarea fluorica	For the appearance of flickering lights.
Calcarea sulfurica	For discharge from any kind of infection.
Calendula officinalis	For general dryness associated with irritants.
Carboneum sulfuratum	For any kind of swelling.
Causticum	For purifying any kind of tissue.
Chamomilla	For calming any kind of tissue.
Cinchona officinalis	For dilated pupils.
Cineraria maritima	For red, irritated eyes.
Cocculuc	For floaters.
Conium	For the heavy-eye feeling.
Cyclamen	For tense eye muscles.
Euphrasia officinalis	For any kind of burning and irritation.
Ferrum phosphoricum	For the early stage of any kind of inflammation; red eyes.
Gelsemium sempervirens	For tired eyes; aching all over the body.
Glonoinum	For red eyes.
Graphites	For light sensitivity.
Hyoscyamus	For double vision.
Hypericum perforatum	For eye injuries; any kind of shooting pain.
Ignatia amara	For severe headaches; emotional stress.
Kali muriaticum	For the "gritty" feeling in eyes.
Kali sulfuricum	For red eyes.
Lac caninum	For blurred vision.
Lachesis	For dull vision.
Ledum palustre	For eye pain if Arnica montana fails to relieve it.
Lycopodium	For eye pain; tearing.
Magnesia carbonica	For red, inflamed, burning eyes.

Remedy	Indications
Magnesia phosphorica	For a general feeling of tiredness; double vision.
Mercurius corrosivus	For eye discharge.
Mercurius vivus	For swollen glands; red eyes with no discharge.
Natrum muriaticum	For eye pain.
Natrum sulfuricum	For light sensitivity.
Nitricum acidum	For tearing.
Nux vomica	For light sensitivity; headaches.
Petroleum	For eyelid inflammation.
Physostigma	For tense eye muscles.
Pulsatilla	For sticky eyelids; yellowish discharge.
Rheum	For any kind of muscle twitching.
Rhus toxicodendron	For light sensitivity; tearing.
Ruta graveolens	For eyestrain followed by headache; red eyes.
Sanguinaria	For eye pain.
Senecio	For any kind of muscle weakness.
Sepia	For excessive tearing.
Silicea	For eye pain accompanied by light sensitivity.
Spigelia	For eye pain.
Staphysagria	For any kind of infection.
Stramonium	For dilated pupils.
Sulphur	For red eyelids.
Symphytum	For injuries to the eyeball; pain from a blow to the eye.
Veratrum album	For dry eyes; cold sweats.
Zincum metallicum	For general dryness; foggy vision.

also be ineffective at treating a disorder. This is why it is important to work in conjunction with a trained homeopathic physician.

HOMEOPATHY AND THE EYES

Although we have been emphasizing that the eyes are an integral part of the body and, like the body, respond to nutritional influences and environmental factors, there are not very many homeopathic remedies specifically for the disorders that afflict them. Many of the recommendations in Part Two may be considered general—that is, prescribed for general symptoms. The remedy may not be directed at the specific eye disorder or even at the chief complaint, but at the person as a whole. The correct remedy may act instantaneously, like an electric spark, upon the defense mechanism or vital force; and the effects of one dose may last for a month.

Homeopathic remedies come in pellets, tablets, and liquids. The liquid form is an alcohol-based extract of a specific remedy and therefore should not be used directly on the eye. The liquid generally is placed under the tongue with an eyedropper, which usually comes with the bottle. The liquid can also be used to make a cream, ointment, or salve. This is done by mixing the liquid with a cream or gel base. Creams, ointments, and salves are almost never used on the eye tissue itself. Tablets and pellets, which are made with a base of lactose (sweet milk sugar), are dissolved in the mouth, usually under the tongue, without chewing. They are excellent for use with children. However, they should not be touched, as this may decrease their effectiveness. For infants, dissolve a pellet or tablet in water and administer it to the child using an eyedropper. Since the oral liquid remedies contain alcohol, they should be given to children only in small doses.

The best time to take a homeopathic treatment is thirty minutes before or after eating. Strong flavors such as mint or camphor, odors from perfumes and paints, and caffeine are believed to decrease the effectiveness of homeopathic remedies. Homeopathy requires personal observation to determine the length of treatment. If no change occurs in a chronic ailment after a week, switch to another remedy. If improvement is noted, continue with the remedy until all the symptoms disappear. It is very important to continually be aware of the symptoms because the remedy should be changed as the symptoms change. For example, a sore throat may turn into a headache, which may turn into sneezing or coughing, which may lead to a runny nose. Each of these symptoms has a separate remedy that is specific for that symptom. For a list of common homeopathic remedies and the symptoms for which they can be used, see the table on page 59.

Homeopathic treatment is different from traditional Western medicine in many ways. Homeopathic remedies treat the series of symptoms as unique, without necessarily assigning a "syndrome" name to the condition. You might be tempted to try to treat your own symptoms based on the conditions listed in this book and the remedies given for each. However, a homeopathic practitioner may see a whole other set of symptoms, based on further questioning, that might indicate you should take a different remedy. He or she will also take your physical characteristics, personality, and emotional state into consideration. It is best to consult a trained homeopathic practitioner before attempting any treatment on your own. It can save you some time, maybe money, and possibly your eyesight!

Part Two

Disorders of the Eye
and Visual System

Introduction

The same as with any other organ system, things can go wrong with your eyes. But your eyes are unique in that they can be "healthy" and still not function properly. In Part Two, we will discuss a good number of the conditions that can affect your eyes' health as well as your visual function. Each entry is broken down into several sections—an overview of the disorder; discussions of the conventional treatments and possible self-treatments; tables detailing effective nutritional supplements, herbs and herbal supplements, and homeopathic remedies; and a listing of general recommendations. Please note that you should consult your eye doctor or homeopathic physician before using any of the recommended homeopathic remedies because the specific remedy appropriate for you will be selected not only according to your symptoms, but also your physical, emotional, and mental profiles.

Part Two starts off with a troubleshooting guide that lists twenty-eight of the most common symptoms of eye trouble and the conditions that often cause them. This is followed by a first-aid guide to eight common eye emergencies and nine contact-lens emergencies. Please be sure to read the first-aid guide carefully and follow the steps as closely as possible if you have an eye emergency.

It is important to note that people's responses to the various eye disorders are very individualistic, so your symptoms may not exactly match the specific ones noted. Part Two is offered solely to aid you in deciding what you can do to help yourself plus assist your doctor in solving your problem. Be careful when attempting to diagnose your own condition—a missed diagnosis can cost valuable time and possibly valuable eyesight.

Troubleshooting Guide

You will most likely never notice an eye problem, then simply walk into your doctor's office and offer a complete and accurate diagnosis of your own condition. However, if you do have an eye problem, it would be helpful if you had a general idea of what your symptoms are, what conditions they might indicate, and what requires immediate attention. The following table lists some of the more common visual symptoms and the conditions that are generally associated with them. It is not meant to serve as a substitute for professional diagnosis. Although you may experience one or more of the symptoms listed, you may not have any of the conditions cited. Also, the conditions are not listed in any order of significance. Rather, they are in alphabetical order.

SYMPTOMS AND THEIR POSSIBLE CAUSES	
Symptom	**Possible Condition**
Blind spots	Glaucoma, lazy eye (from tobacco or alcohol), optic atrophy, retinitis pigmentosa (progressive degeneration of the retina).
Blinking, frequent	Accommodative insufficiency, anxiety, contact-lens irritation, dry-eye syndrome, farsightedness, foreign body in eye, Parkinson's disease, stroke.
Blurred distance vision	Astigmatism, cataracts, lazy eye, macular degeneration, nearsightedness.
Blurred near vision	Accommodative insufficiency, computer vision syndrome, convergence insufficiency, lazy eye, presbyopia.
Blurred vision	Astigmatism, central serous retinopathy, keratoconus.
Burning	Chemical burn, computer vision syndrome, dry-eye syndrome, pinkeye.
Color vision, disturbed	Acute optic neuritis, medication allergy, primary optic atrophy.
Discharge, sticky	Dry-eye syndrome, pinkeye (bacterial).
Discharge, watery	Allergy, blocked tear duct, foreign body in eye, pinkeye (viral).
Double vision	Binocular-vision disorder, convergence insufficiency, diabetes, Grave's disease (hyperthyroidism), high astigmatism, optic-nerve defect, orbital (eye-socket) fracture.
Drooping eyelid	Aging, botulism, diabetes, eyelid or head injury, hypothyroidism, muscle weakness, optic-nerve defect.
Dryness	Hormone imbalance, keratoconjunctivitis sicca (inflammation of cornea and conjunctiva), Sjögren's syndrome (salivary-gland disorder), Stevens-Johnson syndrome (hivelike rash on mucous membranes), xerophthalmia (dry, thickened, wrinkled cornea and conjunctiva).

Symptom	Possible Condition
Eye movements, involuntary	Acute optic neuritis, albinism (absence of pigment in skin, hair, and eyes), alcohol intoxication, lupus erythematosus.
Eyelid, swelling around	Blunt trauma, excessive salt consumption, pinkeye (allergic), smoking.
Eyelid, swelling of	Chalazion, stye.
Flashing lights	Blunt trauma, migraine headache, retinal detachment, vitreous-humor detachment.
Headaches	Astigmatism, computer vision syndrome, convergence insufficiency, farsightedness, migraine headache.
Itching	Dry-eye syndrome, pinkeye (allergic), trichiasis (irritation of eyeball by eyelashes).
Light sensitivity	Computer vision syndrome, eyestrain, iritis (inflammation of the iris), pinkeye.
Night blindness	Nearsightedness, retinitis pigmentosa, vitamin-A deficiency.
Pain, sharp	Corneal abrasion, corneal ulcer, foreign body in eye, torn or broken contact lens.
Protruding eyes	Grave's disease, intra-orbital tumor.
Pupils, different-sized	Glaucoma, intracranial tumor, iritis, meningitis, nearsightedness, nerve defect.
Redness	Computer vision syndrome, corneal abrasion, iritis, pinkeye, subconjunctival hemorrhage.
Tearing	Acute optic neuritis, blocked tear duct, dry-eye syndrome, iritis, pinkeye.
Tired eyes	Accommodative insufficiency, computer vision syndrome, convergence insufficiency, presbyopia.
Yellow eyes	Jaundice.
Yellow spot in eye	Pinguecula (yellow patch on sclera).

First Aid

Things happen, and things happen to the eyes. However, not everything that happens to the eyes is an emergency. Therefore, it is important to know which conditions are true emergencies, requiring prompt or immediate attention, and whether you should see an optometrist, ophthalmologist, or emergency-room physician. Of course, the best way to handle an eye emergency is to prevent it from happening in the first place through the use of appropriate safety procedures and protective eyewear. But, accidents happen, and you should know how to recognize the kinds of problems they can cause.

FIRST AID FOR EYE EMERGENCIES

In most states, optometrists can handle minor eye injuries, such as a foreign body superficially imbedded in the eye. In most states, optometrists also can prescribe certain medications, such as topical antibiotics, to treat minor eye injuries. In all states, optometrists know ophthalmologists to whom they can refer patients with serious injuries, such as those requiring surgery. So, if you think you have a serious injury, but don't know an ophthalmologist, contact your optometrist for a referral. Of course, if you know you have a serious injury—one involving obvious major eye damage, loss of vision, or extensive bleeding—go to your nearest hospital emergency room immediately. A chemical burn is really the only type of serious injury you should try to treat *before* going to the emergency room. (See "Burn.")

Black Eye

For a bruising injury from a blunt object—otherwise known as a black eye—apply an ice bag or cold compress during the first twenty-four to forty-eight hours following the injury. This will help to constrict the damaged blood vessels in and around the eye, and to reduce further bleeding and swelling. This is probably why applying a steak to an injured eye is so popular—a frozen or refrigerated steak is cold.

Once the swelling has subsided, apply heat to the eye. Heat will cause the blood vessels to dilate (open) and to absorb the fluid that is causing the swelling. The dilated blood vessels will also bring in infection-fighting cells from elsewhere in the body. One way to make a hot compress that stays hot is to boil an egg and then wrap it in a towel. Hold the hot compress *gently* against your eye.

Burn

Since the blink reflex is one of the fastest reflexes we have, the eye is rarely burned by fire. Most eye burns are caused by chemicals or radiation. Chemical burns fall into two categories—acid burns and alkali burns. Acid substances that burn the eyes include battery acid, such as car-battery acid; industrial chemicals; and liquid bleach. Alkali burns are most often caused by lye-based drain cleaners. Both acid and alkali substances can splash into unprotected eyes and do a great deal of damage in a short time. Alkali burns, however, are a lot worse than acid burns. Acids "eat through" the eye more slowly than do alkali chemicals and can more often be washed out before doing any major damage.

Speed is crucial with a chemical burn. Immediately begin flushing the eye with water. Rinse the eye, continually and gently, for at least fifteen minutes. If possible, hold the eye open under slowly running water. If you do not have water available, use anything, even milk, tea, or soda pop. *Do not* call for assistance until after you have flushed your eye for fifteen minutes.

During the time you call for help, significant damage can occur to the eye. In addition, *do not* use an eye cup for flushing. An eye cup will allow the chemical to remain in contact with the eye, therefore reversing any of the positive effects of the flushing. For the same reason, *do not* bandage the eye. Leave the eye uncovered, since a bandage will also keep the chemical in contact with the eye. When you have finished flushing the eye, get to an emergency room. The doctor will probably complete irrigating the eye, as well as apply an antibiotic ointment, and give you medications to reduce the inflammation and pain. Your eye will be closed and patched under pressure to help relieve the pain and to allow healing to take place.

The other type of burn that affects the eyes is a radiation burn. This type of burn can come from too much exposure to radiation such as UV, infrared, nuclear, and X-ray radiation. The same as for other injuries, prevention is the best medicine. Never stare directly at the sun, even during an eclipse or as reflected off glass or water. You can permanently damage your retinas and cause complete loss of your central vision this way. When I was a Navy optometrist, one young sailor thought he could get an easy discharge by causing himself some "minor" eye damage by staring at the sun. He ended up nearly blind, although he did get his discharge—a psychiatric one. Rather, make sure you always protect your eyes. Wear appropriate eyewear if you work around excessive UV, infrared, or other radiation. If you indulge in sunbathing, whether in natural sunlight or in a tanning booth, be sure to wear opaque goggles.

Radiation burns leave the eyes feeling gritty and tearing excessively for several hours after exposure to the source of the radiation. You may also experience spasming of the eyelid muscles that makes it difficult to open your eyes. Your eyes will be sensitive to light. The medical treatment will consist of pain medication, bed rest, cold compresses, and topical antibiotics.

Corneal Abrasion

A corneal abrasion is a scrape on the cornea, most often caused by a foreign body such as a grain of sand, piece of dirt, ill-fitting contact lens, baby's fingernail, twig, or mascara wand. Patients with scraped corneas often tell their doctor that something is under their upper eyelid. Usually, the foreign body is no longer present, but the patient feels discomfort whenever the upper eyelid passes over the damaged part of the cornea.

If you have a corneal abrasion, you will probably feel a good deal of pain. Generally, when the injury first occurs, your eye will tear profusely, washing out the foreign body that caused the abrasion, which may have become trapped in your eye. You can try washing out your eye further with purified water or a commercial eyewash. *Do not* use commercial eye-whitening drops. If you or someone else can see the cause of the problem, such as a speck of dirt, you can try to remove it with a *clean* handkerchief.

Scratches on the cornea usually cannot be seen with the naked eye. Your eye doctor will examine the injury under magnification and may also use a fluorescein (FLOOR-ess-seen) stain to make the abrasion visible. You may be given a topical antibiotic, in the form of an ointment or drops, to help prevent infection. I tell my patients to get plenty of rest and to take an over-the-counter pain medication for any discomfort.

Doctors used to routinely patch an eye with a corneal abrasion, but many now feel that the eye is better off healing without a patch. One reason is that a patch keeps the eye warm, which increases the chance of an infection developing. Also, it is easier to monitor progress and apply medication if the eye is not covered. On the other hand, patching makes the eye more comfortable.

Most corneal abrasions heal within a few days, although those from a plant material such as wood or a very dirty substance may take longer.

Corneal Ulcer

A corneal ulcer is an open sore on the cornea and involves a deeper invasion of the corneal tissue than an abrasion. (See "Corneal Abrasion.") It may start with a corneal abrasion that becomes infected, or with a bacterial or viral infection that was not preceded by an injury.

Complications from contact lenses are a frequent cause of corneal ulcers today. Wearing lenses that were improperly disinfected or improperly fitted, or leaving daily-wear lenses in while sleeping can cause corneal ulcers. But any injury, such as from a twig or fingernail, can result in a corneal ulcer. One very serious type of corneal ulcer results from the herpes simplex virus, which is the virus that causes cold sores and genital ulcers. You can transmit a herpes infection to the eye if you touch a herpes sore and then your eye.

Most corneal ulcers are painful, and some can be seen with the naked eye as a round depression or white spot. Corneal ulcers resulting from the herpes virus actually cause the cornea to lose sensitivity in the area of the ulcer, so you may not have pain as a clue that something is seriously wrong. However, your eye will be red and sensitive to light. Your vision in the affected eye also will be blurred, but this is hard to notice unless the unaffected eye is temporarily covered for some reason. Under magnification, an ulcer from a herpes virus has a distinctive branching pattern, but this cannot be seen without special instruments and sometimes even a fluorescein stain.

Corneal ulcers must be treated, or scarring or loss of vision can result. Generally, the treatment includes an antibiotic or antiviral medication. Usually, corneal ulcers are treated by ophthalmologists, although in most states, they can also be treated by optometrists.

If the cornea is irreparably damaged, a corneal transplant may be performed. (The cornea is the actual part of the eye that is donated to eye banks.) In a corneal transplant, the central eight to ten millimeters of the cornea are cut out. The new cornea is then cut into the same diameter and sewn onto the eye. The thread used for this procedure is extremely thin and strong. Rejection is possible, though not as common as in other kinds of transplants. Most corneal transplants are successful, and vision can go from extremely poor to extremely good.

Cuts Around the Eye

Cuts around the outside of the eye bleed a lot and look very frightening, but they heal well, as do cuts in the conjunctiva. See your doctor if the cut is large and near the eye to be sure that you have no hidden damage to your eye. For general lacerations around the eye, bandage the cut lightly and seek a doctor at once. *Do not* wash the eye out with water. Any penetration into the eyeball opens the eye to infection, and tap water contains bacteria. In addition, *do not* attempt to remove the penetrating object from the laceration.

Hyphema

A hyphema (high-FEE-mah) is a condition in which blood sits in the anterior chamber of the eye, in front of the iris. A hyphema almost always is a result of being struck in the eye with a blunt object, such as a racquetball. You don't feel the hyphema itself. Rather, you feel the pain from the injury that caused it.

A hyphema is a true eye emergency, requiring immediate patching of the eye and bed rest for up to a week. Both these measures are intended to minimize your eye movements, promote absorption of the blood, and prevent further bleeding. Without treatment, your eye may be stained with blood, resulting in permanent loss of vision. Glaucoma or a serious inflammation of the iris can also be a consequence of an unsuccessfully resolved hyphema. If you suspect you have a hyphema, or if you have sustained any kind of blunt injury to your eye, see an ophthalmologist right away. Have someone drive you to the doctor, taking care not to make any excessive head or eye movements en route.

Retinal Detachment

Retinal detachment is the peeling away of the retina from the back of the eye, the way wallpaper might peel away from a curved surface. The retina detaches when it has a hole or tear that allows fluid to collect between it and the back of the eye. The separation that results is similar to what happens when water gets behind wallpaper.

Retinal detachment can occur for many reasons, not all of them injuries, although a blunt or penetrating injury to the eye is a common cause. Nearsighted eyes and prominent eyes are more prone to retinal detachment, probably because their retinas are more tautly stretched. Recent cataract surgery is another risk factor.

The retina can be reattached by an ophthalmologist if the detachment is caught in time. If there is only a small hole in the retina, a laser can be used to seal it. If there is a large tear and the retina is actually peeling away from the eye, a freezing probe will be used to make the retina adhere to the eye again.

It is vital to know the symptoms of retinal detachment because failure to seek treatment in time can result in blindness in the affected eye. A developing retinal detachment is heralded by flashes of light that look like sparks or flickers, a large number of floaters in the field of vision, and a shadow or curtain that spreads from the edge of the visual field to the central vision. A shimmering effect—similar to what you would see if you looked through gelatin—may also be noticed in the visual field. No pain will arise from the retina itself because the retina does not contain pain receptors. (You may, of course, feel pain from elsewhere in the eye if the detachment was caused by an injury.)

Subconjunctival Hemorrhage

A subconjunctival (SUB-con-junk-TIE-val) hemorrhage is bleeding from broken blood vessels under the conjunctiva of the eye, between the conjunctiva and the sclera. This is a case where the problem looks much more serious than it is. Subconjunctival hemorrhages can occur from a jarring injury, such as a blow to the head, or from anything that increases the pressure in the delicate blood vessels of the conjunctiva, such as intense coughing, sneezing, vomiting, or labor contractions. The area where the bleeding occurs appears as a bright red patch on the white sclera. There is no pain, and vision is not affected. The blood will be absorbed, and the eye will return to normal within one to three weeks. Of course, if you have any symptoms that concern you, such as pain or visual disturbances, see your eye doctor.

FIRST AID FOR CONTACT-LENS EMERGENCIES

Problems with contact lenses can be a special type of concern because of the close proximity of the contacts to the eye tissue. Although many of the following problems can arise even if you don't wear contacts, they require special attention if you do.

Adherent Lenses

Contact lenses must be wet, especially when riding on the tear film of your eyes. If they dry out, they will adhere, or stick, to the eyes themselves. If your lenses are soft lenses and they dried out due to heat, infrared radiation, wind, or a low-humidity environment, do not attempt to remove them before they are rehydrated. Use a lubricant specifically designed for your type of lenses or an artificial-tear solution. Gas-permeable lenses can also dry out, but don't adhere to the eye quite as easily. Wet these types of lenses with the appropriate eye drops.

Blunt Trauma

Any trauma to the eye can be significant and cause severe damage. In one sense, having a contact lens on the eye affords a certain level of protection from external blows. However, if the lens is a rigid lens and it is broken while in the eye, the eye can be cut. Soft lenses are less likely to break, but they also offer less protection to the eye. No matter what type of lens you wear, if you suffer a blunt trauma that results in a broken lens, see your eye doctor. Swelling or lacerations may make removal of the lens or lens pieces difficult.

Blurred Vision

Contact lenses are designed to clear up the vision. They should not make your vision more blurry or distorted. If your vision becomes worse when you wear your contacts, the first thing you should do is remove them and clean them. If you reinsert the lenses and your vision is still blurred or distorted, check to make sure the lenses are sitting correctly on your eyes. If the lenses are clean and positioned correctly on your eyes, and you still cannot see properly, contact your eye doctor.

Chemical Splash

Contact lenses are permeable to gases and liquids, but absorb liquids. If a chemical splashes into your eye while you are wearing your contacts, remove the affected lens *immediately*. If you don't, the lens will hold the chemical in contact with your eye tissue for an extended period of time, making the problem worse. After removing the lens, hold the lids apart and irrigate the eye continuously for at least fifteen minutes. If you are alone, irrigate your eye *before* calling for help because rinsing the chemical from your eye is more important than getting assistance with transportation. (For more information on how to handle a chemical splash, see "Burn" on page 69.)

Dry Eyes

Dry eyes can be caused by a dry-eye condition or a dry environment. If you are in a low-humidity or air-conditioned environment, you are more likely to experience dry eyes. Use your lens lubricant as needed and, if possible, increase the humidity in the room. Ask your doctor for the best type of eye drops to use.

Dust

Dust particles are notorious for becoming trapped underneath contact lenses, especially the smaller gas-permeable lenses. If your eyes become red or uncomfortable, remove your lenses and irrigate your eyes. If your eyes clear up, clean the lenses and reinsert them. If your eyes remain red or uncomfortable, consult your eye doctor before reinserting the lenses.

Exposure to a Welding or Other Arc

Many tales have been passed down about contact lenses becoming "fused" to the eyes of welders. These stories are not true; this has never happened. However, welding arcs can cause several other types of damage. If you are exposed to an arc of any kind and do not have protective filters in place, remove your lenses before your eyes begin to become inflamed. (Inflammation is usually a delayed reaction.) If no symptoms develop within twenty-four hours, you can reinsert your lenses. If symptoms do develop, consult your eye doctor first.

Lost Lens

If you fear that you may have lost a contact lens, first check the eye itself. The lens may be displaced on the conjunctiva or caught up under the upper lid. If it is, carefully recenter the lens. If the lens was not displaced, check your clothing and the surrounding floor. If you find the lens, clean it and evaluate it for damage. Soft lenses that are not cracked can be rehydrated and successfully worn again. Just soak the lens for at least four hours before attempting to reinsert it. If the lens feels uncomfortable in your eye, remove it immediately and call your doctor.

Red, Sore Eyes

Redness and soreness are indications of some type of eye problem. If your eyes become red or sore, and the problem persists, remove your lenses. If the condition clears, try to reinsert the lenses. If the redness or soreness return, remove the lenses and contact your eye doctor. Never wear lenses when your eyes are red or sore.

Eye emergencies can be serious. It is better to err on the side of caution if you suspect an eye problem. Fortunately, nature has provided us with a sure-fire alarm system for eye emergencies—*pain*! If you feel any pain around your eyes, it is best to play it safe and have an eye doctor check it out.

Ocular Side Effects
of Systemic Medications

It should be obvious by now that the eyes are an integral part of the human body. Whatever we eat or ingest in any way affects all the parts of our body, including our eyes. This is especially true of medications.

The following table lists some of the more common medications taken today for a number of different physical conditions. Included in the table are the brand name and generic name of each medication, as well as what it is used for and how it affects the eyes. Some of these medications may have variations and updated formulas on the market. Therefore, please check with your physician before taking any medication so that you are aware of any possible visual effects.

COMMON MEDICATIONS AND THEIR OCULAR SIDE EFFECTS			
Brand Name	**Generic Name**	**Indications**	**Ocular Side Effects**
Accutane	Isotretinoin	Difficult cases of cystic acne; keratinization disorders; folliculitis; psoriasis.	Redness, tearing, dryness, light sensitivity, contact-lens intolerance.
Achromycin	Tetracycline	Acne; chlamydia.	Retinal hemorrhage, decreased vision, nearsightedness, enlarged blind spot.
Actifed	Pseudoephedrine	Allergic rhinitis; allergic conjunctivitis and skin manifestations; motion sickness.	Hallucinations, decreased eye pressure, dilated pupils.
Adipex	Phentermine	Weight control.	Decreased vision, cataracts, hallucinations, double vision, disturbed accommodation.
Atrovent	Ipratropium bromide	Rhinitis.	Worsened narrow-angle glaucoma, blurred vision, pain.
Benadryl	Diphenhydramine	Allergic rhinitis; allergic conjunctivitis and skin manifestations; motion sickness.	Visual-field constriction, hallucinations, retinal hemorrhage.
Betoptic	Betaxolol	Open-angle glaucoma.	Hallucinations, decreased tear flow, redness, double vision, drooping eyelids.
Cardizem	Diltiazem	Angina due to coronary-artery spasm; mild to moderate hypertension.	Pain, redness, hallucinations, tearing.
Catapres	Clonidine	Hypertension.	Eye irritation, hallucinations, dilated pupils.

Brand Name	Generic Name	Indications	Ocular Side Effects
Coumadin	Warfarin sodium	Venous thrombosis; atrial fibrillation with embolization; pulmonary emboli; coronary occlusion.	Tearing, cataracts, decreased vision.
Desyrel	Trazodone	Depression.	Optic neuritis, lazy eye, retinal or subconjunctival hemorrhage, light sensitivity, dryness, decreased vision.
Detrol	Tolterodine tartrate	Bladder control.	Headaches, dryness, blurred near vision.
Diabinese	Chlorpropamide	Diabetes.	Optic neuritis, disturbed color vision, retinal hemorrhage, light sensitivity, double vision.
Dilantin	Phenytoin	Epilepsy.	Retinal hemorrhage, double vision, disturbed accommodation, flashing lights, glare sensitivity, disturbed color vision.
Dimetapp	Brompheniramine	Coughs and upper respiratory symptoms, including nasal congestion, associated with allergy or common cold.	Different-sized pupils, visual-field constriction, hallucinations, dryness, double vision.
Diuril	Chlorothiazide	Hypertension; edema associated with congestive heart failure, cirrhosis, or corticosteroid or estrogen therapy.	Edema, retinal hemorrhage, disturbed accommodation, nearsightedness, yellow vision.
Donnatal	Phenobarbital	Epilepsy; anxiety.	Blind spots, hallucinations, lazy eye, optic neuritis, involuntary eye movements.
Elavil	Amitriptyline	Depression.	Hallucinations, retinal hemorrhage, lazy eye, optic neuritis.
Enduron	Methyclothiazide	Hypertension; edema associated with congestive heart failure, cirrhosis, premenstrual tension, or corticosteroid or estrogen therapy.	Edema, retinal hemorrhage, decreased vision, disturbed accommodation, redness, light sensitivity.
Ergomar	Ergotamine	Migraines.	Spasming and constriction of blood vessels in all parts of the eye.
Humulin	Insulin	Diabetes.	Decreased pupil reaction, double vision, involuntary eye movements.
Inderal	Propranolol	Hypertension.	Drooping eyelids, double vision, decreased vision, hallucinations.
Ismelin	Guanethidine	Hypertension.	Light sensitivity, burning, double vision, accommodative spasming, flashing lights.
Lamictal	Lomtrigine	Seizures.	Dizziness, ataxia, sedation, involuntary eye movements, double vision.
Lanoxin	Digoxin	Congestive heart failure; atrial fibrillation or flutter; atrial tachycardia.	Optic neuritis, disturbed color vision, hallucinations, glare sensitivity, halos around lights, double vision.
Librium	Chlordiazepoxide	Anxiety.	Disturbed depth perception, retinal hemorrhage, disturbed accommodation.

Brand Name	Generic Name	Indications	Ocular Side Effects
Lithobid	Lithium	Manic phase of bipolar disorder.	Blind spots, retinal or subconjunctival hemorrhage, light sensitivity, involuntary eye movements.
Mellaril	Thioridazine	Psychosis.	Night blindness, blind spots, cataracts, hallucinations, lazy eye, optic atrophy.
Mevacor	Lovastatin	Elevated cholesterol.	Cataracts.
Motrin	Ibuprofen	Osteoarthritis; pain; fever.	Blind spots, visual-field constriction, lazy eye, retinal hemorrhage, optic neuritis.
Niaspan	Niacin	Elevated cholesterol.	Blurred vision, toxic lazy eye, central blind spot, glaucoma, protruding eyes.
Norpramin	Desipramine	Depression.	Hallucinations, lazy eye, optic neuritis, dryness, disturbed accommodation.
Ortho-Novum	Norethindrone	Birth control.	Optic neuritis, blind spots, halos around lights.
Orudis	Ketoprofen	Rheumatoid arthritis.	Decreased vision, retinal or subconjunctival hemorrhage, hallucinations, visual-field constriction.
Pepcid	Famotidine	Duodenal ulcer; benign gastric ulcer.	Decreased vision, hallucinations, retinal or subconjunctival hemorrhage, light sensitivity.
Plaquenil	Hydroxychloroquine	Malaria; rheumatoid arthritis; lupus erythematosus.	Cataracts, halos around lights, hallucinations, night blindness, flashing lights.
Premarin	Estrogen	Menopause; osteoporosis; female hypogonadism; atrophic vaginitis; breast cancer; prostate cancer.	Optic neuritis, blind spots, disturbed color vision, nearsightedness, fluctuations in vision, contact-lens intolerance.
Prozac	Fluoxetine	Depression.	Pain, light sensitivity, dryness, iritis, cataracts, double vision, drooping eyelids.
Restoril	Temazepam	Insomnia; anxiety, tension, agitation; skeletal-muscle spasms.	Pain, disturbed accommodation, hallucinations, tearing, burning, light sensitivity.
Retin-A	Tretinoin	Acne.	Skin dryness, light sensitivity, red eyes, red eyelids.
Ritalin	Methylphenidate	Attention deficit hyperactivity disorder.	Retinal or subconjunctival hemorrhage, dilated pupils, hallucinations.
Rogaine	Minoxidil	Hair regrowth.	Increased eye pressure, decreased vision, optic neuritis.
Seldane	Terfenadine	Allergic rhinitis.	Dryness, different-sized pupils, disturbed accommodation, decreased vision.
Synthroid	Levothyroxine	Hypothyroidism.	Decreased vision, double vision, drooping eyelids.
Tagamet	Cimetidine	Ulcers.	Hallucinations, light sensitivity.
Tavist	Clemastine	Mild allergy symptoms.	Decreased vision, dryness, light sensitivity, hallucinations, different-sized pupils.

Brand Name	Generic Name	Indications	Ocular Side Effects
Tegretol	Carbamazepine	Epilepsy.	Hallucinations, blurred vision, dizziness, involuntary eye movements, retinal hemorrhage, light sensitivity.
Tenormin	Atenolol	Hypertension.	Decreased vision, hallucinations, dryness, burning.
Timoptic	Timolol maleate	Glaucoma.	Dryness, burning, nearsightedness, hallucinations.
Tylenol	Acetaminophen	Fever; mild pain.	Hallucinations, disturbed color vision, double vision, redness.
Voltaren	Diclofenac	Rheumatoid arthritis; osteoarthritis.	Blurred vision, night blindness, lazy eye, blind spots.
Xanax	Alprazolam	Anxiety; depression.	Disturbed color vision, disturbed accommodation, pain, hallucinations.
Zantac	Ranitidine	Gastric ulcers.	Disturbed color vision, hallucinations, redness.
Zocor	Simvastatin	Elevated cholesterol.	Blurred vision, worsened cataracts, eye-muscle weakness.

Accommodative Insufficiency

One of the most fascinating aspects of the eye is its ability to change focal power. This changing of focal power enables us to see things clearly at a distance (twenty feet or more away) and also at a near point (sixteen inches or less away). This changing is called accommodation.

The eye's ability to accommodate usually follows a normal pattern of degeneration, being at its maximum when we are young and gradually decreasing as we age. If you are over forty years old and your eyes are beginning to lose their ability to accommodate, you have presbyopia, a different condition than what is discussed here. (For a discussion of presbyopia, see page 187.) Occasionally, the focal power of the eyes is not up to par for the age of the person. This is most commonly seen in school-aged children who have difficulty focusing on their reading materials. In this case, the condition is called accommodative insufficiency.

CONVENTIONAL TREATMENT

There are two methods that should be considered for treating accommodative insufficiency. The first is the conventional method of reading glasses. The lenses in reading glasses are designed to mimic the shapes of the lenses inside the eyes. In this way, the glasses take over much of the work of near-point vision, allowing the lenses in the eyes to relax and making near-point work easier to do.

The theory behind reading glasses sounds fine, but glasses really accomplish little in the way of helping people to overcome accommodative insufficiency. The eyes and their lenses *should* be worked in a normal viewing environment. Glasses may simply allow the eyes to relax *too* much, making them more dependent on glasses for clear near-point viewing.

The second treatment method is vision therapy. (For a complete discussion of vision therapy, see page 235.) Although vision therapy is considered to be much more than simply eye exercises, in this case exercises are used to work the lenses together with their associated muscles in an effort to increase their functional abilities. Vision therapy helps people learn how to better control their eyes so that they can use them more efficiently.

Occasionally, and depending on the severity of the problem, a doctor may prescribe glasses *and* vision therapy. This combination treatment may be the ideal remedy if the person's accommodative system is so weak that the vision therapy might be prolonged. The reading glasses will help the person to do normal near-point viewing, and the vision therapy will teach the person how to better control his or her eyes. If this combination treatment is successful, the glasses eventually are not needed.

SELF-TREATMENT

The core of the vision-therapy program for accommodative insufficiency is a technique called the accommodative rock. This technique helps to improve the eyes' ability to change focus, and to see clearly at near and at a distance. For complete instructions for doing the accommodative rock, see page 237.

NUTRITIONAL SUPPLEMENTS

Supplement	Directions for Use	Comments
Vitamin B_2	Take 75 mg daily.	Good for the nerves, muscles, and fatigue.
Vitamin C	Take 500 mg twice daily.	Nourishes the lens within the eye.
Vitamin E	Take 200 IU daily.	An antioxidant.

HOMEOPATHIC REMEDIES

Remedy	Directions for Use	Comments
Cocculuc 6c	Place 3–4 pellets under the tongue 3–4 times daily.	Good for accommodative insufficiency associated with nausea.
Gelsemium sempervirens 6c	Place 3–4 pellets under the tongue 3–4 times daily.	Good for accommodative insufficiency associated with headache.
Natrum muriaticum 6c	Place 3–4 pellets under the tongue 3–4 times daily.	Good for accommodative insufficiency associated with anger or irritability.

RECOMMENDATIONS

■ Get a thorough eye examination that includes near-vision testing.

■ If your child is having difficulty with school due to accommodative insufficiency, don't hesitate to get glasses for the child as well as vision therapy. If the child won't cooperate with the vision therapy, then he or she can use just the glasses to at least make reading easier. When the child matures somewhat, the therapy can still be used as a long-term treatment.

■ Don't confuse accommodative insufficiency with presbyopia. If you are near or past your fortieth birthday and are having difficulty focusing at the near point, your condition is probably presbyopia.

Age-Related Farsightedness

See PRESBYOPIA.

Age-Related Macular Degeneration

See MACULAR DEGENERATION.

Albinism

The word "albinism" refers to a group of conditions resulting from the presence of little or no pigment in the eyes, skin, and hair. In some cases, only the eyes are affected. People with albinism have inherited genes from their parents that do not work correctly. These genes do not allow their bodies to make the usual amounts of the pigment melanin. Melanin is a dark-brown to black pigment.

Worldwide, 1 in 17,000 people has some type of albinism. About 18,000 people in the United States are affected. Albinism can be found in every race. The majority of those afflicted were born to parents with normal hair and eye colors.

The eye needs pigment to develop normal vision. People with albinism have impaired vision because their eyes do not have the normal amount of pigment. People with albinism also sunburn easily, since the skin needs pigment for protection against sun damage. In tropical areas, many people with albinism who do not protect their skin get skin cancer. People with albinism often have several problems:

■ *They are very far- or nearsighted, or have astigmatism.* Their visual acuity ranges from 20/30 (nearly normal) to 20/400 (legally blind).

■ *They have nystagmus (nis-TAG-mus), which is an involuntary back-and-forth movement of the eyes.* (For a complete discussion of nystagmus, see page 175.)

■ *They have strabismus (strah-BIZZ-muss), which is an inability of the eyes to fix and track together.* Despite having this condition, people with albinism have some depth perception, although at close distances it is not as sharp as when the eyes work together.

■ *They are light sensitive.* Their irises allow "stray" light to enter the eyes and cause sensitivity. Contrary to popular belief, light sensitivity does not prevent people with albinism from going out in the sunlight. (For a complete discussion of light sensitivity, see page 161.)

It is a common notion that people with albinism have red eyes. In reality, the color of their irises varies from dull gray to blue to brown. (Brown irises are common in races with darker pigmentation.) In some types of albinism and under certain lighting conditions, a reddish or violet hue may be reflected through the iris. The reddish reflection comes from the retina, which lines the inner surface of the eye. It is similar to what occurs when a flash photograph is taken of a person looking directly at the camera—the eyes appear red. In some types of albinism, the red color can reflect back through the iris as well as through the pupil.

The key changes of the eye in albinism involve a lack of development of the fovea and a change in the development of the nerves that connect the eye to the brain. It is not clear why the fovea does not develop in persons with albinism. The developing eye seems to need melanin to organize the fovea, as well as to route the nerves from the retina to the areas of the brain where vision is processed. Studies have shown that the nerve impulses of people with albinism follow an unusual route from the eye. The nerve connections from the eye to the vision areas of the brain are disorganized. This unusual route probably prevents the eyes from working well together, plus causes strabismus.

CONVENTIONAL TREATMENT

Ophthalmologists and optometrists can help people with albinism to compensate for their eye problems, but they cannot cure the problems. To help with visual acuity, eye doctors experienced with low vision can prescribe a variety of devices. (For a discussion of low vision, see page 162.) No one device serves the needs of every patient, since different occupations and hobbies require the use of vision in different ways. Low-vision clinics often prescribe glasses with telescopic lenses, called bioptics, which can be adapted for near-point work as well as for distance vision. Many people with albinism use ordinary glasses or bifocals with a strong reading correction.

For nystagmus, research has not yet found an effective treatment. Although attempted treatments to control nystagmus have included biofeedback, contact lenses, and surgery, research has not proven any specific treatment to be effective for all people.

For strabismus, ophthalmologists normally treat infants starting at about six months of age, before the functioning of the eyes has developed fully. They may recommend that one eye be patched to encourage the use of the nonpreferred eye. This doesn't correct the strabismus, but it does help the "lazy" eye. Neither surgery nor injection of medicine into the muscles around the eyes completely corrects the inability to fix the eyes on one point. Although these treatments may improve the appearance of the eyes, they cannot correct the problem of improper routing of the nerve impulses.

Optometrists, on the other hand, usually take a more functional approach toward strabismus. Their method is to teach the growing child techniques to aid visual development and coordination. (For a discussion of these techniques, see "Vision Therapy" in Part Three.) Vision therapy is certainly more complicated in cases of albinism, but it usually does soften the effects of the condition.

For light sensitivity, eye doctors can prescribe dark glasses, which shield the eyes from bright light, or photochromic lenses, which darken as the light becomes brighter. There is no proof that dark glasses improve vision, however, even when used at a very early age, but they can improve comfort. Many children with albinism do not like tinted glasses.

Most children with albinism can function in a mainstream-classroom environment, provided the school addresses their special visual needs. The majority do not require Braille. Rather, children with albinism often prefer to read with their head tilted and the page held close to their eyes. Sometimes, it is difficult to get them to use their glasses.

RECOMMENDATIONS

■ If your child has low vision, ask his or her teacher to use high-contrast written materials. Children with low vision often have a hard time reading low-contrast materials such as the purple-on-white dittos used as worksheets in many classrooms. Black on white is better, and photocopying low-contrast dittos to make them black on white often makes reading easier.

■ Ask your child's school to order large-print textbooks. Schools can obtain large-print editions of most of their regular textbooks directly from the publishers.

■ Because children with albinism often have difficulty keeping track of their place on the page when shifting back and forth between a textbook and a worksheet, request permission for your child to write in his or her textbooks.

■ Ask the teacher to provide your child with a paper copy of all the board notes. Your child can then read the notes up close while the rest of the class reads from the board.

■ Request that the school purchase some optic devices to make reading assignments easier for your child. Hand-held monoculars, telescopic lenses mounted on eyeglasses, video-enlargement machines, and other types of magnifiers often help children with low vision.

■ The prescription of appropriate classroom visual aids requires teamwork among the student, parents, classroom teacher, vision-resources teacher, and an optometrist or ophthalmologist experienced in working with children with low vision. The American Foundation for the Blind maintains a directory of low-vision clinics in the United States. (To contact this organization, see "Resource Organizations" on page 255.)

Amblyopia

See LAZY EYE.

Anisocoria

Anisocoria (an-is-oh-KOR-ee-ah) is a condition in which the pupils of the two eyes are unequal in size. This has potentially dangerous implications because the size of the pupils is controlled by nerves in the brain. Both pupils should be equal in size and response. In fact, when a light is shined into just one eye, both pupils should react.

It is possible for there to be a slight difference in the sizes of the two pupils. Pupil size can be affected by a number of physical, psychological, environmental, and emotional conditions. Therefore, if you notice a slight difference, don't be alarmed. However, unequal size warrants a thorough evaluation, so be sure to get a professional opinion as soon as possible. Anisocoria is actually just a sign that there may be a disorder affecting the nerves within a certain part of the brain.

CONVENTIONAL TREATMENT

Testing pupil response is part of all routine eye examinations. Pupil response is a good indicator of how well the central nervous system is functioning. If there is any question regarding the size or reaction of the pupils, your doctor will probably order a visual-field test. The retinal nerve fibers, some of which branch off to the control centers for pupil response, can be evaluated by testing the visual field of each eye.

A visual-field test is something like a mapping of the side vision to determine if all of the nerves are functioning properly. It can be a somewhat tedious test, but it is well worth the trouble, since good results indicate that there is no problem with nerve or brain function.

SELF-TREATMENT

To test yourself for anisocoria, stand in front of a mirror and flash a small light into one of your eyes. Look at the pupil of that eye to see if it constricts (closes) when the light enters it. Shine the light into that same eye again, but this time look at the other eye. The pupil of the other eye should also constrict.

Next, shine the light into both eyes, one at a time, alternating between the two eyes using a steady motion of the flashlight. Both pupils should remain constricted. If there is a problem with the transfer of information along one of the optic nerves, one pupil may actually dilate (open) when the light is shined into it. If one of your pupils dilates, immediately phone your eye doctor for an appointment.

HOMEOPATHIC REMEDIES		
Remedy	**Directions for Use**	**Comments**
Argentum nitricum 6c	Place 3–4 pellets under the tongue 3–4 times daily.	Good for dilated pupils.
Belladonna 6c	Place 3–4 pellets under the tongue 3–4 times daily.	Good for dilated pupils.
Calcarea fluorica 6c	Place 3–4 pellets under the tongue 3–4 times daily.	Good for dilated pupils.
Cinchona officinalis 6c	Place 3–4 pellets under the tongue 3–4 times daily.	Good for dilated pupils.
Gelsemium sempervirens 6c	Place 3–4 pellets under the tongue 3–4 times daily.	Good for dilated pupils.
Stramonium 6c	Place 3–4 pellets under the tongue 3–4 times daily.	Good for dilated pupils.

RECOMMENDATIONS

■ Periodically check your pupil reaction with a flashlight to make sure your pupils constrict properly.

Anisometropia

Anisometropia (an-is-oh-met-ROH-pee-ah) is a visual condition in which the refractive error of each eye is different. Most people's eyes have slightly different refractions, but in anisometropia, the difference is great.

In anisometropia, one eye may be farsighted and one nearsighted. Or, both may be farsighted or nearsighted, but of unequal amounts. Additionally, one eye may have some astigmatism while the other doesn't, or both may have astigmatism, but of differing amounts. Anisometropia has many variations.

Because the eyes send their images to the brain independent of each other and the brain must fuse the two images together so that we see only one picture, it is important for both images to be approximately equal in size and clarity. If there is a significant difference between the two images, the brain cannot put them together properly and will either suppress one or cause double vision. (For complete discussions of double vision and suppression, see pages 123 and 201, respectively.) While suppression results in seeing just one picture again, it is not a desirable state for proper visual function. The proper situation is to have both eyes seeing clearly and both images fused into one picture.

CONVENTIONAL TREATMENT

Depending on the amount of the anisometropia, many doctors simply prescribe glasses with the correct prescription for each eye. However, as the refractive error of an eye becomes greater, the thickness of the eyeglass lens increases. With lenses of two significantly different thicknesses, the result is images of two different sizes, even if both eyes are corrected to 20/20. The brain may then have difficulty fusing the two images into a single picture. So, for significant anisometropia, glasses are not an ideal solution.

Contact lenses have shown to be a much more viable solution to anisometropia. Because contact lenses are much thinner than the lenses in eyeglasses and also rest directly on the eyeball, the images seen by the eyes are almost identical. These identically sized images are easier for the brain to fuse, therefore facilitating more comfortable vision.

SELF-TREATMENT

The type of treatment you should self-administer depends on what type of anisometropia you have. In most cases, you might consider a program of vision therapy. With a vision-therapy program, you may be able to correct your problem, as well as learn how to coordinate both your eyes. Ask a doctor who does vision therapy if the techniques outlined in "Vision Therapy" on page 235 would be appropriate for you.

RECOMMENDATIONS

■ If your child is very young, make sure to alternate the side on which he or she sleeps. This will assure that while the child is in the crib, each eye receives adequate visual stimuli.

■ If your child is school-aged, make sure that he or she does not tilt the head significantly while reading or writing. Also, check if the child holds a hand over one eye while doing near-point tasks.

Arcus Senilis

The condition of arcus senilis (ARK-us see-NIL-us) most often develops during the later years, but it is not uncommon in middle age or even younger. In arcus senilis, an opaque white ring encircles the corneas' periphery. If you look closely, you can see a clear section of cornea between the edge of the ring and the sclera. This is due either to the deposition of fat granules in the cornea or to hyaline degeneration. Hyaline degeneration is a type of tissue degeneration that results in rounded masses or broad bands of translucent tissue.

Arcus senilis generally is not considered to be of pathological importance, but from a biochemical viewpoint, it represents a specific metabolic disturbance and is a valuable indication of fat and cholesterol metabolism. The physiology, obviously disturbed, is not clear here. The general consensus among eye doctors is that arcus senilis is normal in older adults, but can be a sign of elevated cholesterol in middle-aged or younger individuals.

CONVENTIONAL TREATMENT

Since arcus senilis is cosmetically unappealing but not sight-threatening, it is most often noted but not treated by eye doctors.

NUTRITIONAL SUPPLEMENTS

Supplement	Directions for Use	Comments
Chromium picolinate	Take 400–600 mcg daily.	Lowers the cholesterol level, and improves the HDL–LDL ratio.
L-carnitine	Take 1,000 mg 3 times daily with meals.	Supports cholesterol metabolism, transports essential fatty acids, and aids liver and gallbladder function.
Lecithin	Take 1,200 mg 3 times daily before meals.	Emulsifies fat in the body.
Phosphatide	Take 1,500 mg daily.	Emulsifies fat in the body.

HERBS AND HERBAL SUPPLEMENTS

Herb	Directions for Use	Comments
Garlic	Take as directed on the label.	Reduces the cholesterol level.
Ginger	Take as directed on the label.	Reduces the cholesterol level.

ARMD

See MACULAR DEGENERATION.

Asthenopia

See EYESTRAIN.

Astigmatism

Astigmatism (ah-STIG-mah-tis-em) is a refractive error of the eye in which the image focused on the retina is distorted. In Latin, *a stigma* means "without point." The distortion of astigmatism comes most often from the cornea being shaped more like a barrel than a ball. The light rays in the vertical orientation focus in one area while the light rays in the horizontal orientation focus in a different area. There is a blur between the two points, and the resulting picture is distorted.

It has been reported that up to 80 percent of the American population has some degree of astigmatism. However, not all of these cases are severe enough to require an optical correction. Slight astigmatism is often of no consequence and just an example of the imperfections in nature. Yet, for many people, the degree of astigmatism can be severe enough to cause headaches and other symptoms. The unique aspect of this problem is that you may have significant astigmatism and not be aware of it. This is due to the fact that the optical disparity is a distortion rather than a blur. Because of the distortion, the brain, when it receives the image, makes a perceptual adjustment, so you *think* that everything is clear and properly orient-ed. This is part of the brain's attempt to make our visual world comfortable. I have seen cases in which young people thought that their vision was "pretty good" when in fact it was tested at 20/60!

CONVENTIONAL TREATMENT

The most conventional way to treat astigmatism is with eyeglasses. The curvatures of the eyeglass lenses roughly correspond to the curvatures of the eyes, and the optical distortion is resolved back into a "point image." This can be very effective, allowing you to see very clearly. However, there are a few things that you need to understand about the vision with new glasses for astigmatism.

First, since your brain has already adjusted to compensate for the distortion in your vision, new glasses may make things seem rather strange. This is because the images your eyes are seeing are now being realigned by the glasses, and your brain must readjust its perception. This may take some time, and until the readjustment is complete, your vision through the glasses will be disorienting. You may notice the floor sloping up, and straight lines may appear curved. These distortions will disappear with time, usually a week or so. To make the readjustment easier, simply wear your new glasses as much as is comfortable initially, and gradually increase your wearing time as you adapt.

Second, the correction for astigmatism is in the central portion of the eyeglass lens—that is, the part through which you look when looking straight ahead. However, when you look off to the side, up, or down, these thicker portions of the lens will create different types of astigmatism and may cause additional distortion. You may feel as if your whole world is moving as you move your head around. This condition will also disappear as you adapt to the lens prescription.

Another treatment for astigmatism is contact lenses. Contact lenses have a few advantages over eyeglasses for most optical corrections and for astigmatism as well. The different types of contacts and the different problems for which they are effective are discussed in detail in "Contact Lenses" on page 211. In recent years, advances in contact lenses have made the use of both the gas-permeable and soft varieties routine for astigmatism.

There is also a surgical option for the treatment of astigmatism. Radial keratotomy (RK), a procedure designed to reduce nearsightedness, can be modified to treat astigmatism. A more recent advance is the use of lasers to correct for astigmatism, as well as for nearsightedness. In addition, a new laser-assisted intrastromal keratomileusis (LASIK) procedure has also been approved recently to correct for astigmatism. These procedures are discussed in more detail in "Refractive Surgery" on page 228.

SELF-TREATMENT

Since most types of astigmatism are related to the curvature of the cornea, conventional wisdom holds that nothing (short of surgery) can effectively correct the condition. However, though this may be true in some cases, many times astigmatism can be dealt with successfully using a program of vision therapy. For complete details of how astigmatism can be addressed using such a program, see "Vision Therapy" on page 235.

Orthokeratology, a corrective program utilizing a series of contact lenses to reshape the eye, can also have an effect on the curvature of the cornea. This program is covered in detail in "Orthokeratology" on page 228.

RECOMMENDATIONS

■ Have a complete eye examination to determine if you have astigmatism and, if you do, if it's enough to warrant correction.

■ Discuss all of the treatment options—including eyeglasses, contact lenses, vision therapy, orthokeratology, and surgery—with your doctor.

Blepharitis

The word "blepharitis" (blef-ar-EYE-tis) comes from *blepharon*, the Greek word for "eyelid," and "itis," a suffix that means "inflammation." In blepharitis, the tiny glands and hair follicles that open onto the surface of the eyelids are inflamed. The eyelids are red, sore, and sticky. There may be little ulcers on the eyelids, and some eyelashes may fall out. Styes, chalazia, and dandruff of the scalp often occur along with blepharitis. (For complete discussions of chalazia and styes, see pages 101 and 198, respectively.)

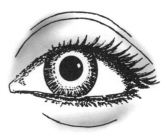

Blepharitis

CONVENTIONAL TREATMENT

Blepharitis has two primary causes. When the blepharitis is accompanied by ulceration (open sores) of the eyelid skin, the cause usually is a bacterial infection. In the presence of such an infection, the blepharitis needs to be promptly treated with a topical antibiotic. You may also be advised to apply warm compresses or to scrub your eyelids with a special solution.

Another cause of blepharitis is a waxy, greasy form of dandruff that affects the scalp and can also involve the eyelids, eyebrows, external ears, and the area around the nose and lips. If this is the cause of your blepharitis, you may be instructed to scrub your eyelids frequently using a washcloth or cotton-tipped applicator dipped in a solution of warm water and baby shampoo. This treatment will remove the crusty material and mucus from the eyelids. An antidandruff shampoo is usually recommended to bring the scalp condition under control. There are now specific eyelid "scrubs" that are recommended to treat this form of blepharitis.

Occasionally, eye doctors recommend that the tear ducts be plugged to prevent them from draining too rapidly. This is most often recommended for dry-eye conditions, but has also been shown to be effective in blepharitis.

SELF-TREATMENT

Blepharitis can also be caused by exposure to dust, smoke, irritating chemicals, or allergens. Antibiotics won't help in these situations, but you can remove yourself from the irritating environment, plus use warm compresses. If these recommended self-treatments bring no improvement, ask your doctor about anti-inflammatory medications.

FIRST AID FOR BLEPHARITIS

✚ Avoid rubbing your eyes.

✚ Apply a warm wet washcloth as a compress to the affected eye and hold it in place until cool. Do this three to four times daily, if possible.

✚ Use a commercial lid "scrub" or baby shampoo on a cotton swab to wash your lids.

NUTRITIONAL SUPPLEMENTS		
Supplement	Directions for Use	Comments
Vitamin A	Take 25,000 IU daily.	Good for dry skin.
Vitamin-B complex	Take 75 mg daily.	Promotes healthy skin and proper circulation. Aids in cellular reproduction.
Vitamin C with bioflavonoids	Take 6,000 mg daily in divided doses.	An antioxidant. Protects the eyes, and reduces inflammation. *Note:* Use powdered buffered ascorbic acid.

Supplement	Directions for Use	Comments
Zinc (OptiZinc)	Take 50 mg daily. *Caution:* Do not take more than 100 mg daily.	Enhances immune function.

HERBS AND HERBAL SUPPLEMENTS

Herb	Directions for Use	Comments
Dulse	Apply as a compress.	High in iodine.
Goldenseal	Apply as a compress.	Soothing for the tissues. *Caution:* Do not take internally for more than 1 week. Do not use during pregnancy.
Horsetail	Apply as a compress.	Tones the skin.
Rosemary	Apply as a compress.	Stimulates the skin.
Sage	Apply as a compress.	An astringent.

HOMEOPATHIC REMEDIES

Remedy	Directions for Use	Comments
Antimonium crudum 6c	Place 3–4 pellets under the tongue 3–4 times daily.	Good for all skin conditions.
Apis mellifica 6c	Place 3–4 pellets under the tongue 3–4 times daily.	Good for all skin conditions.
Argentum nitricum 6c	Place 3–4 pellets under the tongue 3–4 times daily.	Good for all skin conditions.
Arsenicum album 6c	Place 3–4 pellets under the tongue 3–4 times daily.	Good for blepharitis associated with anxiety or burning.
Calcarea sulfurica 6c	Place 3–4 pellets under the tongue 3–4 times daily.	Good for all skin conditions.
Carboneum sulfuratum 6c	Place 3–4 pellets under the tongue 3–4 times daily.	Good for all skin conditions.
Euphrasia officinalis 6c	Place 3–4 pellets under the tongue 3–4 times daily.	Good for blepharitis associated with soreness.
Graphites 6c	Place 3–4 pellets under the tongue 3–4 times daily.	Good for all skin conditions.
Hepar sulphuris 6c	Place 3–4 pellets under the tongue 3–4 times daily.	Good for all skin conditions.
Lycopodium 6c	Place 3–4 pellets under the tongue 3–4 times daily.	Good for all skin conditions.
Petroleum 6c	Place 3–4 pellets under the tongue 3–4 times daily.	Good for all skin conditions.
Rhus toxicodendron 6c	Place 3–4 pellets under the tongue 3–4 times daily.	Good for all skin conditions.
Sulphur 6c	Place 3–4 pellets under the tongue 3–4 times daily.	Good for all skin conditions.

RECOMMENDATIONS

■ Do not rub your eyes, even if they feel itchy.

■ Apply a warm compress to your eyes a few times a day, for at least ten minutes each time. To enhance the effect, make a tea of your chosen herb, soak a clean cloth in the tea, and apply the cloth as the compress. When finished, gently wipe your eyelids with the compress to remove any excess debris. Never re-use a compress.

■ Stay away from irritants such as smoke, wind, excessive sunlight, and bright lights.

■ Eat a well-balanced diet that emphasizes fresh raw vegetables, plus grains, legumes, and fresh fruits.

■ Get sufficient sleep, and avoid eyestrain.

Blepharospasm

Blepharospasm (BLEF-ar-ro-spaz-em) is a condition involving uncontrollable closing of the eyelids. It is a dystonia—that is, a postural disorder caused by abnormal involuntary sustained muscle contractions and spasms. It is both cranial, because it involves the head, and focal, because it is confined to one specific part of the head. "Blepharo" comes from the Greek word for eyelid. Patients with blepharospasm have normal eyes. The visual disturbance is solely the repeated forced closure of the eyelids.

Blepharospasm usually begins gradually with excessive blinking and/or eye irritation. In the early stages, it may occur only in the presence of specific stressful conditions, such as bright lights, fatigue, and emotional tension. As the disorder progresses, it occurs more frequently during the day. The spasms disappear during sleep, and some people find that after a good night's slumber, the spasms don't appear for several hours. Concentrating on a specific task often reduces the frequency of the spasms. As the condition progresses further, the spasms may intensify so that when they occur, the patient is functionally blind. The eyelids may even remain forcefully closed for several hours.

CONVENTIONAL TREATMENT

Botulinum toxin is an approved treatment for blepharospasm in the United States and Canada. This toxin is produced by the bacteria *Clostridium botulinum*. It weakens the muscles by blocking the nerve impulses transmitted from the nerve endings of the muscles. When it is used to treat blepharospasm, it is injected in minute doses into muscles above and below the eyes. The sites of the injections vary slightly from patient to patient and according to physician preference. The injections are usually given in the eyelid, the brow, and the muscles under the lower lid. They are given with a very fine needle. The benefits begin one to fourteen days after the treatment and last for an average of three to four months. Long-term follow-up studies have shown the treatment to be very safe and effective, with up to 90 percent of patients obtaining almost complete relief from their blepharospasm. The side effects include drooping of the eyelids, blurred vision, and double vision. Excessive tearing may occur. All these side effects are transient, caused mainly by excessive muscle relaxation. Providing the dose is kept small and the injections are given no less than three months apart, this method is effective over a long period of time.

Drug therapy for blepharospasm is difficult. Different medications have different mechanisms of action and generally produce unpredictable and short-lasting benefits. One medication may work for some patients and not for others. When one medication becomes ineffective, replacement with another medication sometimes helps. There is, therefore, no fixed or best regimen. Finding a satisfactory treatment regimen requires patience on the part of both the physician and the patient. The medications to try include amantadine (Symmetrel), baclofen (Lioresal), benztropine (Cogentin), bromocriptime (Parlodel), carbamazepine (Tegretol), clonazpam (Klonapin), diazepam (Valium), levodopa (Sinemet or Modopar), and trihexyphenidyl (Artane). This list is by no means complete, especially since there are new medications constantly being developed. The use of medication for blepharospasm requires close supervision by a neurologist.

Another treatment option is surgery. However, before considering surgery, it is advisable to try potentially effective nonsurgical therapies such as the botulinum-toxin injections. Functionally impaired patients with blepharospasm who cannot tolerate or do not respond well to medication or botulinum toxin are candidates for surgical therapy. At present, the removal of some or all of the muscles responsible for eyelid closure has proven to be the most effective surgical treatment for blepharospasm, though it is certainly also a last resort. Current experience has found that this procedure has improved visual disability in 75 to 80 percent of cases of blepharospasm.

SELF-TREATMENT

One method of self-treatment for blepharospasm is stress reduction. Consider seeking out professional assistance to determine if you have excessive stress in your life and how you can best deal with it. Typical modalities are meditation, breathing techniques, visualization, and counseling. Acupuncture is also a viable alternative to traditional medical treatments. (For a complete discussion of acupuncture, see page 209.)

NUTRITIONAL SUPPLEMENTS

Supplement	Directions for Use	Comments
Calcium	Take 1,000 mg daily.	Good for nerve function.
Folic acid	Take 400 mcg daily.	Good for proper nerve-cell production.
Phosphorus	Take 800 mg daily.	Good for proper nerve-cell growth.
Potassium	Take 2,500 mg daily.	Rebalances the nerves.
Vitamin-B complex	Take 100 mg daily.	Good for stress.
Vitamin B$_5$	Take 100 mg daily.	Improves the body's resistance to stress.
Vitamin C with bioflavonoids	Take 500 mg every 3 hours up to 4 times daily.	An antioxidant. *Note:* Use powdered buffered ascorbic acid.

HERBS AND HERBAL SUPPLEMENTS

Herb	Directions for Use	Comments
Lobelia	Apply as a compress.	Relieves muscle cramping. *Caution:* Do not take internally.
Valerian	Take as directed on the label. Take at bedtime.	Good for relaxation.

HOMEOPATHIC REMEDIES

Remedy	Directions for Use	Comments
Agaricus 6c	Place 3–4 pellets under the tongue 3–4 times daily.	Good for eyelid twitching.
Calcarea carbonica 6c *and* Magnesia phosphorica 6c	Place 3–4 pellets of each remedy under the tongue 3–4 times daily.	Good for blepharospasm associated with mineral deficiency.
Hypericum perforatum 6c	Place 3–4 pellets under the tongue 3–4 times daily.	Good for blepharospasm affecting the right eye only.
Ignatia amara 6c	Place 3–4 pellets under the tongue 3–4 times daily.	Good for eyelid twitching.
Nux vomica 6c	Place 3–4 pellets under the tongue 3–4 times daily.	Good for eyelid spasm after drinking coffee.
Physostigma 6c	Place 3–4 pellets under the tongue 3–4 times daily.	Good for eyelid twitching.
Rheum 6c	Place 3–4 pellets under the tongue 3–4 times daily.	Good for eyelid twitching.
Sulphur 6c	Place 3–4 pellets under the tongue 3–4 times daily.	Good for eyelid twitching.

RECOMMENDATIONS

■ If the patient is your child, consider emotional counseling.

■ Very often a stressful situation will initiate an episode of blepharospasm. Talking and releasing your feelings may make a significant difference.

Blood Vessels in Cornea

See CORNEAL NEOVASCULARIZATION.

Bloodshot Eyes

TREATMENT FOR BLOODSHOT EYES

■ If the redness is accompanied by discharge, use a warm wet washcloth as a compress.

■ If the redness is accompanied by itching, use a cold compress.

■ If your eyes are red without discharge, use a cool-water eyewash.

■ Call your eye doctor as soon as possible.

Redness can come from a variety of eye conditions. Eye inflammations, infections, and irritations of all kinds can cause the blood vessels of the conjunctiva to dilate. The eyes then appear red, or bloodshot.

If your eyes are constantly bloodshot, look for an obvious cause, because redness is more a sign that something is amiss than a condition in itself. If your eyes also itch, you are probably allergic to something in your environment. If you have pain, the problem is likely to be an infection. If the redness occurs only in certain situations, such as while cleaning the oven or cutting onions, it is likely due to irritating fumes. If the problem persists or you suspect an infection that needs treatment, see your eye doctor.

A bloodshot appearance can also result from a deficiency of vitamin B_2 or B_6, or the amino acid histidine, lysine, or phenylalanin. Once your body receives the nutrients it needs, the congestion in the blood vessels should disappear.

CONVENTIONAL TREATMENT

Most eye doctors look for the cause of the redness before recommending a treatment. There are dozens of causes for eye redness, and misdiagnosis can make the situation worse. If the cause of the redness is pinkeye, oftentimes no treatment is needed if proper hygiene is followed because the cause of pinkeye is usually self-limiting. Many doctors like to prescribe antibiotics and/or steroid combinations to be cautious. (For a complete discussion of pinkeye, see page 184.)

SELF-TREATMENT

If you experience redness in your eyes without any other symptoms (for example, burning, itching, discharge, or grittiness), then begin your self-treatment with warm compresses of plain water or of some of the herbs recommended below. If the compresses do not reduce the redness within a few days, consult an eye doctor. *Do not* use commercial eye-whitening drops, as they often tend to make the condition worse, which requires more drops.

NUTRITIONAL SUPPLEMENTS		
Supplement	**Directions for Use**	**Comments**
Free-form amino-acid complex	Take as directed on the label.	Provides the proper overall nutrition to the tissues. *Note:* Use a formula containing both the essential and nonessential amino acids.
Vitamin A	Take 50,000 IU daily.	Good for all eye conditions.
Vitamin-B complex	Take 100 mg 3 times daily.	Deficiencies have been linked to bloodshot eyes.

HERBS AND HERBAL SUPPLEMENTS

Herb	Directions for Use	Comments
Eyebright	Apply as a compress or use as an eyewash.	Good for all eye conditions.
Ming mu shang qing pian (Brion)	Take 4 pills twice daily.	Reduces "heat" in the body. *Caution:* Do not use during pregnancy.
Niu huang shang qing wan (Brion)	Take 10 pills daily.	Reduces "heat" in the body. *Caution:* Do not use during pregnancy.
Raspberry	Apply as a cool compress. Apply for 10 minutes.	Alleviates redness and irritation.
Shi hu ye guang wan (Brion)	Take 1 pill twice daily.	Good for red or itchy eyes.

HOMEOPATHIC REMEDIES

Remedy	Directions for Use	Comments
Aconite 6c	Place 3–4 pellets under the tongue 3–4 times daily.	Alleviates redness caused by an eye injury.
Allium cepa 6c	Place 3–4 pellets under the tongue 3–4 times daily.	Alleviates redness caused by a cold.
Apis mellifica 6c	Place 3–4 pellets under the tongue 3–4 times daily.	Alleviates redness, and reduces swelling.
Argentum nitricum 6c	Place 3–4 pellets under the tongue 3–4 times daily.	Alleviates redness caused by a cold.
Arsenicum album 6c	Place 3–4 pellets under the tongue 3–4 times daily.	Alleviates redness caused by a cold.
Belladonna 6c	Place 3–4 pellets under the tongue 3–4 times daily.	Alleviates redness caused by a cold.
Euphrasia officinalis 6c	Place 3–4 pellets under the tongue 3–4 times daily.	Alleviates redness, and reduces the size of blood vessels.
Glonoinum 6c	Place 3–4 pellets under the tongue 3–4 times daily.	Alleviates redness.
Kali sulfuricum 6c	Place 3–4 pellets under the tongue 3–4 times daily.	Alleviates redness accompanied by itching.
Natrum muriaticum 6c	Place 3–4 pellets under the tongue 3–4 times daily.	Alleviates redness accompanied by discharge.
Nux vomica 6c	Place 3–4 pellets under the tongue 3–4 times daily.	Alleviates redness accompanied by headache.
Sulphur 6c	Place 3–4 pellets under the tongue 3–4 times daily.	Alleviates redness.

RECOMMENDATIONS

■ If your eyes are red, avoid visually intense activities such as reading, computer work, and sewing. This will allow you to blink more often, thereby refreshing your eyes.

Cataracts

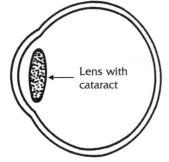

Cataract

Lens with cataract

A cataract (CAT-ah-rackt) is a clouding of the lens within the eye. This clouding can be partial or complete, so not all cataracts interfere with vision to a severe extent. However, the type of cataract that occurs with advancing age is generally progressive. Therefore, a cataract that today is small and not causing much of a problem will probably at some point, perhaps in a few years, become a large cataract that obscures vision.

Cataracts are not limited to the aged, although the so-called senile cataract is the most common type of cataract. Between the ages of sixty-five and seventy-four, about 23 percent of the population is expected to have a cataract. After the age of seventy-five, about 50 percent of people will have one.

Cataracts can also be present at birth, although this is pretty rare. This type of cataract is called congenital, and is sometimes caused by the mother's having contracted German measles, mumps, chickenpox, or any of certain other infectious diseases during pregnancy. Congenital cataracts can also be inherited.

Some diseases and injuries, as well as a class of anti-inflammatory medications called steroids, can also cause cataracts at any point in life. In addition, you can develop a cataract after being exposed to radiation (from having a large number of X-rays taken, for example), from being hit in the head by a high-voltage current (due to lightning or electrocution), or from constant exposure to infrared light. The cataract caused by infrared light is called a glass blower's cataract because these artisans used to work with infrared light without eye protection. Recent research suggests that many years of extreme exposure to UV light, which is part of sunlight but beyond the human visible spectrum, can also play a part in the development of cataracts. This is because the lens is a UV filter and absorbs most of the UV light entering the eye to prevent it from reaching the retina. Another study suggests that cigarette smoking is linked to the formation of cataracts. The eye damage seems to be from certain chemicals that are transported internally to the lens while smoking. Secondhand smoke (smoke in the environment) does not have this effect. In Spain, a recent study found that women who took estrogen for more than four years had a reduced number of opacities in the lenses of their eyes. This is the only study that has looked at the effects of estrogen on cataract formation, but this connection might be worth a further look.

So, are cataracts an inevitable consequence of advancing age, or are they the result of some action that can be changed? Researchers in the field of aging are asking this question about many conditions previously thought to be an unavoidable price of living a long life. The answer in the case of cataracts, as for most conditions, is that they probably are a combination of the aging process and environment. Years of exposure to UV light, radiation, and various as-yet-unidentified environmental insults such as smoking eventually catches up with us as we age. At the same time, the eye's lens fibers begin to break down and are more vulnerable to stresses from the outside world. You may be able to prevent or postpone the development of a cataract by protecting your eyes from UV light with a good pair of sunglasses, eating a nutritious and balanced diet, limiting your exposure to infrared light and radiation from X-rays and other sources, and not smoking.

CONVENTIONAL TREATMENT

When a cataract begins to interfere significantly with your vision and your life, it's usually time to consider surgery. Cataract surgery is the most common surgery in the United States today, with more than 1 million procedures performed every year. You may have heard that you have to wait until a cataract is "ripe" before it can be surgically removed. This was true years ago, but new surgical techniques have made it possible to remove a cataract at any time, as long as your doctor feels that you are in good enough shape to undergo the surgery. A few different surgical techniques can be used, and you and your surgeon can decide which one is best for you. Sometimes, cataract surgery can be done as an outpatient procedure.

For more information on cataract surgery, see page 210.

SELF-TREATMENT

If you have a cataract, you don't necessarily need surgery, at least not right now. What you may be noticing with your cataract is that light is being refracted differently and doesn't look the same as it did before. You may see just a general sort of cloudy haze in your visual field, or you may see a "dazzling" air show of light bouncing off your cataract. Changes in how you see are almost always due to changes in the lighting around you.

Outdoors on a sunny day, wear a hat with a brim to reduce the dazzle effect of the bright sunlight. Sunglasses will help with this, too. Indoors, experiment with the room lighting. You'll find reading easier if you have a small reading lamp that you can move around and adjust for your comfort instead of a ceiling fixture that is bright and immovable. You may want to keep the room lights low (but not off) when you watch television.

There have been many studies conducted on nutrition and cataracts. It has been shown, for example, that diets low in vitamin B_2 can produce cataracts in animals. In horses, cataracts, which are a common cause of blindness in these animals, can be reduced when large amounts of vitamin B_2 are added to the diet. Galactose, a type of milk sugar, increases the need for vitamin B_2. In infants who cannot utilize galactose normally, blindness from cataracts has been corrected by removing milk sugar from the diet and adding vitamin B_2. A 1997 study found a significant reduction in cataracts in a group of nurses who took vitamin-C supplements. It is apparent that, except in those cases of cataracts that are completely congenital, the major factor in the development of the disorder is nutrition. Although the lens can now be replaced with an artificial one, the best lens to have in your eye is the one with which you were born!

NUTRITIONAL SUPPLEMENTS

Supplement	Directions for Use	Comments
Copper *and* manganese	Take 3 mg of copper and 10 mg of manganese daily.	Retard the growth of cataracts.
Glutathione	Take as directed on the label.	An excellent free-radical scavenger.
Grape-seed extract	Take as directed on the label.	A powerful antioxidant.
L-lysine	Take as directed on the label.	Important in collagen formation. Repairs the lens.

Supplement	Directions for Use	Comments
Selenium	Take 400 mg daily.	A free-radical scavenger.
Superoxide dismutase (SOD)	Take as directed on the label.	A free-radical scavenger. Shown to be very effective at reducing cataract density.
Vitamin A	Take 25,000–50,000 IU daily.	Good for all eye conditions.
Vitamin-B complex with extra B_1, B_2, and B_5	Take 50 mg of vitamin-B complex daily.	Important for eye metabolism.
Vitamin C	Take 3,000 mg 4 times daily.	A free-radical scavenger.
Vitamin E	Take 400 IU daily.	A free-radical scavenger.
Zinc	Take 50 mg daily. *Caution:* Do not take more than 100 mg daily.	Protects against light-induced damage.

HERBS AND HERBAL SUPPLEMENTS

Herb	Directions for Use	Comments
Bilberry	Take 180 mg daily.	Boosts the circulation. Supplies bioflavonoids, which remove toxic chemicals. *Note:* Use the extract form.
Eyebright	Use as an eyewash.	Maintains the elasticity of the lens.
Ming mu di huang wan (Brion)	Take 10 pills 3 times daily.	Good for red or itchy eyes.
Nei zhang ming yan wan (Brion)	Take 8 pills 3 times daily.	Clarifies the vision. *Caution:* Contains aluminum, so limit its use.
Shi hu ye guang wan (Brion)	Take 1 pill twice daily.	Valuable during the early stages of cataract formation.
Visioplex Eye Concentrate With Eyebright	Take 3 pills daily as directed on the label.	Promotes the transfer of nutrients to the lens.

HOMEOPATHIC REMEDIES

Remedy	Directions for Use	Comments
Calcarea fluorica 6c	Place 3–4 pellets under the tongue 3–4 times daily.	Supports the connective tissue. Restores the integrity of the elastic fibers.
Calcarea sulfurica 6c	Place 3–4 pellets under the tongue 3–4 times daily.	Supports the connective tissue.
Causticum 6c	Place 3–4 pellets under the tongue 3–4 times daily.	Good for the elastic fibers.
Magnesia carbonica 6c	Place 3–4 pellets under the tongue 3–4 times daily.	Regulates the acidity of the body fluids.
Pulsatilla 6c	Place 3–4 pellets under the tongue 3–4 times daily.	Good during the early stages of cataract formation.
Silicea 6c	Place 3–4 pellets under the tongue 3–4 times daily.	Good for inflammation.
Sulphur 6c	Place 3–4 pellets under the tongue 3–4 times daily.	Good for cortical cataracts.

RECOMMENDATIONS

■ Avoid dairy products, saturated fats, and any fats or oils that have been subjected to heat, whether during cooking or processing. These foods promote the formation of free radicals, which can damage the lens. Use cold-pressed vegetable oils only.

■ Avoid antihistamines.

■ Spinach contains a carotenoid that has been shown to be effective in preventing cataracts.

■ Diabetics are especially prone to cataracts. Fortunately, diabetic cataracts are reversible. Therefore, careful monitoring of the blood-sugar level is critical.

Central Serous Retinopathy

Central serous retinopathy (CSR) involves a collection of fluid under the retina that causes visual distortion. As the name suggests, the fluid affects the central (macular) vision, which it disturbs the most. CSR patients often complain of a blind spot, decreased or blurred vision, and distortion of shapes. The vision may be minimally to significantly affected, with the visual acuity ranging from 20/20 (normal) to 20/200.

CSR affects primarily adults aged twenty to forty-five. Men are affected ten times more frequently than women. Many patients with CSR live under high levels of stress. The exact cause of CSR is highly controversial. However, there appears to be an imbalance in the amount of fluid that enters the space under the retina and the amount that leaves it, resulting in a net accumulation there. Some experimental evidence suggests that high blood levels of epinephrine and selected hormones may be responsible.

Most CSR patients spontaneously recover their visual acuity within about six months. The average recovery time is three to four months. Many patients have some residual symptoms, such as distortion of shapes and disturbed color vision, contrast sensitivity, and night vision. Despite an overall good prognosis, 40 to 50 percent of patients experience one or more recurrences of the disorder.

CONVENTIONAL TREATMENT

No medical therapy has been proven to be effective against CSR. Laser treatment can shorten the duration of the disease, but does not appear to alter the final visual acuity or the recurrence rate. Treatment with laser is controversial because of the potential complications and lack of apparent long-term benefits.

SELF-TREATMENT

The most practical thing that you can do for yourself if you develop CSR is to relax. Since the condition tends to be associated with high stress, reducing your stress level will be helpful. Consider meditation or tai chi, both of which are effective against stress.

Externally, there is not much that you can do because the cause of CSR is internal. Eyewashes, eye drops, and other external treatments are all of limited value.

NUTRITIONAL SUPPLEMENTS

Supplement	Directions for Use	Comments
Vitamin A	Take 25,000 IU daily.	Good for all eye conditions.
Vitamin-B complex	Take 75 mg daily.	Good for stress.
Vitamin B_6	Take 50–200 mg daily.	Reduces fluid retention.
Vitamin C	Take 2,000–5,000 mg daily.	Fortifies the blood-vessel walls.
Vitamin E	Take 200 IU daily.	Reduces fluid retention.
Zinc	Take 50 mg daily.	Good in combination with vitamin A.

HERBS AND HERBAL SUPPLEMENTS

Herb	Directions for Use	Comments
Alfalfa	Drink as a tea.	Good for relaxation. Good for chemical imbalance.
Chamomile	Drink as a tea.	Good for relaxation.
Gotu kola	Drink as a tea.	Good for relaxation.
Lady's slipper	Drink as a tea.	Good for relaxation.
Lobelia	Drink as a tea.	Good for relaxation. *Caution:* Do not take internally on an ongoing basis.
Passion flower	Drink as a tea.	Good for relaxation.
Valerian	Drink as a tea.	Good for relaxation.

HOMEOPATHIC REMEDIES

Remedy	Directions for Use	Comments
Apis mellifica 6c	Place 3–4 pellets under the tongue 3–4 times daily.	Alleviates swelling.

RECOMMENDATIONS

■ Use an Amsler Grid to monitor your visual distortion. (For a sample Amsler Grid and directions for using it, see page 118.)

■ Practice a relaxation technique such as tai chi, yoga, or meditation.

■ Palming is a good technique for relaxing the muscles around the eyes. (For a discussion of palming, see "Vision Therapy," page 235.)

■ Practice deep, relaxed breathing.

Central Vision, Deterioration of

See MACULAR DEGENERATION.

Chalazion

A chalazion (sha-LAY-zee-ohn) is the next step up from a stye in seriousness. The word "chalazion" comes from the Greek word for hailstone. "Chalazion" is the singular form, and "chalazia" is the plural form.

A chalazion results when one of the glands in the eyelid known as a meibomian (my-BOHM-ee-an) gland becomes plugged. Chalazia are therefore also known as meibomian cysts. Under normal circumstances, the meibomian glands, which number twenty or thirty in each eyelid, secrete an oily substance that delays the evaporation of tears and prevents the eyes from drying. Sometimes, one or more of these glands become plugged, and the resulting blockage causes the swelling known as a chalazion. The reason for the plugging usually is some kind of infection that makes the oily fluid thicker than normal.

Chalazia are larger than styes and are located some distance from the lid margin. They're usually not painful, while styes often are painful. If you're not sure whether you have a stye or a chalazion, pull the skin of the eyelid near the bump. If the skin moves and the bump doesn't, you have a chalazion. If the bump moves with the skin, you've probably got a stye. (For a complete discussion of styes, see page 198.)

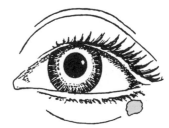

Chalazion

CONVENTIONAL TREATMENT

Many doctors start their treatment of a chalazion with antibiotic eye drops to attack the bacteria that may be causing the condition. They often also recommend applying a hot compress to the chalazion to soften it and help it to drain. Chalazia occasionally grow large enough to obscure vision. At this point, they can be opened and drained by a doctor. The procedure is done using a local anesthetic.

SELF-TREATMENT

Small chalazia often disappear by themselves within six to eight weeks. To help a small chazion resolve, bring it to a head by steaming it. One way to do this is to cover a wooden spoon with gauze and then dip the spoon into boiling water. Hold the spoon so that the steam rises to the eye, but *do not* touch the eye with the spoon. When the spoon has cooled, repeat the procedure. You can also use a washcloth soaked in warm water or herb tea.

FIRST AID FOR CHALAZIA

✚ Apply a warm wet washcloth as a compress to the affected eye as soon as possible after first noticing the chalazion. Use a compress often.

✚ Gently massage the chalazion lump right after using a warm compress.

✚ Check with your eye doctor to confirm that the lump is a chalazion.

HERBS AND HERBAL SUPPLEMENTS

Herb	Directions for Use	Comments
Eyebright	Apply as a hot compress.	Opens the pores to allow drainage.
Goldenseal	Apply as a hot compress.	Good for eye infections. *Caution:* Do not take internally for more than 1 week. Do not use during pregnancy.

HOMEOPATHIC REMEDIES

Remedy	Directions for Use	Comments
Hepar sulphuris 6c	Place 3–4 pellets under the tongue 3–4 times daily.	Good for abscesses, boils, and similar problems.
Mercurius vivus 6c	Place 3–4 pellets under the tongue 3–4 times daily.	Good for swollen glands, boils, and similar problems.
Staphysagria 6c	Place 3–4 pellets under the tongue 3–4 times daily.	Good for extremely emotional persons with chalazia.
Sulphur 6c	Place 3–4 pellets under the tongue 3–4 times daily.	Good for red eyelids.
Thuja occidentalis 6c	Place 3–4 pellets under the tongue 3–4 times daily.	Good for chalazia associated with warts.

RECOMMENDATIONS

■ Do not rub your eyes with dirty hands, since this can lead to infection.

Clouded Lens

See CATARACTS.

CMV Retinitis

See CYTOMEGALOVIRUS RETINITIS.

Color Deficiency

See COLORBLINDNESS.

Color Vision, Deficient

See COLORBLINDNESS.

Colorblindness

For approximately 8 percent of men and .5 percent of women in the United States (the numbers vary somewhat for other countries), something goes wrong with color perception. The color-connection mechanism doesn't work properly, and the afflicted people are colorblind. Actually, the term "color*blind*" is a misnomer because nearly every person with this disorder has only a deficiency in, not a total absence of, the ability to see the full range of colors.

People who are color deficient, the term I prefer, are either missing a certain type of color cone in their retina or have cones that are deficient in the ability to process color signals. When the red-receiving cones do not function properly or are absent, the person has a defect in his or her perception of the color red. The technical term for red blindness is protanopia (proh-tan-OH-pee-ah). When the green-receiving cones do not function or are absent, there is green blindness, which is called deuteranopia (doo-ter-an-OH-pee-ah). Deficiencies in perceiving yellows and blues also occur, but are extremely rare.

Although color deficiency can develop during childhood or adulthood as a result of certain diseases or a side effect of certain medications, it is more often genetically inherited and present at birth. Men are about fifteen times more likely than women to be color deficient because of the way in which the disorder is inherited. (For a discussion of color deficiency as a hereditary trait, see "Before Birth" on page 15.)

You can have your color vision quickly and simply tested by your eye doctor. If your doctor determines that you have some form of color deficiency, fear not. Color problems do not affect visual acuity, and even the most color-deficient person can have 20/20 vision. Electrical workers and pilots need excellent color discrimination, but people in most other occupations can learn to cope with the disorder. Of course, color deficiency can be inconvenient. One of my patients told me that she always knew when her color-deficient coworker had had a disagreement with his wife because he would come to work in clothes that clashed!

CONVENTIONAL TREATMENT

Since colorblindness does not involve an eye or vision disease or aberration in the clarity of eyesight, the treatment of the disorder is very limited. Most often, the "treatment" consists of jotting a note in the patient's record, making sure that the patient is aware of the problem, and counseling the patient to be cautious of taking jobs that require the ability to accurately identify colors.

RECOMMENDATIONS

■ Be sure to have your child's color vision checked as early as possible, especially if your child is a boy. The best time is just before the child enters kindergarten.

■ Although no definitive studies have been conducted on vitamin A and color deficiency, it is always important for the cones of the retina to be well-supplied with this important vitamin.

■ While there is no treatment for colorblindness, there are several ways to make living with it easier. For a thorough discussion of colorblindness and a list of methods for compensating for the disorder, see *Coping With Colorblindness* by Odeda Rosenthal and Robert H. Phillips (Garden City Park, NY: Avery Publishing Group, 1997).

Computer Vision Syndrome

REDUCING THE SYMPTOMS OF COMPUTER VISION SYNDROME

■ When working at a computer, blink often because this rests and re-wets the eyes.

■ Breathe fully, since taking complete breaths is important in relaxing the muscles.

■ Take breaks from the computer. Use the 20/20/20 rule—every twenty minutes, take twenty seconds and look twenty feet away.

Because computer work visually is such a highly demanding task, vision problems and symptoms are very common. Most studies indicate that computer operators report more eye-related problems than do paper-oriented office workers. A 1994 study by the National Institute of Occupational Safety and Health showed that 88 percent of computer users complained of computer-related eyestrain. The symptoms generally affecting computer users are now collectively known as computer vision syndrome (CVS). CVS most often occurs when the viewing demand of the task exceeds the visual abilities of the computer user. The American Optometric Association defines CVS as that "complex of eye and vision problems related to near work which are experienced during or related to computer use." The symptoms can vary, but usually include eyestrain, headaches, blurred vision (distance and/or near), disturbed accommodation, neck pain and/or backache, light sensitivity, double vision, disturbed color vision, and dry, irritated eyes.

The causes of the inefficiencies and the visual symptoms are a combination of individual visual problems and poor office ergonomics. Poor office ergonomics can be further divided into poor workplace conditions and improper work habits. Many people have marginal vision disorders that do not cause symptoms when performing less demanding visual tasks. In other words, you must address your working environment as well as your visual condition when treating CVS.

CONVENTIONAL TREATMENT

Most likely, your doctor will prescribe glasses for you to help reduce the eyestrain caused by your computer work. What the doctor will recommend is a pair of glasses designed to help you see the computer monitor without having to overfocus your eyes. What the doctor may not recommend is making adjustments to your workspace to help improve the conditions that are contributing to your vision problems.

Very often, environmental conditions may lead to eye problems. If your computer monitor is too high in your visual field, you may have to lift up your eyes or head to see it properly, especially if you wear bifocals. Putting the monitor off to one side can cause neck problems. Using reading glasses that were designed for seeing things sixteen inches away may cause blurriness when looking at a monitor twenty-five inches away, so you may lean toward the monitor, creating a back problem. Proper ergonomics must be addressed along with the proper visual correction.

SELF-TREATMENT

Since there are many different environmental and visual corrections that can be made to achieve the proper balance for computer use, giving overall recommendations is difficult. However, I have often recommended a "3-B" approach to reducing eyestrain from computer use. The three Bs are blink, breathe, and break.

Blinking is extremely important for maintaining clarity of vision and eye health. Blinking spreads tears over the eye and cleans the surface. These new tears also facilitate oxygen transmission to the cornea, allowing the cornea to stay clear and healthy. Research has shown that we blink less when we read and even less when we work at computers. I could recommend that you remember to blink, but that is sort of silly, since your mind has too many other things to remember and blinking should be automatic. However, just by being aware of the problem you will be better off. You might try putting a small sticky-note with the word "blink" on the corner of your computer screen as a reminder.

Breathing controls the stress level of many of the muscles. Imagine a weight lifter attempting to lift a very heavy weight. He inhales deeply and holds his breath while lifting the weight. Once he has achieved the lift, he quickly exhales. This is a simple illustration of how we hold our breath while confronting stressful conditions. Without your knowledge, computer use can be a very stressful situation. Awkward posture, glaring lights, unreasonable deadlines, low humidity, and other stresses can affect you while using a computer. Breathing regularly and deeply can help to alleviate the resulting symptoms.

The eyes are designed to see mostly at distance and occasionally at near. However, today we do much more near-point work, especially since computers showed up on our desks at work. We must take more *breaks* to ease the stress on the focusing system. These breaks can be simple visual breaks—just looking into the far distance or closing your eyes for a few minutes—or they can be full breaks—getting up and moving around. In either case, varying your viewing distance is critical to maintaining comfortable vision. And remember, when you take a visual break, don't do needlepoint or read or do any other near-point activity.

For eye techniques to use during breaks and for general improvement of your visual abilities, see "Vision Therapy" on page 235.

NUTRITIONAL SUPPLEMENTS

Supplement	Directions for Use	Comments
Vitamin A	Take 25,000 IU daily.	Good for all eye conditions.
Vitamin-B complex	Take 75 mg daily.	Good for stress.
Vitamin C	Take 5,000 mg daily.	An antioxidant. Good for stress.
Vitamin E	Take 200 IU daily.	An antioxidant.

HERBS AND HERBAL SUPPLEMENTS

Herb	Directions for Use	Comments
Eyebright	Take 3–4 drops daily or apply as a compress.	Good for the eye tissues.
Goldenseal	Apply as a compress.	Soothing for the tissues. *Caution:* Do not take internally for more than 1 week. Do not use during pregnancy.

HOMEOPATHIC REMEDIES

Remedy	Directions for Use	Comments
Euphrasia officinalis 6c	Place 3–4 pellets under the tongue 3–4 times daily.	Alleviates redness.
Nux vomica 6c	Place 3–4 pellets under the tongue 3–4 times daily.	Good for eyestrain associated with overwork.
Ruta graveolens 6c	Place 3–4 pellets under the tongue 3–4 times daily.	Good for eyestrain followed by headache. Heals the tendons and ligaments.
Sulphur 6c	Place 3–4 pellets under the tongue 3–4 times daily.	Alleviates redness following near-point work.

RECOMMENDATIONS

■ Lower your monitor so that when you hold your head in the normal position, you can look straight ahead and see just over the top of it.

■ Make the background illumination of the screen and the illumination of your immediate work area approximately equal.

■ The best screen "colors" to use are black letters on a white background. This combination simulates paper and ink, and provides the highest contrast between the letters and the background.

■ Make sure the screen does not have a glare. To check for this, turn the computer off and look for any reflections of lights or lightly colored articles in the screen.

■ Make sure there is no other light hitting your eyes, either directly from a window or lamp, or by reflection off a shiny surface.

Conjunctiva, Bleeding Under

See SUBCONJUNCTIVAL HEMORRHAGE.

Conjunctivitis

See PINKEYE.

Convergence Excess

Convergence is the process in which the two eyes turn in toward one another in order to view an object that is within twenty feet away. In convergence excess, the eye muscles that control this process are not coordinated and the eyes turn inward too far. However, convergence excess does not actually occur in the eye muscles, but rather in the brain, since that is where the signals to converge originate.

There are a number of possible causes of convergence excess. The most common is an overstimulation to focus, or accommodate. The two systems of convergence and accommodation are tied together in the brain. Therefore, when we accommodate, we converge; and when we converge, we accommodate. If there is too much stimulus to accommodate, the eyes will be forced to overconverge. This creates a stressful situation and makes it difficult to read comfortably.

CONVENTIONAL TREATMENT

The most popular conventional treatment for convergence excess is glasses. Glasses prescribed for this disorder are intended to reduce the need of the eyes to overfocus. This allows the eyes to realign easier. Glasses are often very effective at achieving the desired results of straight eyes and comfortable vision.

SELF-TREATMENT

There are a number of techniques that you can do as part of a vision-therapy program to treat your own convergence excess. For sample techniques, see "Vision Therapy" on page 235. In most cases of convergence excess, relaxation is an important part of the treatment. Among the relaxation techniques I recommend are meditation and tai chi, both of which are extremely effective at reducing stress.

NUTRITIONAL SUPPLEMENTS		
Supplement	Directions for Use	Comments
Vitamin-B complex	Take 75 mg daily.	Good for nerve function.
Vitamin C	Take 3,000 mg daily.	Good for stress.

RECOMMENDATIONS

■ Make sure your near-point vision is tested during your next eye examination.

Convergence Insufficiency

As explained in "Convergence Excess" on page 107, the two eyes must turn in toward one another while viewing an object within twenty feet away. This process is called convergence. If, for some reason, the eye muscles are not able to smoothly or efficiently achieve adequate convergence to view the desired object, the visual system will experience convergence insufficiency.

The main symptom of convergence insufficiency is tiring of the eyes when doing near-point work. This can manifest as a preference to read while trying to go to sleep (in other words, using reading as a method to bring on sleep) or as difficulty remaining focused on the reading material. You may get headaches or eyestrain, or often lose your place while reading.

CONVENTIONAL TREATMENT

There are a few different treatments for convergence insufficiency. One is glasses, usually used just for reading. The lenses of these glasses might have some power to reduce the focusing requirement of your eyes, but they may also just contain prism. Prism helps to displace the image laterally so that the eyes don't have to converge as much as normal. This might be good for relieving the symptoms of convergence insufficiency, but it does not really cure the disorder. If you are satisfied with your glasses and the glasses relieve your symptoms, however, you may not need to do anything else.

In some cases, the doctor will recommend a program of vision therapy. The aim of therapy for convergence insufficiency is to teach you to better coordinate your eyes so that they can converge more efficiently. This is more than just eye-muscle exercising. It's actually a form of visual biofeedback that can enhance your ability to see more effectively. (For a complete discussion of vision therapy, see page 235.)

Since some of the nerves that control convergence travel through the spinal column, chiropractic adjustment may have an effect on convergence ability.

SELF-TREATMENT

There are a number of techniques usually used in vision therapy that you can do by yourself. They are among the easiest and most effective techniques to do. Included are the Brock string technique and convergence stimulation. For descriptions of these techniques, see "Vision Therapy" on page 235.

NUTRITIONAL SUPPLEMENTS		
Supplement	Directions for Use	Comments
Vitamin-B complex	Take 75 mg daily.	Good for nerve function.

RECOMMENDATIONS

■ Make sure your near-point vision is tested during your next eye examination.

■ Test your convergence ability with this technique: Hold your fingertip or a pencil straight out in front of your face. Slowly move the finger or pencil toward your nose, following it with both your eyes. Watch it until it splits in two. It should be closer than four inches away when you begin to see double.

Cornea, Barrel-Shaped

See ASTIGMATISM.

Cornea, Cone-Shaped

See KERATOCONUS.

Corneal Abrasion

A corneal abrasion is a scrape on the cornea, most often from a foreign body such as a grain of sand, a piece of dirt, or an ill-fitting contact lens. Patients with scraped corneas often tell the doctor that something is under their upper eyelid. Oftentimes, the foreign body is no longer present, but the patient feels some discomfort when the eyelid passes over the scrape. Usually, it is the first few layers of the cornea that are affected, and since these layers have the most nerve endings, the prominent sensation is pain.

EMERGENCY TREATMENT FOR CORNEAL ABRASION

✚Gently pull your upper eyelid away from the eyeball by grasping the lashes, and shake the eyelid from side to side.

✚ Flush the eye with a sterile saline solution, if available, or cool clean water.

✚ Avoid blinking excessively.

✚ If the pain is severe, take a pain reliever.

✚Call your eye doctor as soon as possible.

CONVENTIONAL TREATMENT

Scratches on the cornea usually cannot be seen with the naked eye. Your eye doctor will examine the injury under magnification and may also use a green stain called fluorescein to make the abrasion visible. You may be given a prescription for a topical antibiotic, in the form of an ointment or drops, to help prevent an infection.

Doctors once routinely patched eyes with corneal abrasions, but many now feel the eye is better off healing without a patch. One reason is that a patch keeps the eye warm, which increases the chance of an infection developing. Also, it's easier to monitor the eye's healing and apply medications if your eye is not covered. On the other hand, a patch makes the healing eye more comfortable.

Most corneal abrasions heal within a few days, although injuries from a plant material such as wood or a very dirty substance may take longer.

SELF-TREATMENT

If you suffer a corneal abrasion, your eye will generally tear profusely when the injury first occurs. This tearing may wash out the foreign body that caused the abrasion, which may have become trapped in your eye. If you or someone else can see the foreign body, you can try to remove it with a handkerchief or facial tissue. Make sure that the handkerchief or tissue is clean and wet, and be *very* gentle!

The first thing you should do, though, is to look down and gently grasp the upper eyelashes between your thumb and forefinger. Gently pull the lid away from the eyeball and "shake" it in a side-to-side motion. This will hopefully dislodge the foreign body. Be careful not to shake the lid hard enough to pull out any of the lashes. You can try washing out your eye with purified water or a commercial eyewash. However, *do not* use commercial eye-whitening drops. Always make sure you use a sterilized eyewash cup or a very clean hand when washing out your eye. Although this condition is self-limiting, you must use caution to prevent an infection.

NUTRITIONAL SUPPLEMENTS

Supplement	Directions for Use	Comments
Vitamin A (Viva-Drops)	Take 1–2 drops 3–4 times daily for 2 days.	Supports the corneal tissue as it heals.
Vitamin C	Take 500 mg twice daily for 2 days.	Builds collagen tissue.

HERBS AND HERBAL SUPPLEMENTS

Herb	Directions for Use	Comments
Bayberry, eyebright, *and* goldenseal	Use as an eyewash twice daily.	Good for all eye conditions. *Caution:* Do not take goldenseal internally for more than 1 week. Do not use goldenseal during pregnancy.
Comfrey	Use as an eyewash.	Promotes healing.
White willow bark	Take 400 mg as needed.	Good for pain.

HOMEOPATHIC REMEDIES

Remedy	Directions for Use	Comments
Aconite 6c	Place 3–4 pellets under the tongue 3–4 times daily.	Good for general eye discomfort.
Aurum 6c	Place 3–4 pellets under the tongue 3–4 times daily.	Good for pain.
Belladonna 6c	Place 3–4 pellets under the tongue 3–4 times daily.	Good for pain.
Bryonia 6c	Place 3–4 pellets under the tongue 3–4 times daily.	Good for pain.
Chamomilla 6c	Place 3–4 pellets under the tongue 3–4 times daily.	Good for pain.
Cinchona officinalis 6c	Place 3–4 pellets under the tongue 3–4 times daily.	Good for pain.
Hypericum perforatum 6c	Place 3–4 pellets under the tongue 3–4 times daily.	Good for nerve injury.
Lycopodium 6c	Place 3–4 pellets under the tongue 3–4 times daily.	Good for pain.
Mercurius vivus 6c	Place 3–4 pellets under the tongue 3–4 times daily.	Good for corneal abrasions accompanied by discharge.
Natrum muriaticum 6c	Place 3–4 pellets under the tongue 3–4 times daily.	Good for pain.
Nitricum acidum 6c	Place 3–4 pellets under the tongue 3–4 times daily.	Good for pain.
Sanguinaria 6c	Place 3–4 pellets under the tongue 3–4 times daily.	Good for pain.
Staphysagria 6c	Place 3–4 pellets under the tongue 3–4 times daily.	Good for corneal abrasions associated with anger.
Spigelia 6c	Place 3–4 pellets under the tongue 3–4 times daily.	Good for pain.

RECOMMENDATIONS

■ Get plenty of rest, including a good night's sleep.

■ Take an over-the-counter pain medication if the homeopathic remedies aren't effective enough or if your eye is still very uncomfortable.

■ Use a cool compress to calm the eye and to reduce the inflammation.

■ If your eye doesn't feel "normal" again in twenty-four to thirty-six hours, see your eye doctor. Both optometrists and ophthalmologists are qualified to deal with corneal abrasions that don't respond to self-treatment.

Corneal Abrasion, Nonhealing

See RECURRENT CORNEAL EROSION.

Corneal Lesion

See CORNEAL ULCER.

Corneal Neovascularization

Yes, this is quite a mouthful to pronounce. However, corneal neovascularization (NEE-oh-vas-que-ler-eh-ZAY-shun) is a potentially serious problem of which you should be aware.

The cornea is normally a clear membrane that contains no blood vessels. It receives its oxygen and nourishment from the tear film, which covers the front surface of the eye. There are, however, blood vessels in the conjunctiva, the thin tissue covering the eye. These blood vessels travel to the edges of the cornea and then turn back to feed the other parts of the eye. As long as the cornea continues to receive an adequate supply of oxygen from the tears, it does not need any blood vessels to grow through it. However, if there is a significant decrease in the oxygen flow to the cornea, the body responds by growing new blood vessels into the cornea. This new growth of blood vessels is called neovascularization, which literally means "new blood-vessel growth."

Even a slight amount of blood-vessel growth into the edges of the cornea indicates that the amount of oxygen reaching the cornea has decreased. This most commonly occurs with excessive contact-lenses wearing. A small amount of growth is not normally considered significant or a threat to eyesight. However, if left unchecked, the growth will continue until blood vessels have grown throughout the cornea. This will cause the clear cornea to become clouded and block light from passing through, causing blindness. The possibility of blindness should be enough to encourage all contact-lens wearers to get regular checkups.

CONVENTIONAL TREATMENT

There is really only one conventional treatment recommended for corneal neovascularization—to remove your contacts! Depending on how severe the condition is and how you are wearing your lenses, this discontinuation may be temporary. However, once blood vessels have grown into the cornea, they are there for good. If you remedy the situation causing the problem and more oxygen is again diffused to the cornea in the proper manner, your body will not need to send blood into those new vessels and the vessels will become dormant. Be warned, however, that if the amount of oxygen reaching the cornea is decreased again, the vessels will fill with blood very quickly, and the process will start over.

SELF-TREATMENT

The best way to avoid corneal neovascularization is to take proper care of your contact lenses. If you use daily-wear soft lenses, be sure to remove them nightly, clean them properly, use an enzyme cleaner weekly, and follow your doctor's recommendations. If you sleep with your contacts on, be sure to remove them weekly and give them a very thorough cleaning. The best way to assure that you always wear clean lenses is to use disposable lenses, which are thrown away every week or two. Disposable lenses have a reputation for being the healthiest for the eye because there is less chance for debris to build up on them and block oxygen transmission.

Whichever type of contact lens you use, make sure to continually check in with your doctor and follow his or her recommendations. In addition, review the information in "Contact Lenses" on page 211.

NUTRITIONAL SUPPLEMENTS		
Supplement	Directions for Use	Comments
Vitamin A	Take 25,000 IU daily.	Good for all eye conditions.
Vitamin C	Take 3,000 mg daily.	Maintains eye stability.
Vitamin E	Take 200 IU daily.	Fortifies the blood-vessel walls.

HERBS AND HERBAL SUPPLEMENTS		
Herb	Directions for Use	Comments
Eyebright	Use as an eyewash.	Good for all eye conditions.

HOMEOPATHIC REMEDIES		
Remedy	Directions for Use	Comments
Aconite 6c	Place 3–4 pellets under the tongue 3–4 times daily.	Alleviates redness.
Apis mellifica 6c	Place 3–4 pellets under the tongue 3–4 times daily.	Alleviates swelling.

RECOMMENDATIONS

■ Don't wait until your contact lenses start to irritate your eyes before getting them evaluated.

■ Check with your doctor at the first sign of redness in your eyes.

■ Shark cartilage has been shown to reduce neovascularization in tumors. Therefore, it might be useful for corneal neovascularization.

Corneal Ring

See ARCUS SENILIS.

Corneal Scratch

See CORNEAL ABRASION.

Corneal Ulcer

An ulcer of any kind is a very serious condition. It usually starts as a break in the surface tissue. This leads to progressive erosion and death of the tissue. The main symptoms of a corneal ulcer are extreme pain, tearing, and redness. If you experience these symptoms and see what looks like a small white dot on the cornea, you probably have an ulcer, or at least a corneal infiltrate. An untreated corneal infiltrate will lead to an ulcer.

The most common cause of corneal ulcers today is excessive contact-lens wearing. The lens being in constant contact with the corneal surface, combined with poor lens hygiene and/or long wearing time, can lead to a break in the surface of the cornea. Once a break occurs, there is an increased likelihood that bacteria, which are normally dormant in the tears, will infect the tissue and create an ulcer.

CONVENTIONAL TREATMENT

The first course of treatment for a corneal ulcer is a combination antibiotic-steroid medication, which is designed to kill bacteria and reduce inflammation. Depending on the severity of the condition and the type of bacteria, the medication may be used as often as every fifteen minutes during the first few hours. Its use is tapered as the condition improves. The eye may be patched to reduce excess irritation. The doctor may want to see you every day to gauge the effectiveness of the treatment.

SELF-TREATMENT

The best thing you can do if you have a corneal ulcer is to follow your doctor's advice exactly. Ulcers can cause permanent vision loss if they are not dealt with quickly and effectively, so pay attention to all of your doctor's instructions. Keep excessive makeup away from the eye area, and be sure not to touch the eye area with unwashed fingers. Once the main episode has resolved and the healing process has begun, you can use some supplemental support to speed up the healing.

NUTRITIONAL SUPPLEMENTS

Supplement	Directions for Use	Comments
Folic acid	Take 5 mg 3 times daily.	Aids tissue healing.
Vitamin A	Take 50,000 IU daily.	Good for all eye conditions.
Vitamin B_2	Take 400 mg daily.	Aids nerve healing.
Vitamin C	Take 3,000 mg daily.	Aids tissue healing.
Vitamin E	Take 800 IU daily.	Aids tissue healing.

HERBS AND HERBAL SUPPLEMENTS

Herb	Directions for Use	Comments
Eyebright	Take 1–2 drops 4–5 times daily.	Good for overall eye healing. *Note:* Begin taking after you have finished taking other drops.

HOMEOPATHIC REMEDIES

Remedy	Directions for Use	Comments
Aconite 6c	Place 3–4 pellets under the tongue 3–4 times daily.	Alleviates pain and inflammation in the early stages of corneal-ulcer formation.
Apis mellifica 6c	Place 3–4 pellets under the tongue 3–4 times daily.	Good for inflammation.
Calcarea sulfurica 6c	Place 3–4 pellets under the tongue 3–4 times daily.	Reduces light sensitivity.
Euphrasia officinalis 6c	Place 3–4 pellets under the tongue 3–4 times daily.	Good for all eye conditions.
Mercurius corrosivus 6c	Place 3–4 pellets under the tongue 3–4 times daily.	Good for pain.

RECOMMENDATIONS

■ If you experience sharp pain and discomfort around the eyes, see your eye doctor immediately.

■ If you wear contact lenses and feel discomfort, remove the lenses immediately and don't re-insert them until your eyes feel comfortable again. If your eyes continue to feel uncomfortable, see your doctor.

Crossed Eyes

See STRABISMUS.

CSR

See CENTRAL SEROUS RETINOPATHY.

CVS

See COMPUTER VISION SYNDROME.

Cytomegalovirus Retinitis

Cytomegalovirus (CMV) retinitis is the disease that most often causes people with acquired immune deficiency syndrome (AIDS) to go blind. AIDS is an immune-system disorder in which the body's ability to defend itself is greatly diminished. When human immunodeficiency virus (HIV), the virus that causes AIDS, invades key immune cells and multiplies, it causes a breakdown in the body's immune system, which eventually leads to overwhelming infection and/or cancer. Most of the deaths among people with AIDS are not caused by the AIDS, but by one of the many infections or cancers to which the syndrome makes the body vulnerable.

The eye is not exempt from AIDS-related conditions. It is most often infected with cytomegalovirus, a herpes virus. CMV is a virus that usually causes illness in the retinas or the intestines of people with HIV. However, it can also infect the whole body, as well as cause illness in the lungs, throat, brain, kidneys, gallbladder, liver, and other organs. CMV of the eyes is called CMV retinitis.

People with CMV retinitis have blurred vision, undergo unusual changes in their eyesight, or see small moving spots called floaters. Floaters are transparent or dark spots floating or moving in the field of vision. They are especially apparent when looking at a light or bright background. While it is normal to see a certain number of floaters when looking at, for instance, the sky on a sunny day, an obvious and sudden increase in the number of these floaters is a danger signal. (For a complete discussion of floaters, see page 134.)

Any distortion or absence of a section of the field of vision is also dangerous. This may appear as an area of blurred vision or a spot of vision that is missing altogether. It can also resemble a curtain or veil blocking your vision. The particular type of vision problem you have will depend on what part of your retina has been damaged by the virus. To learn what the specific damage is, you must consult an eye specialist.

If the damage to your retina is along the edges, your peripheral vision will be affected. Peripheral vision is indirect vision—that is, what you see on the edges of your vision. It is important because it is what you use to determine the position of things other than what you are looking at directly. Without adequate peripheral vision, you would have problems driving a car or playing a sport, for example. This is because you need to concentrate on one thing, such as the road ahead of you when you are driving, but must also be aware of the other things happening around you, such as cars approaching from your side. While you could see without full peripheral vision, your vision would be limited. If the damage is to the center of the retina, your central vision will be affected. Central vision is direct, line-of-sight vision, the vision used to read and do close work. It is the most important part of vision. Self-tests for both peripheral and central vision are easy to do. (See "Self-Treatment," on page 118.)

Early detection of vision changes can greatly minimize the total amount of damage done by CMV by alerting both you and your doctor to the presence of the virus at the earliest possible stage, and by speeding diagnosis and treatment. CMV responds to treatment in the vast majority of cases, and while the treatment is certainly no picnic, it's much better than going blind! Most patients seem to tolerate the CMV medications pretty well. Hopefully, in the near future, advances in the tests and treatments for CMV will make this disease more manageable and perhaps even preventable.

CONVENTIONAL TREATMENT

There are no medications that can prevent illness from CMV. Although some people take acyclovir (Zovirax) to prevent CMV illness, studies have shown that it does not really work. Other medications to prevent CMV illness are being studied in clinical trials. Most people already have the CMV virus in their bodies, but it does not make them sick, even if they are HIV-positive. The majority of people who develop illness from CMV have very low T-cell counts. Your doctor can perform a blood test to see if you have been exposed to CMV.

Treatment for CMV infection today consists mainly of using the antiviral medication foscarnet (Foscavir) or ganciclovir (Cytovene), both of which are given intravenously (into the vein). This treatment method can be severely limiting for many people, but must be endured indefinitely in order to successfully treat the disease. Sadly, these treatments are both costly and toxic to the bone marrow. Recently, several new modes of ganciclovir administration, including an oral formulation and intraocular pellets (time-release pellets that are placed inside the eyeball), have shown promise as well. While research is being conducted into new drug treatments for CMV, it will be some time before any are approved for use. So, at present, the best way to slow and/or minimize the eye damage from CMV infection is a system of early detection and prompt, aggressive treatment.

Recently, the Food and Drug Administration (FDA) approved a new medication called fomivirsen (Vitravene) for the treatment of CMV retinitis in AIDS patients. Fomivirsen is an antisense inhibitor of CMV replication—that is, it is a type of antiviral medication that prevents the virus's genetic instructions from being read. Administered locally into the eye by intravitreal (into the vitreous humor) injection, fomivirsen has been shown to be well-tolerated. The most frequently observed ocular side effects are transient increased intraocular pressure and generally mild to moderate, reversible intraocular inflammation. The retinal-detachment rate overall has been considerably lower than normal, and there has been no evidence of systemic toxicity.

Many doctors recommend that HIV-positive persons with very low T-cell

Amsler Grid.
Cover one eye, look at the dot with the other eye, and note any distortions in the surrounding lines or rectangles.

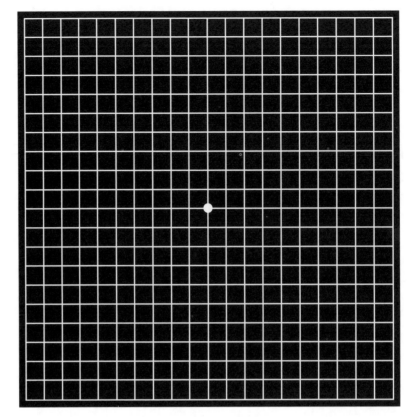

counts have an eye examination at least every six months. However, because CMV retinitis can develop very rapidly and unexpectedly, many eye specialists with AIDS experience also recommend a system of regular blood tests and self-examinations for everyone whose T-cell count is below 100.

While there is a test that can detect the presence of CMV in the blood, there is no test that can detect the development of CMV disease before it begins to actually cause physical damage to the eyes or other organs. However, several lab tests can offer early warnings that CMV infection is likely. One of these tests is the CMV culture, which looks for virus particles that were shed into the blood or urine. New DNA-based tests also offer some hope of more accurate diagnoses of CMV disease, although they are still being developed. At present, one of the best methods for the early detection of eye damage from CMV is the self-test. (See "Self-Treatment," below.)

SELF-TREATMENT

There are two tests that can detect the effects of CMV retinitis. They are the peripheral-vision test and the Amsler Grid. Both of these tests evaluate the retina for subtle defects.

The peripheral-vision self-test, described on page 9, is a cursory test and will uncover only gross, long-standing defects in the visual field. Eye doctors do a peripheral-vision test that is much more complete and much more accurate. An accurate peripheral-vision test is critical for the proper evaluation of CMV, as well as of such conditions as glaucoma, lattice degeneration, retinal detachment, and brain tumor.

A more critical test of the central visual field is the Amsler Grid. An Amsler Grid consists of a small-grid pattern with a central dot. (For a sample Amsler Grid, see page 118.) To test your central vision, simply cover one eye and hold the grid away from your face at a comfortable viewing distance and look directly at the central dot. At the same time, use your peripheral vision to be aware of the lines all around the dot. Note if any of the surrounding lines are wavy or distorted, or disappear; or if the rectangles formed by the lines are not perfectly square. If so, there may be a defect in your retina that requires further evaluation.

NUTRITIONAL SUPPLEMENTS		
Supplement	**Directions for Use**	**Comments**
Acetyl-L-carnitine	Take as directed on the label.	An energy carrier, metabolic facilitator, and cell-membrane protector. Also protects the heart.
Acidophilus	Take as directed on the label 3 times daily.	Supplies friendly bacteria to the digestive tract. *Note:* Use a high-potency, nondairy formula.
Carotenoid Complex (Betatene)	Take as directed on the label.	A powerful antioxidant, free-radical scavenger, and immune enhancer.
Bovine colostrum	Take as directed on the label.	Enhances immune function, and controls AIDS-related diarrhea.
Coenzyme Q$_{10}$	Take 100 mg daily.	A powerful antioxidant. Boosts the circulation and energy, and protects the heart.
Colloidal silver	Take as directed on the label.	A broad-spectrum antibiotic that subdues inflammation and promotes the healing of skin lesions.
Egg lecithin	Take 20 g daily in divided doses. Take on an empty stomach.	Protects the cells.
Free-form amino-acid complex	Take as directed on the label.	Supplies protein for the repair and rebuilding of body tissues. *Note:* Use a formula containing both the essential and nonessential amino acids.
Germanium	Take 200 mg daily.	Improves tissue oxygenation and interferon production.
Glutathione	Take as directed on the label. Take on an empty stomach.	An excellent free-radical scavenger. Enhances the integrity of the red blood cells, and protects the immune cells.
Pine bark extract (Pycnogenol)	Take as directed on the label 3 times daily.	A unique bioflavonoid. A potent antioxidant and immune enhancer.
Selenium	Take 400 mcg daily.	A free-radical scavenger and powerful immune enhancer.
Shark cartilage	Take as directed on the label. Take on an empty stomach.	Inhibits tumor growth. *Note:* Be sure to use 100% pure, dried shark cartilage.
Superoxide dismutase (SOD)	Take as directed on the label.	A free-radical scavenger needed for cell protection.
Vitamin-B complex	Take as prescribed by your physician.	Good for stress. Especially important for brain function. *Note:* Most effective by injection.
Vitamin C with bioflavonoids	Take 10,000–20,000 mg daily in divided doses.	Boosts the immune system. *Note:* Use powdered buffered ascorbic acid.

HERBS AND HERBAL SUPPLEMENTS

Herb	Directions for Use	Comments
Aloe vera	Drink 2 C twice daily.	Contains carrisyn, which appears to inhibit the growth and spread of HIV.
Astragalus	Take as directed on the label.	Boosts the immune system. *Caution:* Do not use if fever is present.
Black radish, dandelion, *and* silymarin (milk-thistle extract)	Take as directed on the label.	Protect and repair the liver.
Burdock, echinacea, goldenseal, mullein, red clover, *and* suma	Take as directed on the label.	Good for cleansing the blood and lymph, and for boosting the immune system. *Caution:* Do not use during pregnancy. Do not take goldenseal internally for more than 1 week.
Cat's claw	Take as directed on the label.	Enhances immune function. *Caution:* Do not use during pregnancy.
Garlic	Take 200 mg 3 times daily with meals.	A powerful immunostimulant that also aids digestion, endurance, and strength.

RECOMMENDATIONS

■ Pay special attention to meeting your nutritional needs, and keep in mind that you will most likely require a higher-than-normal nutrient intake.

■ Increase your consumption of fresh fruits and vegetables. Concentrate on eating more raw foods, organically grown, if possible.

■ Eat plenty of cruciferous vegetables, such as broccoli, Brussels sprouts, cabbage, and cauliflower. Also, consume yellow and deep-orange vegetables, such as carrots, pumpkin, squash, and yams.

■ Eat onion and garlic, or take garlic in supplemental form.

■ Avoid diet cola, foods with additives or colorings, junk food, peanuts, processed foods, saturated fats, salt, sugar, white flour, animal protein, and caffeine.

■ Educate yourself. HIV and AIDS are complicated conditions, and the treatment options are constantly changing and expanding. In order to stay well, you must remain as informed as possible.

Diabetic Retinopathy

Diabetic retinopathy is a complication of diabetes mellitus. In diabetes mellitus, the body is unable to produce enough insulin or, in some cases, to use the insulin it produces, which causes sugar (glucose) to stay in the blood instead of entering the cells of the body, where it is needed. The disorder is controlled through diet and medication, which normalize the blood-sugar level and the way the cells utilize the sugar. For reasons that are not completely understood, diabetes, even when controlled, also affects the blood vessels, especially in the kidneys and eyes.

There are two types of diabetes mellitus—type I, formerly called juvenile diabetes because it strikes mainly children and young adults, and type II, formerly called adult-onset diabetes because it strikes mainly adults. In type I diabetes, the body's immune system destroys the insulin-producing beta cells in the pancreas. Therefore, type I diabetics must give themselves insulin—either by injection or pump—on a daily basis to keep their blood sugar from rising to dangerous levels, which can cause coma and death. The classic symptoms of type I diabetes are frequent urination, excessive thirst and hunger, and weight loss. The disorder affects about 700,000 Americans.

Type II diabetes mellitus has nothing to do with the immune system. It is caused by a combination of insulin resistance and improper secretion of insulin. In the beginning, it usually can be controlled with diet, exercise, and oral medications. Eventually, however, 40 percent of type II diabetics require insulin injections. The symptoms—including blurred vision; frequent or recurring infections of the skin, gums, or bladder; and tingling and numbness in the hands or feet—appear more gradually than do the symptoms of type I diabetes, so many people with type II diabetes only become aware that they have the disorder when they develop one of its life-threatening complications.

Early in diabetes, before the blood sugar is brought under control, diabetics often experience blurred vision. This is because the high blood sugar causes changes in the lens within the eye. Blurred vision may, in fact, be the first sign of diabetes. After the proper insulin dosage is determined and the disease is stabilized, the blurred vision from the lens change resolves, although it may recur if the blood sugar rises again.

Diabetic retinopathy, a more serious complication of diabetes, occurs about ten to twelve years into the disorder. Diabetic retinopathy involves dilation of and small hemorrhages in the blood vessels of the retina. These can occur without any symptoms, unless the macula is affected. If the macula is affected, you may see spots or streaks in your vision that correspond to the blood-vessel leaks in the retina. If left unchecked, these hemorrhages and fluid leaks will eventually spill into the vitreous of the eye. Once in the vitreous, they can scar and pull on the retina, often causing retinal detachment and blindness. Diabetes is the second-leading cause of adult blindness. Not all diabetics develop diabetic retinopathy.

CONVENTIONAL TREATMENT

If you have diabetes, you should be checked regularly by an optometrist experienced with the disorder. Your optometrist should be qualified to follow the progression of the disease and be able to counsel you on appropriate care. However, when it comes time for treatment of diabetic retinopathy, you will need to see an ophthalmologist, who will have to perform surgery. The hemorrhages of diabetic retinopathy can be stopped with a laser in a painless outpatient procedure that takes about half an hour. A medical laser is directed at the retina, where it "spot welds" the hemorrhages. The laser administers hundreds to thousands of flashes of light to the affected eye. Anesthesia is unnecessary, although your eyes will be dilated by drops and you may feel somewhat "dazzled" afterwards.

SELF-TREATMENT

The best treatment for diabetes is to prevent it from beginning in the first place.

There is evidence that staying in good diabetic control—that is, keeping the blood-sugar level normal through diet and insulin—minimizes the long-term, as well as short-term, complications of the disorder. There is also a hereditary factor, so if you have a parent with diabetes, you are automatically at high risk and should be especially careful to eat a healthy diet and get regular medical checkups.

NUTRITIONAL SUPPLEMENTS

Supplement	Directions for Use	Comments
Chromium picolinate	Take 400–600 mcg daily.	Improves insulin efficiency.
Magnesium	Take 500 mg daily.	Protects against arterial spasm.
Manganese	Take 4 mg daily.	An enzyme activator.
Potassium	Take 300 mg daily.	Maintains the proper fluid balance.
Vitamin A	Take 5,000 IU daily.	Recommended for diabetics, who often have difficulty converting beta-carotene to vitamin A.
Vitamin B$_1$	Take 10 mg daily.	Boosts the circulation.
Supplement	Directions for Use	Comments
Vitamin B$_2$	Take 10 mg daily.	Boosts the circulation.
Vitamin B$_3$	Take up to 100 mg daily.	Boosts the circulation.
Vitamin B$_6$	Take 50–100 mg daily.	Boosts the circulation.
Vitamin B$_{12}$	Take 25 mcg or more daily.	Boosts the circulation. *Note:* Use the sublingual form.
Vitamin C with bioflavonoids	Take 1,000–3,000 mg daily.	Reduces the chance of vascular problems developing. *Note:* Use powdered buffered ascorbic acid.
Vitamin D	Take 400 IU daily.	Necessary for proper blood clotting.
Vitamin E	Take 400–1,200 IU daily.	Aids tissue healing.

HERBS AND HERBAL SUPPLEMENTS

Herb	Directions for Use	Comments
Comfrey	Drink as a tea.	Strengthens the blood.
Dandelion	Drink as a tea.	Boosts the activity of the pancreas.
Ginseng	Drink as a tea.	Normalizes the blood.
Yarrow	Drink as a tea.	Controls bleeding.

HOMEOPATHIC REMEDIES

Remedy	Directions for Use	Comments
Lachesis 6c	Place 3–4 pellets under the tongue 3–4 times daily.	Restores vascular integrity.
Natrum sulfuricum 6c	Place 3–4 pellets under the tongue 3–4 times daily.	Supports pancreatic function.
Phosphorus 6c	Place 3–4 pellets under the tongue 3–4 times daily.	Improves metabolism of the vascular tissue.

Remedy	Directions for Use	Comments
Syzygium jambolanum 6c	Place 3–4 pellets under the tongue 3–4 times daily.	Supports sugar metabolism.
Uranium nitricum 6c	Place 3–4 pellets under the tongue 3–4 times daily.	Acts as a glucose stabilizer.

RECOMMENDATIONS

■ Since diabetes is a systemic disease, even the control of diabetic eye changes is initially done using general treatments such as diet and exercise.

■ Have your blood-sugar level checked regularly, especially if diabetes runs in your family.

■ If you notice any fluctuations in your vision, either day-to-day or within the day, request that you be tested for diabetes.

■ Once you are diagnosed with diabetic retinopathy, you should have a dilated eye exam once a year, and more often if recommended by your doctor.

Diplopia

See DOUBLE VISION.

Double Vision

As discussed in "The Eyes and the Visual System" in Part One, the eyes act as a team, working together to create one picture from two images. This process is called fusion and occurs in the back part of the brain. If the eyes have a breakdown of coordination, they will aim at different points in space, and the two images they receive will be dissimilar. Two different images will be transmitted to one single brain cell, and this brain cell will attempt to see them both and will experience double vision.

Double vision, also known as diplopia (di-PLO-pee-ah), is not desirable, so the brain will actually supress, or tune out, one of the images. This will have the beneficial effect of the brain receiving one image again. However, the visual system will lose some of its function because it will be seeing with just one eye instead of both. (For a complete discussion of suppression, see page 201.)

Looking at the disorder from this perspective, you might think that double vision is the worst of all possible situations. (It can be if it happens while you're driving!) Yet, there are times when double vision is actually good. If you have a lazy eye or crossed eyes, you will suppress one of the images your eyes see. Using vision therapy, your doctor will attempt to get both your eyes working at the same time, even though they may still be pointing in different directions. In this instance, double vision is a step in the right direction.

CONVENTIONAL TREATMENT

The treatment for double vision depends on the cause of the condition, and the causes range from convergence insufficiency, convergence excess, and accommodative insufficiency to strabismus, trauma, intracranial tumor, and even cataracts. Assuming there is no pathological reason for the double vision, the cause is likely poor coordination of the eyes. This coordination difficulty actually does not occur in the eye muscles, but in the brain. Therefore, a therapy program to improve eye coordination is really more a "brain training" program than just eye-muscle exercises.

If therapy proves ineffective, your doctor may prescribe glasses with prism. Prism relocates the image of one eye so that the two eyes see the same image at the same location. However, prism most often is used in conjunction with a therapy program.

Sometimes, if no other treatment is effective, patching one eye will achieve single vision. Wearing a patch, however, is not an ideal solution because it is superficial and temporary. If you are in a vision-therapy program designed to encourage the use of both of your eyes, then patching one of the eyes doesn't really make sense. Patching is normally reserved for lazy eye.

In extreme cases of double vision that cannot be corrected by any other means, surgery to reposition the eye muscles is sometimes necessary. However, surgery is useful only in getting the eyes more closely aligned and very often requires a number of procedures, none of which may be totally successful. Remember that the muscles are controlled by the brain, so if the muscles are manually repositioned, the brain may not be able to successfully control them anymore. In some cases, however, success has been achieved with a combination of surgery and follow-up vision therapy that reinforces the effects of the surgery. I recommend surgery as a last resort, to be used only if all other attempts at fusion fail.

SELF-TREATMENT

If your double vision is a symptom of another condition, see the appropriate section in Part Two for the self-treatment options for that condition. In addition, see "Vision Therapy" in Part Three for a vision-therapy program to do at home to augment your doctor's program.

NUTRITIONAL SUPPLEMENTS		
Supplement	Directions for Use	Comments
Manganese	Take 4 mg daily.	Stimulates the nerve-muscle connection.
Vitamin-B complex	Take 75 mg daily.	Good for nerve function.

HOMEOPATHIC REMEDIES		
Remedy	Directions for Use	Comments
Agaricus 6c	Place 3–4 pellets under the tongue 3–4 times daily.	Good for double vision resulting from overwork.
Arnica montana 6c	Place 3–4 pellets under the tongue 3–4 times daily.	Good for double vision resulting from injury.

Remedy	Directions for Use	Comments
Aurum 6c	Place 3–4 pellets under the tongue 3–4 times daily.	Good for double vision accompanied by flushed feeling and congestion.
Gelsemium sempervirens 6c	Place 3–4 pellets under the tongue 3–4 times daily.	Good for double vision accompanied by general muscle spasm or headache.

RECOMMENDATIONS

■ If you ever see double, note whether the two images are side-by-side or above one another. Also, while keeping both eyes open, cover one eye with your hand and note which image disappears. Report these findings to your doctor.

Drooping Eyelids

Both eyelids should cover the eyes about the same amount. If they cover significantly different amounts of the eyes, you could be suffering from a condition known as ptosis (TOE-sis). Ptosis is simply the drooping of the upper eyelid to lower than its normal position. When the edge of the upper eyelid falls and covers the top part of the pupil, it blocks the upper part of the vision. In severe cases, the head may have to be tilted backward or the eyelid lifted with a finger in order to see out from under the drooping lid.

A certain aging process often appears similar to ptosis, but is really different. After the age of fifty, the skin of the upper eyelids may begin to sag significantly, creating a condition in which the lids appear to droop. This condition is known as blepharochalasis (blef-ah-roh-kal-AY-sis). Rarely, a lid that has blepharochalasis coupled with a significant amount of body fat will droop because of the excessive weight of the fat.

In most cases, a drooping upper eyelid results from the aging of previously normal structures. Typically, the tendon that attaches the levator (leh-VAY-tor) muscle to the eyelid becomes stretched, and the eyelid falls too low. The levator muscle is the major muscle responsible for elevating the upper eyelid. Since the levator muscle has normal strength, surgical correction of the drooping eyelid involves repair of the stretched tendon. It is not uncommon for a person to develop a drooping upper eyelid following cataract surgery. The cataract surgery is apparently the last straw that causes a weak tendon to finally give way.

Ptosis that is present from birth is called congenital ptosis. This ptosis may be mild, with the lid partially covering the pupil, or severe, with the lid completely covering the pupil. While the cause of congenital ptosis is often unclear, the most common reason is improper development of the levator muscle. Children with congenital ptosis may also have lazy eye, strabismus, refractive errors, astigmatism, or blurred vision. In addition, they may have an undesirable facial appearance because of the drooping lid.

CONVENTIONAL TREATMENT

For acquired ptosis, the doctor must first determine the cause of the problem. If the cause is muscle or nerve disease, the doctor will treat the disease first. If the cause is a tumor, the doctor may remove it. If the cause is something else, the doctor will often suggest surgery. The surgical procedure to correct ptosis involves shortening the levator muscle or connecting it to the brow muscles. Surgery to correct ptosis is most commonly performed by ophthalmic plastic and reconstructive surgeons who specialize in diseases and conditions affecting the eyelids, lacrimal (tear) system, orbit (bone cavity around the eye), and adjacent facial structures.

Congenital ptosis is also treated surgically, with the specific operation based on the severity of the ptosis and the strength of the levator muscle. If the ptosis is not severe, the surgery is generally performed when the child is between three and five years of age (during the preschool years). However, if the ptosis interferes with the child's vision, the surgery is performed at an earlier age to allow the vision to develop properly.

SELF-TREATMENT

The self-treatment of ptosis depends on the cause of the condition. If the problem is a torn or stretched tendon, no type of self-treatment can help. However, if the problem is a muscle weakness, and the nerve connection to the muscle is complete, it can sometimes be overcome using exercises.

NUTRITIONAL SUPPLEMENTS

Supplement	Directions for Use	Comments
Manganese	Take 4 mg daily.	Stimulates the nerve-muscle connection.
Vitamin-B complex	Take 75 mg daily.	Good for nerve function.

HOMEOPATHIC REMEDIES

Remedy	Directions for Use	Comments
Causticum 6c	Place 3–4 pellets under the tongue 3–4 times daily.	Aids muscle "heaviness" and facial paralysis.
Gelsemium sempervirens 6c	Place 3–4 pellets under the tongue 3–4 times daily.	Good for drooping eyelids associated with fever or nerve conditions. Good for muscle weakness and anxiety.
Rhus toxicodendron 6c	Place 3–4 pellets under the tongue 3–4 times daily.	Good for rheumatic and muscle pain.
Sepia 6c	Place 3–4 pellets under the tongue 3–4 times daily.	Good for drooping eyelids associated with headache.

Dry-Eye Syndrome

Dry-eye syndrome is a problem with either the quantity or quality of the tear film of the eye, leading to the symptoms of dryness, redness, burning, grittiness, and excessive tearing. The eyes may also be very light sensitive. Dry-eye syndrome is not so much a disease, but a group of symptoms that develops as a result of another condition such as an allergy or arthritis, the use of medication, or an environmental factor such as low humidity.

To understand dry-eye syndrome, we must first understand the function and components of the tear film. There are three layers of tears on the front of the eye. The outermost is the oily layer. It is produced by the meibomian glands, which are located primarily in the eyelids. The oily layer reduces tear evaporation. The second layer is the watery layer, the middle layer that is the major part of the tear film. The watery layer is produced by the lacrimal (LAK-ri-mal) gland, located under the brow bone. It is produced in copious amounts when we cut onions, for example. The innermost layer, which is called the mucin (MEW-sin) layer, is a mucous layer. It is produced by the cells in the conjunctiva.

Many dry-eye sufferers do not understand how their eyes can run with tears when their problem was diagnosed as *dry* eye. Dry eyes may be excessively wet because the tear glands pump extra amounts of watery tears onto the eyes to compensate for the dry condition. Eyes that are constantly watery may also have a blocked tear duct.

Dry-eye syndrome is probably the most common of all the eye problems. A recent Harris Poll indicated that 33 million American adults are affected by dry eyes. At the same time, 89 percent of Americans are unfamiliar with the condition.

Adults who have arthritis or another autoimmune disorder are more likely to have dry-eye syndrome. Dry eyes accompanied by dry mouth (difficulty swallowing) is called Sjögren's syndrome, a condition that occurs most commonly among women over the age of forty. In Sjögren's syndrome, the body's immune system mistakes the moisture-producing glands for foreign invaders. The immune system then attacks and destroys these glands, causing the hallmark symptoms of dry eyes and dry mouth. Like lupus, Sjögren's can also damage vital organs of the body with symptoms that may plateau, worsen, or go into remission. Some people experience only the mild symptoms of dry eyes and mouth, while others go through cycles of good health followed by severe illness.

The eyes produce about 40-percent less moisture with advancing age. Certain medications may also interfere with tear production. (For a list, see "Self-Treatment" on page 128.) In addition, drooping lower eyelids and excessive computer use may expose the surface of the eyes to the air, increasing evaporation and symptoms.

CONVENTIONAL TREATMENT

The first treatment that doctors tend to recommend for dry eyes is the application of artificial tears. There are many types of eye-drop preparations. It is best to avoid those with preservatives, which can eventually make a dry-eye condition worse. Most preservative-free eye drops come in individual-dose vials, which can be conveniently carried in the pocket or purse. Some of the more viscous (thicker) eye drops remain on the eye longer, but your vision is likely to be foggy for the first few minutes after application.

There is no known cure for Sjögren's syndrome. Nonsteroidal anti-inflammatory drugs (NSAIDs), steroids, and disease-modifying medications are often used to treat Sjögren's, and moisture-replacement therapies can ease the symptoms of dryness. Studies indicate that the male hormone androgen may restore lacrimal-gland function and relieve chronic dry-eye symptoms. However, androgen can have side effects, such as virilism (the growth of facial hair and the manifestation of other male characteristics) when used by women. Further studies are being conducted to identify an androgen compound that does not have these side effects.

One of the most practical methods for treating dry eye is to plug the hole in the tear "sink." There are tear-drainage canals on the edges of the upper and lower eyelids near the nose area. Inside these drainage openings are tiny pumps that suck away the fluid from the surface of the eyes. The lacrimal gland behind the eyelid produces the tears. The eyelid spreads the tears across the eye's surface, much like a windshield wiper. The drain at the bottom permits the fluid to drain away. If the drain is plugged, more fluid stays on the surface of the eye. When other methods of treating dry-eye syndrome prove unsatisfactory, closure of the tear drains may be indicated. Many dry-eyed people report dramatic improvement in their dry-eye condition once their tear drains are closed.

SELF-TREATMENT

To help conserve the moisture on the surface of your eyes, consider some of the following measures:

■ *Use humidifiers in your home.* This is especially important if you live in a dry, desert area.

■ *Wear wraparound sun goggles outdoors.* Sunglasses (or even clear goggles) with side shields can help to reduce the evaporation of moisture from the eye by as much as 40 percent.

■ *Blink your eyes.* When you blink, you squeeze out tears from the glands in your eyelids. Waiting twenty to thirty seconds between blinks may cause the tear film to break, which can lead to dehydration of the surface of the eye.

■ *Quit smoking.* Cigarette smoke causes dry spots to develop on the surface of the eye 40-percent faster than when the lids are held open.

■ *Avoid smog and fumes.* Smog and fumes not only cause dry and irritated eyes, they also inactivate the enzyme that acts as an antibacterial agent in the tear fluid.

■ *Check the nose pads on your eyeglasses.* If your lower eyelids are pushed down by the nose pads of your glasses, you may experience increased evaporation of tears. Have an optician adjust the pads.

■ *Reposition your computer monitor.* If you use a computer, position the monitor so that your eyes aim downward when you look at the monitor. This will allow you to keep your eyes partially closed, reducing the surface area of the eye exposed to the air. (For a complete discussion of computer vision syndrome, see page 104.)

■ *Reduce, replace, or avoid eye makeup.* Eye makeup has been shown to thin out the oily layer of the tear film, the outer layer that keeps the eyes from becoming dehydrated. It can harbor bacteria and should be replaced frequently. Gentle removal of all eye makeup every night is essential.

■ *Check your medications.* Some medications can cause dry eyes as a side effect. These medications include antihistamines such as Benadryl and Coricidin; atropine; beta blockers such as Timoptic, Betoptic, Betagan, and Ocupress; cancer medications such as methotrexate; chlorothiazide; codeine; decongestant eye drops such as Visine, Murine, Prefrin, and Clear Eyes; decongestants such as Sudafed; diazepam; morphine; Patanol, prescribed for allergic conjunctivitis; scopolamine; tranquilizers such as Elavil and Valium; and vitamin-A analogs such as isotretinoin. The artificial sweetener aspartame, supplemental vitamin B_3, and the recreational drug hashish can also cause dry eyes.

■ *Check your soft contact lenses.* Soft contact lenses often promote the evaporation of tears from the surface of the eye. In severe dry-eye cases, contact lenses cannot be worn.

■ *Check your diet.* The body requires the consumption of the essential oils for lubrication of the joints and the eyes, and for restoration of normal lubrication to the body. There are good fats and bad fats. The undesired fats, called saturated fats, are found in meats, fried foods, butter, dairy products, and margarine. The good fats, especially the omega-3 oils, are polyunsaturated and are found in cold-water fish, flaxseeds, and walnuts.

NUTRITIONAL SUPPLEMENTS

Supplement	Directions for Use	Comments
Cod-liver oil	Take 3 tbsp daily.	High in vitamin A. Re-moisturizes the eye tissues.
Coenzyme Q_{10}	Take 80 mg daily.	A powerful antioxidant.
Evening primrose oil	Take 3,000 mg daily at bedtime.	Supplies essential fatty acids, which promote circulation.
Vitamin A	Take 25,000 IU daily in tablet form or apply drops directly to the eye.	Maintains the moisture in the eye tissues.
Vitamin B_6	Take 50 mg daily.	Regulates kidney function.
Vitamin C	Take 7,500 mg daily.	An antioxidant.

HERBS AND HERBAL SUPPLEMENTS

Herb	Directions for Use	Comments
Chamomile	Use warm as an infusion or cool as an eyewash.	Supports the eye tissues.
Goldenseal	Use warm as an infusion or cool as an eyewash.	Supports the eye tissues. *Caution:* Do not take internally for more than 1 week. Do not use during pregnancy.
Ming mu di huang wan (Brion)	Take 10 pills 3 times daily or drink as a tea.	Builds "yin" in the kidneys, and "cools" the liver.
Qi ju di huang wan (Brion)	Take 8 pills 3 times daily or drink as a tea.	Builds "yin" in the kidneys, and "cools" the liver.
Shi hu ye guang wan (Brion)	Take 1 pill twice daily.	Good for all eye conditions.

HOMEOPATHIC REMEDIES

Remedy	Directions for Use	Comments
Aconite 6c	Place 3–4 pellets under the tongue 3–4 times daily.	Alleviates dryness.

Remedy	Directions for Use	Comments
Alumina 6c	Place 3–4 pellets under the tongue 3–4 times daily.	Alleviates dryness.
Arsenicum album 6c	Place 3–4 pellets under the tongue 3–4 times daily.	Alleviates dryness.
Belladonna 6c	Place 3–4 pellets under the tongue 3–4 times daily.	Good for dry eyes associated with fever and redness.
Euphrasia officinalis 6c	Place 3–4 pellets under the tongue 3–4 times daily.	Good for dry eyes associated with wind (gas).
Optique 1 (Boiron) 6c	Take 1–2 drops daily as needed for relief.	A good general remedy.
Pulsatilla 6c	Place 3–4 pellets under the tongue 3–4 times daily.	Alleviates dryness.
Similisan No. 1 6c (Millen)	Take 1–2 drops daily as needed for relief.	Good for red, dry eyes.
Sulphur 6c	Place 3–4 pellets under the tongue 3–4 times daily.	Alleviates dryness, and reduces redness.
Veratrum album 6c	Place 3–4 pellets under the tongue 3–4 times daily.	Alleviates dryness.
Zincum metallicum 6c	Place 3–4 pellets under the tongue 3–4 times daily.	Alleviates dryness.

RECOMMENDATIONS

■ Avoid consuming margarine, fried foods, and saturated fats in general.

■ Use preservative-free eye drops.

■ Check your medications for any that may cause dry eyes as a side effect.

■ Wear wraparound sun goggles when you go outdoors.

■ If you have dry eyes, contact your eye doctor before changing your diet. In addition to your specific eye condition, your medical history, prescription medications, and allergies all need to be taken into account.

Eye Pressure, Elevated

See GLAUCOMA.

Eyelid Gland, Plugged

See CHALAZION.

Eyelid Inflammation

See BLEPHARITIS.

Eyelid Spasm

See BLEPHAROSPASM.

Eyestrain

Eyestrain is a concept that doesn't really exist in the minds of eye doctors. In fact, I don't remember ever hearing about eyestrain during my studies at optometry school. The term that professionals use for this type of discomfort is "asthenopia" (as-then-OH-pee-ah). Asthenopia is defined in visual-science dictionaries as eye discomfort or fatigue attributed to uncorrected refractive error, eye-muscle disorder, prolonged use of the eyes, or something similar.

This definition for asthenopia is rather broad and vague, but in general, eyestrain can be thought of as just about any discomfort involving the eyes. The term "eyestrain" really means little because we must delve deeper into the specific complaints to determine the cause of the problem. Most people, you see, have their own personal definition of eyestrain.

CONVENTIONAL TREATMENT

Since eyestrain can result from a variety of causes, the treatment varies with the source of the problem. The conventional treatments for eyestrain that are used most often, however, are eyeglasses and vision therapy.

The glasses used to relieve eyestrain have what are called plus lenses. (For a discussion of plus lenses, see "Minus Lenses and Plus Lenses" on page 218.) If the eyes and/or visual system are not able to perform their functions correctly and efficiently, plus lenses can take over some of the workload and allow the eyes to function with less strain or effort. If your eyes do not react correctly to these lenses, a program of vision therapy can help you learn how to better coordinate your eyes and see more effectively. (For a discussion of vision therapy, see page 235.)

SELF-TREATMENT

There are many things that you can do for yourself to reduce eyestrain. Most often, eyestrain is the result of excessive use of the eyes for near-point tasks. Therefore, simply taking adequate breaks from your near-point chores will allow your eyes to relax, thus relieving much of the tension. These breaks can consist of something as simple as just looking far away for a few seconds or closing the eyes. If you use a computer, taking breaks is especially important. For a complete discussion of computer vision syndrome, see page 104.

If your eyes become irritated with continued use, try an eyewash or lubricating drops to refresh them. Eyebright works well as an eyewash.

NUTRITIONAL SUPPLEMENTS

Supplement	Directions for Use	Comments
Vitamin A	Take 25,000 IU daily.	Good for all eye conditions.
Vitamin-B complex	Take 50–100 mg daily.	Improves intraocular cellular metabolism.
Vitamin B$_2$	Take 25 mg 3 times daily.	Alleviates eye fatigue.
Vitamin C	Take 2,000 mg 3 times daily.	An antioxidant.
Vitamin E	Take 400 IU daily.	An antioxidant.

HERBS AND HERBAL SUPPLEMENTS

Herb	Directions for Use	Comments
Bayberry, cayenne, *and* raspberry	Take in supplement form as directed on the label or drink as a tea.	Boost the circulation around the eyes.
Eyebright	Take in supplement form as directed on the label, drink as a tea, or use as an eyewash.	Rejuvenates the eye tissues.
Goldenseal	Take 200 mg daily for 1 week.	Rejuvenates the eye tissues. *Caution:* Do not take internally for more than 1 week. Do not use during pregnancy.

HOMEOPATHIC REMEDIES

Remedy	Directions for Use	Comments
Nux vomica 6c	Place 3–4 pellets under the tongue 3–4 times daily.	Good for eyestrain associated with overwork.
Ruta graveolens 6c	Place 3–4 pellets under the tongue 3–4 times daily.	Good for eyestrain followed by headache. Promotes healing of the tendons and ligaments.
Sulphur 6c	Place 3–4 pellets under the tongue 3–4 times daily.	Alleviates redness following near-point work.

RECOMMENDATIONS

■ Include broccoli, raw cabbage, carrots, cauliflower, green vegetables, squash, sunflower seeds, and watercress in your diet.

■ Drink fresh carrot juice, the best food source of beta-carotene.

■ Two teaspoons of cod-liver oil a day may also be helpful.

■ Eliminate sugar and white flour from your diet.

■ Get plenty of sleep. Fatigue can lead to eyestrain.

Farsightedness

Farsightedness, also called hyperopia (hy-per-OH-pee-ah), is one of the refractive errors of the eye. Farsightedness, nearsightedness, and astigmatism are all known as refractive errors because they cause distortions in the way light is refracted—that is, deflected from a straight path—as it passes through the eye.

Farsightedness is not exactly the opposite of nearsightedness. For the farsighted person, the image of an object twenty or more feet away is focused behind the retina (if the lens is relaxed) and looks blurred. Farsightedness results when the eye is too short or the cornea too flat, or from some combination of these and other factors. The main difference between farsightedness and nearsightedness is that in farsightedness, the eye can accommodate, or refocus, to adjust for the misplacement of the light, while in nearsightedness, any accommodation of the eye makes the image more blurred.

Because of this difference, the farsighted eye may be able to see clearly at a distance, but must work to do so. This makes it more difficult to test the farsighted eye because there may not be any blurring of the image. In addition, a farsighted eye will fatigue easier, a symptom that a quick eyesight test may not be able to detect.

CONVENTIONAL TREATMENT

The conventional treatment for farsightedness is simply eyeglasses. Most often, these glasses have lenses that approximate the shape of the lens within the eye, thus relieving the internal lens from overworking. This may sound like the glasses act as a crutch that will make the eye lazy and not work enough. However, there are different degrees of farsightedness and different reasons to wear glasses, so one general statement may not apply to all conditions.

Oftentimes, people (mostly children) have difficulty reading due to farsightedness or a similar condition affecting focusing ability. If you have this problem, you may be advised to utilize a combination of reading glasses and vision therapy to improve your visual abilities to perform more efficiently. For a complete discussion of vision therapy, see page 235.

SELF-TREATMENT

If the cause of your farsightedness is a physically short eyeball, there is likely nothing that can be done to change your vision. However, keeping your focusing mechanism in good functional condition will help to overcome the physical problem. One thing you can do is to keep altering your focusing distance on a regular basis. Avoid focusing at a close distance for an extended period of time, and make sure to blink frequently.

NUTRITIONAL SUPPLEMENTS

Supplement	Directions for Use	Comments
Vitamin A	Take 25,000 IU daily.	Good for all eye conditions.
Vitamin C	Take 2,000–5,000 mg daily.	Maintains the flexibility of the lens.

HERBS AND HERBAL SUPPLEMENTS

Herb	Directions for Use	Comments
Eyebright	Take as directed on the label.	Good for all eye conditions.

HOMEOPATHIC REMEDIES

Remedy	Directions for Use	Comments
Argentum nitricum 6c	Place 3–4 pellets under the tongue 3–4 times daily.	Good when doing intense near-point work.

RECOMMENDATIONS

■ If you notice that it takes a second or two to refocus when you look from far to near, then you may be farsighted. Contact your eye doctor, and schedule a complete examination.

■ School vision screenings rarely check for farsightedness, so make a complete eye examination for your school-aged child an annual event.

■ Farsightedness is different from presbyopia, which is a type of farsightedness that manifests after the age of forty. If you are farsighted and over forty, you may notice presbyopia developing earlier than it does in people with normal vision.

Farsightedness, Age-Related

See PRESBYOPIA.

Floaters

People often talk about seeing small dark spots in front of their eyes that seem to move as their eyes do. These spots may look like dots, squiggles, strands, or any of hundreds of other different shapes, and they are very common. They exist because, before birth, the eye develops with the help of blood vessels growing through the center of it. During the last three months of fetal life, these blood vessels dissolve, but sometimes they don't disappear completely. So, what you see after birth are small strands of old blood vessels floating in the vitreous of the eye. These spots are called floaters. Floaters can also occur when protein fibers from the gel in the vitreous clump together. Floaters may be more obvious when you look at bright areas, such as a blank wall or the white pages of a book, and you may even see them when your eyes are closed, especially if you're in a bright light or lying in the sun.

Although floaters do not normally increase in number with age, oftentimes they seem to become more apparent. The reason for this is that the vitreous of the eye becomes less gel-like and slightly more fluid with age. This allows the floaters to move more freely and to more frequently get into your line of sight.

CONVENTIONAL TREATMENT

Floaters are harmless, and there is no practical treatment for them. One word of caution, however—if you become aware of *a lot* of floaters that appear all of a sudden or are associated with flashes of light in your vision, see your eye doctor to make sure there is nothing seriously wrong with your eyes.

SELF-TREATMENT

When you become aware of floaters in your field of vision, try to just quickly look away, then back at what you were viewing. This is often enough to move the floaters out of the way—until they float back into your field of vision later on!

RECOMMENDATIONS

■ Make sure you report any floater activity to your doctor. Note if the spots appeared suddenly and if flashes of light are associated with them.

WHEN TO CALL THE DOCTOR FOR FLOATERS

■ A few floaters are usually normal. However, if you see "dozens" of floaters all of a sudden, call your eye doctor immediately.

■ If you see floaters with flashes of light, call your eye doctor immediately.

Fluid Under the Retina

See CENTRAL SEROUS RETINOPATHY.

Focusing Problem

See ACCOMMODATIVE INSUFFICIENCY.

Giant Papillary Conjunctivitis

Giant papillary conjunctivitis (GPC) is a type of pinkeye that usually occurs in contact-lens wearers. It is a chronic low-grade allergic reaction in the conjunctiva of the upper lid. Sooner or later, many people who wear conventional soft contacts encounter GPC. The disorder can also develop over time from the irritation caused by a surgical suture or other foreign body.

GPC is not a threat to vision or to the health of the eyeball, but it can be a nuisance. In contact-lens wearers, it usually appears after lenses have been worn for a long time, many times with no other problems. The symptoms include:

■ Itching, often more in one eye and worse with the contact lenses on.

■ A white mucous discharge that collects at the lids, especially when you're awake.

■ Contacts that slide around and feel dry, especially when you blink.

■ A milky deposit, sometimes a ringlike stain, that appears on the contacts and won't come off.

The symptoms often continue to worsen until you can no longer wear your contact lenses. When you quit wearing the lenses, the symptoms diminish, then eventually get better. To evaluate your condition, your doctor must look under your upper lids, turning them inside out using a cotton applicator, to see the inner linings of the lids. Everted lids feel funny, but not painful, when this is done correctly.

Under a microscope, the lid membrane is bumpy instead of glassy smooth or finely grained as normal. The lumps are papillae, ashy gray bumps that are giant only in comparison to other common conditions. The papillae are sticky, and they secrete a whitish mucus that collects in the lids and makes contact lenses misbehave. The discharge sometimes leaves a circular chalky stain on soft contacts.

CONVENTIONAL TREATMENT

In most cases, the treatment of GPC involves discontinuing the use of the contact lenses to allow the eye to recover. The contacts may need to be avoided for several days or weeks. Severe cases may take even longer to resolve. Sometimes, the lenses may need to be professionally cleaned and polished to remove the deposits that triggered the allergic reaction. Often, the lenses must be discarded. Changing the type of lenses worn may help—gas-permeable lenses are much less prone to contributing to this condition, as are disposable soft contacts. Also, switching to a contact-lens solution that does not contain preservatives may help. Prescription eye drops can help to alleviate the symptoms, especially the itchiness. Over-the-counter eye drops are generally not recommended, however, since they are not effective enough.

Follow-up care is important. GPC is difficult to control. If the condition is not treated properly and steps are not taken to prevent a recurrence, it can become a chronic condition. It may even prevent the further use of contact lenses.

SELF-TREATMENT

If you wear contact lenses, be sure to pay attention to your doctor's instructions. As the lenses age, it is important to maintain a proper care schedule. If an enzyme cleaner is recommended (it usually is for nondisposable lenses), do not skimp on its use. Weekly use of an enzyme cleaner will assure that protein, which has been shown to be one of the possible causes of GPC, does not build up on the lenses.

If your eyes feel dry, use your recommended contact-lens lubricant. Dirt collects much easier on dry lenses than on moist lenses, and can lead to irritation of the upper-eyelid tissue.

NUTRITIONAL SUPPLEMENTS

Supplement	Directions for Use	Comments
Vitamin A	Take 25,000 IU daily.	Maintains the moisture in the eye tissues.
Vitamin-B complex	Take 50–100 mg daily.	Improves the intraocular cellular metabolism.
Vitamin C	Take 2,000–6,000 mg daily.	Protects the eye from further inflammation.
Zinc	Take 50 mg daily.	Enhances the immune response.

HERBS AND HERBAL SUPPLEMENTS

Herb	Directions for Use	Comments
Eyebright	Use as an eyewash.	Good for all eye conditions.
Goldenseal	Apply as a compress.	Soothing for the mucous membranes. *Caution:* Do not take internally for more than 1 week. Do not use during pregnancy.

HOMEOPATHIC REMEDIES

Remedy	Directions for Use	Comments
Allium cepa 6c	Place 3–4 pellets under the tongue 3–4 times daily.	Relieves mucous discharge.
Apis mellifica 6c	Place 3–4 pellets under the tongue 3–4 times daily.	Alleviates swelling.
Mercurius corrosivus 6c	Place 3–4 pellets under the tongue 3–4 times daily.	Relieves discharge.
Pulsatilla 6c	Place 3–4 pellets under the tongue 3–4 times daily.	Relieves discharge associated with emotions.

RECOMMENDATIONS

■ Change your contact lenses often. Fresh, new lenses promote GPC far less than older ones do.

■ Switch to a different type of lens. Eyes with GPC often tolerate rigid gas-permeable lenses better than they do soft lenses. The vision sometimes improves, too. Some soft-lens materials aggravate GPC more than others do, and hygiene is always a contributing factor. If you wear reusable lenses, the problem usually goes away if you switch to disposable or frequently replaced lenses.

■ Wear your lenses only occasionally. On the night before a special occasion, get them out and change the solution they've been in.

■ A cold compress used several times a day will help to relieve the itching associated with GPC.

■ Since GPC is a form of pinkeye, the same treatments and recommendations are effective. (For the treatments and recommendations for pinkeye, see page 184.)

Glaucoma

Glaucoma (glaw-KO-mah) is a condition in which the pressure inside the eye (intraocular pressure) is markedly elevated, which prevents blood from reaching, nourishing, and circulating through the eye. Glaucoma is deceptive and dangerous. Most sufferers have few or no symptoms of the disease, which occurs in 1 to 2 percent of the over-forty population and is the second-most-common cause of blindness in the United States. A family history of glaucoma or diabetes, a previous eye injury or surgery, or the use of eye drops containing steroids are considered risk factors for developing glaucoma. It is also much more common in African Americans than in Caucasian Americans.

In a normal eye, the aqueous humor is produced and drained into the bloodstream at a constant rate so that you always have a fresh supply and always the right amount. It drains through a little canal between the iris and the cornea. In glaucoma, either too much aqueous humor is produced and the eye can't get rid of it fast enough to maintain a normal intraocular pressure, or the drainage mechanism has broken down and the fluid can't escape fast enough. Either way, the increased pressure interferes with the blood circulation to and from the eye, and the result is damage to the optic nerve with increasing loss of vision. Peripheral vision is the first to go.

Sometimes, the doctor can see the blockage in the drainage channel. In this case, the glaucoma is called narrow- or closed-angle glaucoma. Often, however, the channel appears to be normal despite the elevated pressure. Here, the glaucoma is called open-angle. Prolonged stress and an inadequate diet over a long period of time are considered by many authorities to be the main causative factors in glaucoma. Prolonged stress leads to adrenal exhaustion, and exhausted adrenals are no longer able to produce aldosterone, which stabilizes the salt balance in the body. When too much salt is lost from the body, the tissue fluids build up and often will push into the eyeball, increasing the intraocular pressure, forcing the lens forward, and damaging the optic nerve. This closes off the drainage tubes, causing visual disturbances and distortions.

Unless it is caused by a specific injury or a tumor in one eye, glaucoma usually affects both eyes, but the two eyes may not succumb at the same rate. About 15 percent of glaucoma patients know they have a problem. They have an acute form of glaucoma characterized by extreme eye pain, redness, dilated pupils, blurred vision, and halos around lights. These people, in reality, are lucky because they usually get themselves to an eye doctor promptly. In the remaining 85 percent of glaucoma patients, the disease is chronic and insidious. The symptoms are subtle and may not even be noticed until a significant amount of vision has been lost. Contrary to popular conception, there is no feeling of pressure in the eye with the chronic type of glaucoma.

Fortunately, the test for glaucoma, which checks for increased eye pressure, is very simple and can be easily done in the office by your optometrist or ophthalmologist. In the most common version done today, a puff of air is blown at your eye by a machine. Be sure you have this test done every time you have an eye checkup. Another indication of glaucoma is a change in your peripheral vision or an enlarging blind spot. Unfortunately, people rarely notice these changes early on; rather, they are usually detected by eye doctors during examinations. Your eye doctor should check for these indicators regularly.

As is true for most conditions, there is no single cause of glaucoma. It is suspected that a general stiffening of the sclera and other parts of the eye plays a role in the development of the disorder in people over forty. Other causes are a serious eye injury, eye surgery, some medications (especially steroids), and an eye tumor, to name a few. When glaucoma develops in a child during the first year of life, it is almost always due to an inherited malformation of the aqueous-humor drainage canal.

CONVENTIONAL TREATMENT

Glaucoma can be treated with medications, surgery, or both. The medical treatment involves the use of one or more of the following—eye drops to constrict the pupils (when the pupil is constricted, the angle between the cornea and the iris is increased to allow better drainage of the aqueous fluid); eye drops to reduce the production of the aqueous fluid; and systemic medications to reduce the production of the fluid. Among the medications used are:

■ *The beta blockers.* Most patients take beta blockers without any problems. However, these medications should be used cautiously by patients who have a breathing disorder (asthma, bronchitis, emphysema, or chronic obstructive pulmonary disease) or certain heart problems (congestive heart failure or a pulse rate of less than sixty beats per minute). Occasionally, depression, confusion, and impotence have been reported. Examples of the beta blockers are betaxolol (Betoptic), carteolol (Ocupress), levobunolol (Betagan), metipranolol (Optipranolol), timolol hemihydrate (Betimol), and timolol maleate (Timoptic).

■ *The miotics.* The pupil of the eye becomes small, or miotic, in patients who take these glaucoma medications. When the pupil is miotic, less light gets into the eye, which causes the vision to dim, especially at night and in patients with cataracts. Also, the vision may vary between clear and blurry, especially in younger patients. In addition, it is very common to have a brow- or headache during the first several days of taking the miotic. This discomfort usually disappears within five to ten days. The stronger miotics (for example, phospholine iodide) occasionally cause excess sweating, stomach cramps, or nausea. Pilocarpine, the most common miotic agent, comes as eye drops, an ocular insert similar to contact lenses, and a convenient one-dose-a-day ointment. Your doctor will help you decide which type is the best for you. Examples of the miotics are carbachol (Isopto and Miostat) and pilocarpine (Ocusert, Pilocar, and Pilostat).

■ *The epinephrines.* The epinephrine medications, which come in eye-drop form, commonly cause stinging, tearing, and burning when they are first placed on the eye. They often cause the eye to become red or bloodshot several hours after application, although at first they whiten the eye. Some patients develop true allergies to these medications, occasionally after taking them for years without any problems. Propine, which is more expensive than the basic epinephrine eye drop, is less likely to have these annoying side effects. Patients may find that epinephrine drops dilate their pupils. These drops should be used cautiously by patients whose blood pressure is difficult to control or who have an irregular heart beat or rapid pulse rate. Examples of the epinephrines are epinephrine (Epifrin and Glaucon) and dipivefrin (Propine).

■ *The alpha-agonists.* The alpha-agonists are the newest class of medications developed to control eye pressure. Generally, they are used only by patients whose eye pressure cannot be controlled with any of the other glaucoma medications. The side effects include stinging, tearing, and burning when the drops are first placed on the eye, as well as redness or a bloodshot appearance. These side effects are similar to those of the epinephrine class of glaucoma medications. Additionally, the eyelids may open up slightly. Some elderly patients whose eyelids normally droop find this cosmetic side effect desirable rather than unwanted! Examples of the alpha-agonists are apraclonidine (Iopidine) and brimonidine (Alphagan).

■ *The carbonic anhydrase inhibitors.* These eye-pressure-reducing medications come in pill form and, as you might expect, systemic side effects are therefore more common with them than with the glaucoma eye drops. About half the patients who take carbonic anhydrase medicines must stop because of the side effects, which include tingling in the hands and feet, poor appetite and poor taste of food, stomach upsets and diarrhea, and fatigue and depression. Less common are kidney stones and, very rarely, a serious form of anemia that prevents the body from fighting infection, which could prove fatal. The carbonic anhydrase inhibitors are a type of sulfa medication and should be avoided by patients who have known allergies to these substances. A new eye drop, dorzolamide, should have fewer side effects than the oral forms. Examples of the carbonic anhydrase inhibitors are acetazolamide (Diamox), dorzolamide (Trusopt), and methazolamide (MZM and Neptazane).

■ *The prostaglandin-agonists.* Latanoprost is the first of this entirely new class of glaucoma medications. It works by opening the so-called accessory drainage pathway in the eye. The medicine is administered as one drop on the affected eye at bedtime. Latanoprost has one unusual side effect—in some persons with hazel, green, or bluish brown eyes, the eye color is permanently changed to brown, even if the medication is discontinued. This side effect appears to be only cosmetic, with no known ill effects on the eye. Lantanoprost may help to reduce the eye pressure in patients already taking the maximum doses of other antiglaucoma eye drops. An example of the prostaglandin-agonists is latanoprost (Xalatan).

Much has been made in recent years of the use of marijuana to treat glaucoma. One side-effect of marijuana is the lowering of the intraocular pressure. Therefore, yes, it does the job. However, there are many other medications that achieve this desired effect easier and with less of the euphoric side effect.

Surgery for glaucoma often involves the creation of new channels through which the aqueous fluid can escape. In another procedure, a laser is used to burn little spots into the area around the iris. As these burns heal, they form scars that pull the tissue in toward them. This contracting of the tissue around the burns opens up the meshwork of the eye and reduces the overall intraocular pressure by increasing the drainage of the aqueous fluid. The laser procedures for glaucoma are still being improved.

SELF-TREATMENT

Because of the uncertainty surrounding the causes of the various types of glaucoma, there is no one self-treatment that is appropriate for everyone. However, there are some general guidelines that seem to help most of the people who are afflicted with the disorder.

Since one cause of glaucoma may be adrenal exhaustion, as discussed above, it is important to give the adrenal glands nutritional support. For a list of nutritional supplements that have been found useful in the treatment of glaucoma, see below. Also, avoid consuming refined carbohydrates, such as white bread, which are taxing to the adrenal glands. In general, any disturbance in the metabolism may lead to an increase in the eye pressure.

Exercise has also been shown to be effective at reducing eye pressure. Be sure to check with your primary health-care provider before starting any exercise program.

NUTRITIONAL SUPPLEMENTS

Supplement	Directions for Use	Comments
Choline *and* inositol	Take 1,000–2,000 mg of a combination supplement daily.	Important B vitamins for the eyes.
Glutathione	Take 500 mg twice daily.	A powerful antioxidant.
Manganese	Take 4 mg daily.	An enzyme activator.
Rutin	Take 50 mg 3 times daily.	Works with vitamin C to reduce the eye pressure.
Selenium	Take 100 mcg daily.	Reduces scarring.
Vitamin A	Take 25,000 IU daily.	Aids in mucopolysaccharide metabolism.
Vitamin B$_5$	Take 100 mg 3 times daily.	A stress vitamin needed for the adrenal glands.
Vitamin C	Take 10,000–15,000 mg daily.	Reduces the eye pressure.

HERBS AND HERBAL SUPPLEMENTS

Herb	Directions for Use	Comments
Bilberry	Take as directed on the label.	Protects the eye from further damage.
Er ming zuo ci wan (Brion)	Take 8 pills 3 times daily or drink as a tea.	Reduces congestion.
Eyebright	Take in supplement form as directed on the label or drink as a tea.	Good for all eye conditions.
Ginkgo *and* zinc sulfate	Take as directed on the label.	Slow vision loss.

Herb	Directions for Use	Comments
Ming mu di huang wan (Brion)	Take 10 pills 3 times daily or drink as a tea.	Clarifies the vision.
Nei zhang ming yan wan (Brion)	Take 8 pills 3 times daily.	Clarifies the vision. *Caution:* Contains aluminum, so limit its use.
Rose hips	Take in supplement form as directed on the label or drink as a tea.	A source of vitamin C.
Shi hu ye guang wan (Brion)	Take 1 pill twice daily.	Reduces the eye pressure.

HOMEOPATHIC REMEDIES

Remedy	Directions for Use	Comments
Belladonna 6c	Place 3–4 pellets under the tongue 3–4 times daily.	Relieves the colored halo around lights.
Nux vomica 6c	Place 3–4 pellets under the tongue 3–4 times daily.	Good for high eye pressure.
Phosphorus 6c	Place 3–4 pellets under the tongue 3–4 times daily.	Relieves the colored halo around lights.
Pulsatilla 6c	Place 3–4 pellets under the tongue 3–4 times daily.	Relieves the colored halo around lights.
Sulphur 6c	Place 3–4 pellets under the tongue 3–4 times daily.	Good for glaucoma with pain.

RECOMMENDATIONS

■ It is critical to have your eye pressure checked regularly to monitor the progress of your glaucoma. In addition, be very careful to heed your eye doctor's instructions.

■ Since the peripheral vision is affected first, be sure to have that tested periodically, too.

■ Be careful when drinking large amounts of fluids. Lower amounts are recommended.

■ Avoid tobacco smoke, nicotine, alcohol, and all caffeine.

GPC

See GIANT PAPILLARY CONJUNCTIVITIS.

Grave's Disease

Grave's disease is one of the more common types of hyperthyroidism. It is a disorder in which the thyroid gland produces too much thyroid hormone, resulting in an overactive metabolism. All of the body's processes speed up, so the symptoms may include nervousness, irritability, a constant feeling of being hot, increased perspiration, insomnia, and fatigue. Patients often also present the symptoms of goiter (enlarged thyroid gland), exophthalmos (bulging eyeball), tachycardia (rapid heartbeat), weight loss, hyperactive reflexes, drooping eyelids, and tremor. The thyroid gland may be normal sized in a small number of patients. The eye symptoms may include pain, excessive tearing, blurred vision, and double vision. Other eye findings may be lid retraction, in which the eyes appear to bulge; swelling around the eyes; optic-nerve inflammation; and enlargement of the extraocular muscles.

The thyroid gland is the body's internal thermostat. It regulates the body's temperature by secreting two hormones that control how quickly the body burns calories and uses energy. If the thyroid gland secretes too much hormone, hyperthyroidism results. If it secretes too little, hypothyroidism results. Many cases of hyper- and hypothyroidism are believed to result from an abnormal immune response. The exact cause is not understood, but the immune system produces antibodies that invade and attack the thyroid, disrupting the hormone production.

The age of onset of Grave's disease is most commonly between thirty and forty years old. Females are affected seven times more often than men.

CONVENTIONAL TREATMENT

Grave's disease can be treated with medication or surgery.

The surgery for Grave's disease involves the removal of thyroid tissue to reduce the overall hormone output to normal. Surgery, however, is not the preferred method of treatment because of the complications that may be caused by the general anesthesia and the possibility of nerve damage. Furthermore, too little or too much thyroid tissue frequently is removed.

The medications used to treat Grave's disease are called antithyroidal medications. These medications, such as methimazole (Tapazole) and propylthiouracil (Propylthiouracil Tablets), act by blocking the formation of thyroid hormone. The therapeutic actions of these agents begin as soon as four to twelve hours after administration.

The antithyroidal medications may also alter the thyroid–immune system mechanisms that are central to the cause of Grave's disease. They control the symptoms of hyperthyroidism in 90 percent of patients. Permanent remission is achieved in 10 to 30 percent of patients. Unfortunately, the relapse rates are high, many about 50 percent, even in patients who were treated for more than two years. The relapse rates are even higher, nearly 90 percent, in patients who were treated for less than two years.

The side effects of the antithyroidal medications include fever, rash, itching, and neutropenia (decrease in the white-blood-cell count). Rare but serious side effects are arthritis, blood-vessel inflammation, and hepatitis. The risk of side effects increases as the dose is increased.

SELF-TREATMENT

Because Grave's disease is a metabolic disturbance, it is imperative that you watch your diet closely. Be sure to eat plenty of broccoli, Brussels sprouts, cabbage, cauliflower, kale, mustard greens, peaches, pears, rutabagas, soybeans, spinach, and turnips. These foods help to suppress the production of thyroid hormone.

To help with your eye symptoms, use eyewashes and artificial tears to maintain eye moisture. If your eyes dry out at night, lightly tape them closed (use surgical paper tape).

NUTRITIONAL SUPPLEMENTS

Supplement	Directions for Use	Comments
Multi-vitamin-and-mineral complex	Take as directed on the label.	Increased amounts of all the vitamins and minerals are needed by people with Grave's disease.
Vitamin-B complex	Take 50 mg 3 times daily with meals.	Benefits thyroid function.
Vitamin B_1	Take 50 mg twice daily.	Benefits blood formation and energy levels.
Vitamin B_2	Take 50 mg twice daily.	Necessary for the normal functioning of all the cells, glands, and organs.
Vitamin B_6	Take 50 mg twice daily.	An enzyme activator. Necessary for proper immune function and antibody production.

HERBS AND HERBAL SUPPLEMENTS

Herb	Directions for Use	Comments
Alfalfa	Take as directed on the label.	A good source of vitamin K. Good for relaxation.
Burdock	Take as directed on the label.	A good source of iron.
Eyebright	Use as an eyewash.	Maintains the eye moisture.
Gotu kola	Take as directed on the label.	Good for relaxation.
Kelp	Take as directed on the label.	An infection fighter.
Licorice	Take as directed on the label.	Good for stress.

HOMEOPATHIC REMEDIES

Remedy	Directions for Use	Comments
Aconite 6c	Place 3–4 pellets under the tongue 3–4 times daily.	Good for anxiety.
Arsenicum album 6c	Place 3–4 pellets under thetongue 3–4 times daily.	Good for anxiety.
Belladonna 6c	Place 3–4 pellets under the tongue 3–4 times daily.	Good for restlessness.
Iodium 6c	Place 3–4 pellets under the tongue 3–4 times daily.	Restores iodine intake by the thyroid gland.
Thyroidium 6c (Boiron)	Place 3–4 pellets under the tongue 3–4 times daily.	Regulates the metabolism.

RECOMMENDATIONS

■ Avoid dairy products for at least three months. Also avoid stimulants, coffee, tea, nicotine, and soft drinks.

■ Be wary of treatment with radioactive sodium iodine, which is often recommended for this condition. It has been known to cause severe side effects. Also, do not rush into surgery. Instead, try to improve your diet first.

Headache

The most common complaint among optometric patients is headache. It is very often the first sign of a vision-related problem. However, almost everyone experiences headache at one time or another. Common causes are stress, tension, anxiety, allergies, constipation, coffee consumption, hunger, sinus pressure, muscular tension, hormone imbalance, trauma, nutritional deficiency, alcohol consumption, drug use, smoking, fever, and, of course, eyestrain.

Experts estimate that about 90 percent of all headaches are tension headaches and 6 percent are migraines. Tension headaches, as the name implies, are caused by muscular tension. Migraines result from, most likely, a disturbance in the blood circulation to the brain. Another type of headache is the cluster headache. This is a severe, recurring headache that strikes about 1 million Americans.

Vision-related headaches most often are located toward the front of the head, although there are a few exceptions. They occur most often at the middle or end of the day, are not present upon awakening in the morning, and do not produce visual auras such as flashing lights. They often strike in a different pattern on the weekend than during the week, or not at all on the weekend. They also affect one side of the head more than they do the other, and may be accompanied by a number of more general symptoms.

Because of all the symptoms that accompany headaches, it is important that your doctor obtain a thorough history from you to determine the type of headache you suffer. You should be aware of the time of the headache's onset, location of the pain, frequency, duration, severity, and precipitating factors such as stress, certain foods, and medications. You should also note such associated signs and symptoms as nausea, vomiting, light sensitivity, and sound sensitivity.

The migraine headache is a disorder consisting of localized symptoms that may or may not be associated with headaches. The eye symptoms are similar to those of many other diseases, so you should seek professional care. Migraines have a number of phases that exhibit definite symptoms. The first is called the prodromal or premonitory phase, during which you might suffer irritability, depression, or light or sound sensitivity. These symptoms may show up as early as two days before the actual headache. The second phase is called the aura phase and consists of visual symptoms such as flashing lights, halos around lights, zigzagging of lines, and distortion of shapes and colors. This phase typically evolves over twenty minutes and is commonly, but not always, followed by the headache itself. The headache may throb, be located on one or both sides of the head, and last from four to seventy-two hours. The final phase is called the postdromal phase, which can leave you washed out and exhausted.

Because migraine headaches have a visual aspect to them, eye doctors are often consulted. Light sensitivity, blurred vision, auras, blind spots, flashes of colored lights, tunnel vision, and other disorders are all possible visual effects of migraine headaches.

CONVENTIONAL TREATMENT

Americans tend to be pill poppers. The medical establishment has trained us to expect some type of pill to cure almost every malady. This is no more true than with the common headache. The largest-selling over-the-counter medications in this country today are aspirin and the newer forms of pain relievers. These newer forms include the non-steroidal anti-inflammatory drugs (NSAIDS), which form a billion-dollar business. So, if you call your doctor about a headache, you'll most likely be told, "Take two aspirin and call me in the morning."

SELF-TREATMENT

There are many options for self-treating a headache. Most of them involve discovering the source of the condition that led to the headache, then treating that condition. People who suffer from frequent headaches may be reacting to certain foods or food additives, such as wheat, chocolate, monosodium glutamate (MSG), sulfites, sugar, fermented foods (such as cheese, sour cream, and yogurt), alcohol, vinegar, or marinated foods. Other possible causes are anemia, bowel problems, brain disorders, teeth-grinding, high blood pressure, low blood sugar, sinusitis, spinal misalignment, toxic overdose of vitamin A, deficiency of vitamin B, or a nose, throat, or eye disorder.

Many times, lying down and remaining quiet for a short period of time will alleviate a headache, especially a tension headache. You might also try a cold washcloth over the painful spot to reduce the excessive blood flow to the area.

NUTRITIONAL SUPPLEMENTS

Supplement	Directions for Use	Comments
Bromelain	Take 500 mg as needed.	An enzyme that helps to regulate the inflammatory response.
Calcium	Take 1,500 mg daily.	Relieves muscular tension.
Coenzyme Q_{10}	Take 30 mg twice daily.	Improves tissue oxygenation.
Evening primrose oil	Take 500 mg 3–4 times daily.	Supplies essential fatty acids, which promote circulation.
Glucosamine sulfate	Take as directed on the label.	A natural alternative to aspirin and NSAIDs.
Magnesium	Take 1,000 mg daily.	Relieves muscular tension.
Potassium	Take 100 mg daily.	Maintains the proper balance between sodium and potassium.
Vitamin-B complex	Take 50 mg 3 times daily.	Good for nerve function. *Note:* It is better to take the entire B complex than just isolated B vitamins.

Supplement	Directions for Use	Comments
Vitamin C	Take 2,000–8,000 mg daily in divided doses.	A free-radical scavenger. Good for stress.
Vitamin E	Take 400 IU daily.	Boosts the circulation.

HERBS AND HERBAL SUPPLEMENTS

Herb	Directions for Use	Comments
Burdock	Take as directed on the label.	An excellent detoxifier.
Er ming zuo ci wan (Brion)	Take 8 pills 3 times daily.	Good for headaches accompanied by ear-ringing.
Fenugreek	Take as directed on the label.	Good for headache.
Feverfew	Take as directed on the label.	Good for headache. *Caution:* Do not use during pregnancy.
Goldenseal	Take as directed on the label.	Soothing for the tissues. *Caution:* Do not take internally for more than 1 week. Do not use during pregnancy.
Lavender	Rub essential oil on the temples.	Good for headaches accompanied by stomach upset.
Lobelia	Take as directed on the label.	Good for tension headaches. *Caution:* Do not take internally.
Long dan xie gan wan (Brion)	Take 6 pills twice daily.	Reduces inflammation and "heat."
Marshmallow	Take as directed on the label.	An anti-inflammatory.
Mint	Rub essential oil on the sore area.	Calms the nerves.
Niu huang shang qing wan (Brion)	Take 10 pills daily.	Reduces "heat" and toxins in the body. *Caution:* Do not use during pregnancy.
Qi ju di huang wan (Brion)	Take 8 pills 3 times daily or drink as a tea.	Good for headaches resulting from a "yin" deficiency.
Rosemary	Take as directed on the label.	Boosts the circulation.
Skullcap	Take as directed on the label.	Relieves spasm.
Thyme	Take as directed on the label.	Good for sinus headaches.
White willow bark	Take as directed on the label.	Good for pain.
Xiao yao wan (Brion)	Take 8 pills 3 times daily.	Good for a wide range of symptoms.

HOMEOPATHIC REMEDIES

Remedy	Directions for Use	Comments
Aconite 6c	Place 3–4 pellets under the tongue 3–4 times daily.	Good for throbbing headaches.
Arsenicum album 6c	Place 3–4 pellets under the tongue 3–4 times daily.	Good for head colds.
Belladonna 6c	Place 3–4 pellets under the tongue 3–4 times daily.	Good for colds, flu, sore throats, and similar problems.
Bryonia 6c	Place 3–4 pellets under the tongue 3–4 times daily.	Relieves pressure inside the head.

Remedy	Directions for Use	Comments
Gelsemium sempervirens 6c	Place 3–4 pellets under the tongue 3–4 times daily.	Good for headaches that form a band around the head.
Nux vomica 6c	Place 3–4 pellets under the tongue 3–4 times daily.	Good for headaches at the back of the head or over the eyes. Good for sharp pains. Good for eyestrain resulting from overwork.
Pulsatilla 6c	Place 3–4 pellets under the tongue 3–4 times daily.	Good for "ripe" colds.
Ruta graveolens 6c	Place 3–4 pellets under the tongue 3–4 times daily.	Supports the tendons and ligaments.
Sulphur 6c	Place 3–4 pellets under the tongue 3–4 times daily.	Relieves hot, burning sensations at the top of the head.

RECOMMENDATIONS

■ Eat a well-balanced diet. Avoid chewing gum, ice cream, iced beverages, and salt.

■ Avoid excessive sunlight.

■ Practice deep-breathing exercises. A lack of oxygen can cause headaches.

■ If you use a computer, take breaks often. For more treatments and recommendations, see "Computer Vision Syndrome" on page 104.

■ Always seek and treat the cause of a headache. Long-term reliance on aspirin and other painkillers can make chronic headaches worse by interfering with the brain's natural ability to fight them.

■ Poor vertebral alignment, often caused by flat feet or wearing high heels, can cause a reduced blood flow to the brain. Chiropractic adjustment is helpful.

Herpes Infection of the Eyes

See CYTOMEGALOVIRUS RETINITIS.

High Blood Pressure, Eye Problems Related to

See HYPERTENSIVE RETINOPATHY.

Hordeolum

See STYE.

Hyperopia

See FARSIGHTEDNESS.

Hypertensive Retinopathy

Hypertensive retinopathy is a pathological condition of the retina directly caused by high blood pressure. Because many of the blood vessels of the eye lie within the structure of the retina, any condition that affects the blood vessels can in turn affect the retina.

It is beyond the scope of this book to discuss all of the causes of high blood pressure, which is also called hypertension, but it is certainly worth looking at how to control the disorder. High blood pressure most often has no symptoms. The warning signs associated with advanced hypertension include headache, sweating, rapid pulse, shortness of breath, dizziness, and visual disturbances.

High blood pressure is usually divided into two categories—primary and secondary. Primary hypertension is high blood pressure that is not due to any other, underlying disorder. The precise cause of primary hypertension is unknown, but a number of definite risk factors have been identified. These include cigarette smoking, stress, obesity, excessive use of stimulants such as coffee or tea, drug abuse, high sodium intake, and use of oral contraceptives.

When the blood pressure rises as a result of another health problem, such as a hormonal abnormality or an inherited narrowing of the aorta, it is called secondary hypertension. Secondary hypertension may also result from the blood vessels being chronically constricted or having lost their elasticity due to a buildup of fatty plaque on their inside walls, a condition known as atherosclerosis. Atherosclerosis and arteriosclerosis (thickening of the artery walls due to aging, hypertension, or calcium deposits) are common precursors of hypertension, and both of these conditions can be assessed by viewing the blood vessels inside the eye. In hypertensive retinopathy, the fluids gradually seep out of the weakened blood vessels into the spaces within the structure of the retina. This blood eventually clots and forms scar tissue, which pulls on the structure of the retina, causing blindness in extreme cases.

CONVENTIONAL TREATMENT

The standard treatment of hypertensive retinopathy is directed at both resolving the basic problem (the high blood pressure) and preventing the progression of the disease. Preventing the development of hypertension should be a primary goal of all persons at risk for the disease—that is, those persons with the risk factors discussed above or with a family history of the disease.

The first thing that must be done to treat hypertensive retinopathy is to recognize that the disorder exists. This can be accomplished only by an eye doctor looking into the eye and viewing the blood vessels in the retina. Signs of the condition can show up early in the disease process, so treatment of the disease can reduce the severity of the eye complications.

There are more than a hundred different blood-pressure-lowering medications presently available. Most of these belong to six major classes—the beta blockers, diuretics, alpha blockers, calcium channel blockers, angiotensin-converting enzyme (ACE) inhibitors, and angiotensin antagonists. Within each class are several medications that are very similar to each other. Many physicians start with either a beta blocker or a diuretic because these are the medications that have been the most widely used in the trials demonstrating that lowering of the blood pressure reduces the risk of stroke and heart attack. In other words, they are the tried-and-true medications. Of the newer agents, the calcium channel blockers and ACE inhibitors are very popular, and may have fewer side effects. However, it remains to be seen if they are as good as the beta blockers and diuretics at preventing stroke and heart attack.

Not every medication works well for every patient. It would be wonderful if your doctor could tell you which medication will work the best for you and with the least side effects, but unfortunately, no doctor can do this. There are some medications that you cannot or should not take if you have certain medical conditions; beta blockers, for example, make asthma worse. Beyond that, selecting the most appropriate medication is in good part a hit-or-miss process.

Laser treatment is used on the retina to seal off the leakages in the blood vessels. Usually, it is a spot laser treatment, which targets a specific point of leakage. The leakage is detected using a procedure called fluorescein angiography, in which a dye is injected into the blood vessels and pictures of the retina are taken in a timed sequence. As the dye begins to fill the arteries, the point of leakage can be observed. If there are several points of leakage, a scanning-type of treatment can be effective at targeting the multiple areas.

SELF-TREATMENT

Whether or not you take medication, there are several things that you can do yourself to lower your blood pressure:

■ *Lose weight.* Of all the nondrug methods of lowering the blood pressure, losing weight is definitely the most effective. On average, a ten-pound loss of weight lowers the blood-pressure reading by as much as five points.

■ *Exercise more.* Exercise helps partly by boosting the weight loss, but also is beneficial in its own right. The usual goal is at least thirty minutes of aerobic exercise three times a week. Weightlifting and bodybuilding are not recommended.

■ *If you are a regular drinker, cut down on your alcohol intake.* More than one or two drinks a day raises the blood pressure.

■ *Reduce your salt intake.* This doesn't work for everyone, and it is more likely to be effective if you are more than forty-five years old and have definite hypertension.

In younger people and those with borderline hypertension, losing weight is much more important.

■ *Increase your potassium intake.* Fruits and vegetables are good sources of potassium and are also low in sodium.

■ *Try stress reduction.* In general, however, stress-reduction techniques such as biofeedback and relaxation have been found to be only marginally successful.

■ *Quit smoking.* If you smoke, quitting may be the best thing you ever do. It won't have *much* effect on your blood pressure, but it will greatly reduce your risk of having a stroke or heart attack.

NUTRITIONAL SUPPLEMENTS

Supplement	Directions for Use	Comments
Calcium *and* magnesium	Take 1,500–3,000 mg of a combination supplement daily.	Deficiencies have been linked to hypertension.
Coenzyme Q$_{10}$	Take 100 mg daily.	Improves heart function, and lowers blood pressure.
L-carnitine, L-glutamic acid, *and* L-glutamine	Take 500 mg of a combination supplement twice daily. Take on an empty stomach.	Help to prevent heart disease.
Lecithin	Take 1,200 mg 3 times daily.	Emulsifies fat in the body, and lowers blood pressure.
Selenium	Take 200 mcg daily.	Deficiency has been linked to heart disease.
Vitamin C	Take 3,000–6,000 mg daily.	Improves adrenal function, and reduces blood clotting.
Vitamin E	Take up to 400 IU daily.	Improves heart function.

HERBS AND HERBAL SUPPLEMENTS

Herb	Directions for Use	Comments
Cayenne	Take as directed on the label.	Boosts the circulation.
Fennel	Take as directed on the label.	An anti-inflammatory.
Garlic	Take 250 mg 3 times daily.	Effective at lowering the blood pressure.
Hawthorn	Take as directed on the label.	Boosts the circulation.
Hops	Take as directed on the label.	Promotes relaxation of the smooth muscles.
Lady's slipper	Take as directed on the label.	Good for relaxation.
Parsley	Take as directed on the label.	Relieves mucous discharge.
Passion flower	Take as directed on the label.	Good for relaxation.
Rosemary	Take as directed on the label.	Stimulates the skin.
Scullcap	Take as directed on the label.	Relieves smooth-muscle spasm.
Valerian	Take as directed on the label.	Calms the nerves.

HOMEOPATHIC REMEDIES		
Remedy	Directions for Use	Comments
Crataegus oxycantha 6c	Place 20 drops of tincture in 4 oz of water, and drink. Use daily for 3 months.	Regulates the blood pressure.
Lachesis 6c	Place 3–4 pellets under the tongue 3–4 times daily.	Increases vascular integrity.
Natrum muriaticum 6c	Place 3–4 pellets under the tongue 3–4 times daily.	Good for increased salt intake.

RECOMMENDATIONS

■ Consider lifestyle counseling, a program to revamp your way of living. Lifestyle counseling will address your eating habits, exercise routine, stress level, work habits, and more.

■ People with high blood pressure often have sleep apnea (temporary cessation of breathing while sleeping). If you have this condition, consult your physician.

■ Avoid artificial sweeteners, which contain phenylalanine. Many contain warnings on their packages.

■ Have your blood pressure checked at least every four to six months. If necessary, buy your own blood-pressure-checking equipment. Many pharmacies have self-test equipment available for public use.

Hyperthyroidism

See GRAVE'S DISEASE.

Involuntary Eye Movements

See NYSTAGMUS.

Iris, Inflammation of

See IRITIS.

Iritis

Iritis (eye-RITE-iss) is an inflammation of the iris, and sometimes also of the ciliary body, which is behind the iris. In iritis, microscopic white blood cells from the inflamed area and excess protein that leaked from the small blood vessels inside the eye float in the aqueous fluid between the iris and the cornea. If there are a lot of floating cells, they may become attached to the back of the cornea or settle at the bottom of the area. The cause of iritis is not known. Even when the disorder is treated early, it often recurs. In most cases, however, it eventually disappears completely.

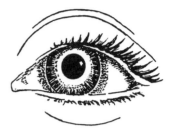

Iritis

In many cases, iritis is related to a disease or infection in another part of the body. Diseases such as arthritis, tuberculosis, or syphilis can contribute to its development. Infection in some parts of the body, such as the tonsils, sinuses, kidneys, gallbladder, or teeth, can also cause inflammation of the iris. In other cases, iritis may follow an injury to the eye or accompany an ulcer or foreign body on the cornea. Often, the exact cause of the disorder remains unknown.

The symptoms of iritis usually appear suddenly and develop rapidly over a few hours or days. Iritis commonly causes extreme pain, tearing, light sensitivity, and blurred vision. Redness often develops. Some patients experience floaters, small specks or dots moving in the field of vision. In addition, the pupil may become smaller in the affected eye.

A careful eye examination is extremely important when the symptoms of iritis occur, as inflammation inside the eye can affect sight and could lead to blindness. A slit lamp, which illuminates and magnifies the structures of the eye, is commonly used to detect any signs of inflammation. Since iritis can be associated with another disease, an evaluation of your overall health is sometimes necessary for proper diagnosis and treatment. In some cases, blood tests, skin tests, and X-rays may be conducted, and other specialists may be consulted to help determine the cause of the inflammation.

CONVENTIONAL TREATMENT

The conventional treatment of iritis is often directed at finding and removing the cause of the inflammation. In addition, eye drops and ointments are recommended to relieve the pain, quiet the inflammation, dilate the pupil, and reduce any scarring that may occur. Both steroids and antibiotics may be prescribed. In severe cases, oral medications and injections may be necessary.

A case of iritis usually lasts six to eight weeks. During this time, you must be observed carefully for side effects from the medications and any complications. Cataracts, glaucoma, corneal changes, and secondary inflammation of the retina may occur as a result of the iritis or the medications.

SELF-TREATMENT

Since iritis is an inflammation inside the eye, the condition is potentially sight-threatening. Proper diagnosis and prompt treatment are essential. To minimize vision loss, you should have a complete eye examination as soon as you notice any symptoms. If diagnosed in the early stages, iritis usually can be controlled with eye drops before any loss of vision occurs. The application of hot packs may also provide relief from the symptoms.

NUTRITIONAL SUPPLEMENTS

Supplement	Directions for Use	Comments
Boron	Take 3 mg daily.	Supports the connective tissue.
Bromelain	Take as directed on the label.	Assists in the production of prostaglandins.
Evening primrose oil *or* salmon oil	Take as directed on the label.	Assist in the production of prostaglandins.
Superoxide dismutase (SOD)	Take as directed on the label.	An antioxidant.
Vitamin B$_5$	Take 500–1,000 mg daily.	Vital for the production of steroids.
Vitamin E	Take 400 IU daily.	An antioxidant.

HERBS AND HERBAL SUPPLEMENTS

Herb	Directions for Use	Comments
Belladonna	Take as directed on the label.	Dilates the pupil.
Cat's claw	Take as directed on the label.	Good for pain. *Caution:* Do not use during pregnancy.
Feverfew *and* ginger	Take as directed on the label.	Good for pain and soreness. *Caution:* Do not use feverfew during pregnancy.

HOMEOPATHIC REMEDIES

Remedy	Directions for Use	Comments
Aconite 6c	Place 3–4 pellets under the tongue 3–4 times daily.	Good for iritis in the early stages.
Allium cepa 6c	Place 3–4 pellets under the tongue 3–4 times daily.	Good for inflammation.
Apis mellifica 6c	Place 3–4 pellets under the tongue 3–4 times daily.	Alleviates swelling.
Belladonna 6c	Place 3–4 pellets under the tongue 3–4 times daily.	Good for inflammation accompanied by dilated pupils.
Calcarea fluorica 6c	Place 3–4 pellets under the tongue 3–4 times daily.	Good for inflammation accompanied by light sensitivity.
Euphrasia officinalis 6c	Place 3–4 pellets under the tongue 3–4 times daily.	Good for all eye conditions.
Mercurius corrosivus 6c	Place 3–4 pellets under the tongue 3–4 times daily.	Alleviates pain and inflammation.
Rhus toxicodendron 6c	Place 3–4 pellets under the tongue 3–4 times daily.	Good for inflammation accompanied by muscle paralysis.

RECOMMENDATIONS

■ If you are diagnosed with iritis, keep your eyes "quiet"—that is, avoid light, wind, dust, sun, and other types of irritations.

Keratoconus

The word "keratoconus" (carrot-oh-CONE-us) is formed from two Greek words—*karato*, meaning cornea, and *konos*, meaning cone. Keratoconus (KC), or conical cornea, is a condition in which the normally spherical shape of the cornea has become deformed. A conelike bulge is present, causing significant visual impairment. The distortion has been compared to viewing a street sign through a car windshield during a driving rainstorm. KC's progression is generally slow and can stop at any stage from mild to severe. As the disease progresses, the cornea bulges and thins, becoming irregular and sometimes developing scars.

KC is not one of the common eye diseases, but it is by no means rare. It has been estimated to occur in 1 out of every 2,000 persons in the general population. The disease usually shows up in young people at puberty or during the late teens. It is found in all the parts of the United States and the rest of the world. It has no known significant geographic, cultural, or social pattern.

The first indication of KC is a blurring and distortion of vision. If caught in the early stages, KC may be corrected with glasses, which require frequent changes in the astigmatism prescription. The thinning of the cornea usually progresses slowly for five to ten years and then tends to stop. Occasionally, it is rapid, and in the advanced stage, the patient may experience a sudden clouding of vision in one eye that clears over a period of weeks or months. This is called acute hydrops and is due to the sudden infusion of fluid into the stretched cornea. In advanced cases of KC, superficial scars form at the apex of the corneal bulge, resulting in more vision impairment.

CONVENTIONAL TREATMENT

In the earliest stages of KC, ordinary eyeglasses may correct the mild nearsightedness and astigmatism that are experienced. As the disease advances, gas-permeable contact lenses are the only way to correct the vision adequately. Most of the time, contact lenses are a permanent remedy.

Contact lenses must be fitted with great care, and most KC patients need frequent checkups and changes in prescription to achieve good vision and comfort. In some instances, the use of one lens on top of another (piggybacking) is an alternative solution. Technological advances in both gas-permeable and soft lenses are being made constantly, offering more and more options to KC patients. For example, a gas-permeable scleral lens was developed in 1994 and has proven to be helpful even in advanced cases of KC. This is why the wearing of contact lenses is the preferred method of managing KC until surgery is necessary.

In only about 10 percent of KC cases, a corneal transplant becomes necessary. In this process, much of the central cornea of the KC patient is removed and is replaced with a healthy cornea. For a complete discussion of corneal transplants, see page 218.

SELF-TREATMENT

Eventually, you will learn to live with your KC whether or not you need surgery. People react differently to the news that they have KC, and you may find a group discussion to be enlightening and reassuring. Lack of knowledge often creates fear. Perhaps there is no better psychological therapy than sharing your experience with others in similar circumstances. The National Keratoconus Foundation maintains a registry of KC patients and organizes self-help groups in various communities. To contact the organization, see "Resource Organizations" on page 255 for the address and phone number.

From a medical standpoint, the most important thing you can do is to keep in touch with your eye doctor and follow his or her instructions. Be alert to any changes in your eye condition and in your vision. If you experience blurring, scratchiness, irritation, tearing, or discharge, contact your eye doctor as soon as possible. These symptoms signal a problem with your eyes' tolerance of the contact lenses or the need for refitting. You should, or course, take normal care of your eyes and avoid the use of any substance not prescribed for you. Women should be careful about the cosmetics they use. Anyone suffering from KC should wear goggles when swimming and safety glasses when engaging in yard work or athletics.

NUTRITIONAL SUPPLEMENTS

Supplement	Directions for Use	Comments
Vitamin A	Take 25,000 IU daily.	Good for all eye conditions
Vitamin C	Take 2,500–3,000 mg daily.	Builds collagen tissue.

RECOMMENDATIONS
■ Inform every health-care professional you see about your eye problem and the medications you take for it.

Lattice Degeneration

Lattice degeneration is a condition in which small areas of the retina are thinner than normal. These thin areas are more prone to developing retinal holes or tears than the areas of normal thickness.

Although we do not know for sure if lattice degeneration is congenital or develops during life, we do know that it slightly increases the risk of retinal holes or tears, and therefore also increases the risk of retinal detachment. No one progresses directly from lattice degeneration to retinal detachment, but sometimes a retinal tear or hole will develop in or near the area of lattice degeneration and progress to retinal detachment.

Lattice degeneration usually has no symptoms, but occasionally it is associated with sudden flashes of light inside the eye, usually at night when the eyes are moved quickly. This is due to the vitreous of the eye tugging on the retina in the area of the degeneration. These flashes are more likely if there is a hole or tear in the retina associated with the degeneration.

If you have lattice degeneration, you should watch for flashes of light or a shower of many floaters in your vision. These symptoms may indicate a retinal tear or retinal detachment, and if you notice either, you will need to call your eye doctor immediately for an appointment. Even without these symptoms, lattice degeneration should be followed and checked on a regular basis.

CONVENTIONAL TREATMENT

Occasionally, lattice degeneration needs to be treated with freezing or a laser in order to prevent the possibility of retinal detachment. These treatments usually are necessary only if there is a very large amount of degeneration. A second reason for these treatments is the presence of an associated hole or tear in the retina. In this circumstance, treatment is often done even if the area of degeneration is small because the tear or hole increases the retinal-detachment risk.

SELF-TREATMENT

Lattice degeneration is much more common in elongated (nearsighted) eyeballs. Therefore, highly nearsighted people should have a dilated eye exam on a regular (yearly!) basis to ascertain that the areas of concern are healthy.

NUTRITIONAL SUPPLEMENTS		
Supplement	Directions for Use	Comments
Vitamin A	Take 25,000 IU daily.	Good for all retinal conditions.
Vitamin C	Take 1,000–5,000 mg daily in divided doses.	Supports all the eye structures.

HOMEOPATHIC REMEDIES		
Remedy	Directions for Use	Comments
Hamamelis virginiana 6c	Place 3–4 pellets under the tongue 3–4 times daily.	Alleviates venous congestion.
Phosphorus 6c	Place 3–4 pellets under the tongue 3–4 times daily.	Improves the metabolism of the retinal tissue.

RECOMMENDATIONS

■ If you have been diagnosed with lattice degeneration, you should avoid high-impact activities (for example, hockey, football, and wrestling) and have your peripheral vision checked regularly.

Lazy Eye

If the visual information to one eye is distorted or dissimilar in any way from the visual information to the other eye, the brain will receive two images that are very different from each other. Double vision is often the result under these circumstances. Since double vision is obviously an undesirable condition, the brain will "turn off" one of the two images it receives in order to see just one image again. (For a discussion of this process, see "Suppression" on page 201.) This double vision followed by turning off of the input from one eye can occur when strabismus causes the eyes to point at two different objects rather than at the same one. It can also occur if the two eyes handle refraction in a dissimilar manner—for example, one eye is nearsighted and the other is astigmatic. If the situation exists for a long time, the eye that is not used will adapt to seeing that way—poorly. After some time, the best obtainable vision in that eye will not be as good as was once possible, even if the proper corrective lens is placed before the eye. This condition of having a healthy eye that cannot be fully corrected to 20/20 is called lazy eye, or amblyopia (am-blee-OH-pee-ah). The lazy eye's vision has been sacrificed to preserve the visual function.

Lazy eye rarely develops in adults. The misinformation between the two eyes most often begins during the first few years of life and occasionally at birth. Once the two eyes have developed their full visual capability—that is, can see 20/20—lazy eye will not develop. However, there are some rare instances of poisons, including tobacco and alcohol, that can create an amblyopia-like condition.

CONVENTIONAL TREATMENT

Amblyopia affects about 4 million people in the United States, but there is no definitive medical treatment for it. The only conventional treatment is trying to encourage the lazy eye to see clearly by patching the good eye. Amblyopia can be prevented almost 100 percent of the time if it is detected early enough (during early childhood) and if the cause is effectively treated.

Vision therapy for amblyopia involves much more than simply patching the good eye. It includes a series of techniques designed to enhance all the visual abilities and to encourage eye teaming. A behavioral optometrist who specializes in vision therapy can offer you a complete program that should be effective at resolving the amblyopia.

SELF-TREATMENT

Most vision-therapy programs include techniques to do at home. It is unlikely that doing therapy techniques for just an hour or so a week at a doctor's office can make a significant difference in your visual abilities. It is critical that you maintain the effect of the therapy throughout your daily routine. Maintaining home vision therapy is essential to a successful program. Be sure to perform the techniques on a daily basis, as prescribed. There are literally dozens of different techniques that you can perform, so vary them as needed to prevent boredom.

One other important point: If you have one good eye and one that is amblyopic, it is strongly suggested that you wear protective eyewear at all times. You never know when an object may come too close for comfort. A pair of plano, or nonprescription, unbreakable polycarbonate lenses are the best protection you can have. Ask your optician about these lenses.

NUTRITIONAL SUPPLEMENTS

Supplement	Directions for Use	Comments
Inositol	Take 500 mg daily.	An antioxidant.
Lutein	Take 6 mg daily.	Increases macular function.
Pantothene	Take 900 mg daily.	An antioxidant.
Selenium	Take 50 mcg daily.	An antioxidant.
Vitamin A	Take 25,000 IU daily.	Good for all retinal conditions.
Vitamin-B complex	Take 75–100 mg daily.	Good for stress.
Vitamin B_1	Take 20 mg daily.	Stimulates nerve transmission.
Vitamin B_6	Take 50–200 mg daily.	Reduces fluid retention.
Vitamin C	Take 2,000–5,000 mg daily.	Fortifies the blood-vessel walls.
Vitamin E	Take 200 IU daily.	An antioxidant. Improves retinal function.
Zinc	Take 50 mg daily.	Good in combination with vitamin A.

HOMEOPATHIC REMEDIES

Remedy	Directions for Use	Comments
Agaricus 6c	Place 3–4 pellets under the tongue 3–4 times daily.	Good for eyelid twitching.
Aurum 6c	Place 3–4 pellets under the tongue 3–4 times daily.	Good for lazy eye accompanied by blind spots.
Calcarea fluorica 6c	Place 3–4 pellets under the tongue 3–4 times daily.	Supports the connective tissue.
Carboneum sulfuratum 6c	Place 3–4 pellets under the tongue 3–4 times daily.	Good for headache.
Causticum 6c	Place 3–4 pellets under the tongue 3–4 times daily.	Good for lazy eye accompanied by strabismus.
Conium 6c	Place 3–4 pellets under the tongue 3–4 times daily.	Good for dizziness.
Gelsemium sempervirens 6c	Place 3–4 pellets under the tongue 3–4 times daily.	Good for lazy eye accompanied by strabismus.
Lachesis 6c	Place 3–4 pellets under the tongue 3–4 times daily.	Good for headache.
Lycopodium 6c	Place 3–4 pellets under the tongue 3–4 times daily.	Good for lazy eye accompanied by blind spots.
Phosphorus 6c	Place 3–4 pellets under the tongue 3–4 times daily.	Good for lazy eye accompanied by exhaustion.
Ruta graveolens 6c	Place 3–4 pellets under the tongue 3–4 times daily.	Good for lazy eye resulting from overexertion of eyes or intense near-point work. Supports the tendons and ligaments.

Remedy	Directions for Use	Comments
Sepia 6c	Place 3–4 pellets under the tongue 3–4 times daily.	Good for lazy eye accompanied by headache.
Sulphur 6c	Place 3–4 pellets under the tongue 3–4 times daily.	Good for lazy eye accompanied by irritation.

RECOMMENDATIONS

■ It is never too early to have a child's eyes examined. In fact, a child's first eye exam should be at six months of age. If your child is six months old or older, make an appointment.

■ The eyes develop in response to visual stimulation, so make sure that your child is surrounded with a full range of colors, lights, shapes, and sizes.

Leber's Primary Optic Neuropathy

See OPTIC ATROPHY.

Legal Blindness

See LOW VISION.

Lens, Clouded

See CATARACTS.

Lens, Hardened

See PRESBYOPIA.

Light Sensitivity

The eyes are designed to respond to light. However, there are a number of conditions that can make them overly sensitive to light. This light sensitivity is also known as photophobia (fo-toe-FO-bee-ah). Among the common causes of light sensitivity are the excessive wearing of contact lenses; poorly fitting contact lenses; eye diseases, injuries, and infections; burns to the eye; migraine headaches; meningitis; acute iritis; corneal abrasion; corneal ulcer; dilated eye examinations; and medications such as amphetamines, atropine, cocaine, cyclopentolate, idoxuridine, phenylephrine, scopolamine, trifluridine, and tropicamide. There are other causes of light sensitivity, too. This list is not inclusive. In fact, light sensitivity is such a general and vague condition—really more a symptom than a condition—that it can be caused by almost anything.

CONVENTIONAL TREATMENT

The treatment for light sensitivity depends upon the cause of the problem. If the cause is an eye disorder covered in this book, see the appropriate section in Part Two for the specific conventional treatments.

SELF-TREATMENT

No matter what the specific cause of your light sensitivity is, keep your eyes shaded from excessive light by wearing sunglasses, keeping the room lights dimmed, or simply closing your eyes. In addition, work on improving your diet. Nutrition has been shown to have a profound effect upon the eyes and visual system. Sensitivity to light and glare, night blindness, and rapid tiring of the eyes are common symptoms of a vitamin-A deficiency. Excessive tearing and severe light sensitivity, along with pain and redness in the eyes, are often part of a B-complex deficiency, in particular of vitamins B_2, B_5, and B_6.

NUTRITIONAL SUPPLEMENTS		
Supplement	Directions for Use	Comments
Vitamin A	Take 25,000 IU daily.	Good for all eye conditions.
Vitamin-B complex	Take as directed on the label.	Supports the eye tissues.

HERBS AND HERBAL SUPPLEMENTS		
Herb	Directions for Use	Comments
Eyebright	Take in supplement form as directed on the label or use as an eyewash.	Good for external eye conditions.
Ming mu di huang wan (Brion)	Take 10 pills 3 times daily.	Clarifies the vision.

HOMEOPATHIC REMEDIES		
Remedy	**Directions for Use**	**Comments**
Argentum nitricum 6c	Place 3–4 pellets under the tongue 3–4 times daily.	Good for light sensitivity after eyestrain. Good for dilated pupils. Maintains healthy nerves.
Arsenicum album 6c	Place 3–4 pellets under the tongue 3–4 times daily.	Good for light sensitivity accompanied by discharge and burning.
Belladonna 6c	Place 3–4 pellets under the tongue 3–4 times daily.	Good for dilated pupils.
Calcarea fluorica 6c	Place 3–4 pellets under the tongue 3–4 times daily.	Good for dilated pupils.
Carboneum sulfuratum 6c	Place 3–4 pellets under the tongue 3–4 times daily.	Good for headache.
Cinchona officinalis 6c	Place 3–4 pellets under the tongue 3–4 times daily.	Good for dilated pupils.
Euphrasia officinalis 6c	Place 3–4 pellets under the tongue 3–4 times daily.	Good for all eye conditions.
Graphites 6c	Place 3–4 pellets under the tongue 3–4 times daily.	Reduces eye sensitivity.
Mercurius vivus 6c	Place 3–4 pellets under the tongue 3–4 times daily.	Good for inflammation.
Natrum muriaticum 6c	Place 3–4 pellets under the tongue 3–4 times daily.	Alleviates redness.
Natrum sulfuricum 6c	Place 3-4 pellets under the tongue 3–4 times daily.	Good for inflammation. Relieves mucous discharge.
Nux vomica 6c	Place 3–4 pellets under the tongue 3–4 times daily.	Alleviates redness.
Rhus toxicodendron 6c	Place 3–4 pellets under the tongue 3–4 times daily.	Alleviates swelling.
Silicea 6c	Place 3–4 pellets under the tongue 3–4 times daily.	Good for chronic light sensitivity. Improves nutrient absorption and metabolism. Maintains healthy nerves.
Sulphur 6c	Place 3–4 pellets under the tongue 3–4 times daily.	Good for inflammation.

RECOMMENDATIONS

■ Light sensitivity is usually a symptom of a more significant condition, so appropriate diagnosis is important. Consult an eye doctor if the condition persists.

Low Vision

If you have been reading this book from page one without any difficulty, your eyes must be working rather well. Congratulations! However, a great number of people cannot do this because they have a visual impairment that is not correctable with traditional treatments. Whether due to a genetic defect, a disease process, an accident, or progressive degeneration, visual impairment is a serious problem for millions of people. However, despite their disadvantage, these people can still be productive members of society and should be offered the opportunity to contribute.

Low vision, as it is often called, is some type of reduction in visual acuity or the visual field that cannot be corrected. There is no clear consensus on what constitutes low vision, but individuals should be considered visually impaired if their vision is not adequate for their individual needs. The term "legal blindness" is bandied about quite often, but it is grossly misunderstood. State and Federal laws dictate that individuals are legally blind when their best corrected vision is 20/200 or less, or their visual field is limited to a maximum of 20 degrees. It is estimated that more than 10 million people in the United States are visually impaired.

CONVENTIONAL TREATMENT

The treatment for low vision depends primarily upon what visual condition is causing the problem. Most often, some kind of device is recommended to enhance the images sent to the eyes.

For impaired near vision, a simple magnifying glass is often of great help. You can also get a magnifying glass with a light attached and a unit that is placed around the neck to allow the hands to remain free for reading, sewing, and other activities.

Extremely high magnification of printed material can be obtained with closed-circuit television. The printed matter is held under the television camera, magnified, and shown on a television screen. For the truly blind, print can actually be "read" by a small camera and converted into a pattern that can be felt with the fingers. Of course, this type of equipment is expensive, but it may be worth the money if it enables you to keep earning a living or doing what you like to do.

For distance vision, small telescopes, which can be adjusted for focus, can be attached to your glasses. They will greatly restrict your visual field, but they may make it possible for you to see clearly within the smaller field. Pocket telescopes are also available to read such things as street signs and bus numbers.

Other devices that are available include binoculars and head-mounted display units.

The appropriateness of these devices in your case can be evaluated by an optometrist who specializes in low vision, the organization Lighthouse for the Blind, or a low-vision center. For the name of a doctor or clinic in your area, contact your local branch of the Optometric Society.

Surgical treatment may also be an option, depending on the specific condition that is causing your loss of vision. There have been many significant advances in eye surgery over the last several years, so consult your ophthalmologist about the options that might best serve your needs.

SELF-TREATMENT

A positive attitude and a little ingenuity can take you a long way in your efforts to adapt to low vision. Among the things you can do yourself is putting a raised dot on your oven at the 350° point to make setting your oven temperature easier. You can learn to dial or punch the numbers on your telephone without having to look.

You can practice using the bottom edge of sheets of paper as a guide for signing your name on a straight line without looking.

Get involved in a regular exercise program, keep good music and audiotaped books on hand, and become familiar with the large-print book collection at your local library. Many communities offer support groups for persons with low vision that can help you with the emotional and practical aspects of your condition.

See "Recommended Suppliers" on page 253 for a list of companies that have devices to assist persons with visual impairments.

RECOMMENDATIONS

■ Join a support group for your particular visual condition. It is always reassuring to know that you're not alone.

Macular Degeneration

The macula (MAC-yoo-lah) is the area of the retina that is used for direct, central vision. It is the most sensitive part of the retina. For one in four people over the age of sixty-five and for one in three over the age of eighty, the macula begins to degenerate (deteriorate). Therefore, this condition is known as age-related macular degeneration (ARMD). Very often, the macular area of one eye shows this degenerative change while the other eye remains perfectly normal. In this circumstance, you may not notice any change taking place because the good eye will dominate your vision.

There are two types of ARMD—the wet and the dry forms. The wet form accounts for only 10 percent of cases. It occurs when tiny new abnormal blood vessels begin to grow behind the retina toward the macula. These abnormal vessels often leak blood and fluid, which damage the macula, causing rapid and severe vision loss. The dry form constitutes the other 90 percent of cases and occurs when small yellowish deposits called drusen (DROO-zin) start to accumulate beneath the macula. These deposits gradually break down the light-sensing cells in the macula, causing distorted vision in the eye.

There are certain risk factors that can increase your susceptibility to ARMD. These risk factors are:

■ *Age.* It is estimated that about 14 percent of people aged fifty-five to sixty-four have some form of ARMD. This rises to about 25 percent of persons aged sixty-five to seventy-five, and up to 37 percent of those over seventy-five.

■ *Diet and nutrition.* The macula's fragile cells are highly susceptible to damage from the oxygen-charged molecules called free radicals. Early research showed that people with a low dietary intake of antioxidants may be at risk for developing ARMD. In addition, alcohol may deplete the body of antioxidants. High levels of saturated fats and cholesterol harm blood vessels and are also involved in producing free-radical reactions.

■ *Sunlight.* The cells of the macula are highly sensitive to sunlight. Cell damage from the sun can lead, over time, to deterioration of the macula. People with light colored eyes may be more prone to damage from sunlight than people with dark eyes, as are individuals who are exposed to UV light for prolonged periods of time.

■ *Smoking.* A recent study showed that smoking, which reduces the amount of protective antioxidants in the eye, more than doubles the risk of ARMD. The study found that ARMD is more than twice as common in people who smoke more than one pack of cigarettes a day than in people who do not smoke, and the risk remains high even up to fifteen years after quitting.

■ *Heredity.* Some studies have shown that ARMD may be in part inherited. This means that if you have one or more immediate relatives with ARMD, you may be at a higher risk for developing the condition.

■ *Gender and race.* Women over the age of seventy-five have double the chance of developing ARMD as men of the same age. Low levels of estrogen in postmenopausal women may also increase the risk for the condition. There is some suggestion that postmenopausal estrogen therapy may protect against ARMD, but more research is needed in this area. Women also live longer than men. Caucasians are much more likely than African-Americans to lose vision to ARMD.

■ *Heart disease.* If you have high blood pressure or another form of heart disease, you may also have a greater chance of getting ARMD because of the poor blood circulation to the eyes.

Macular degeneration does not result in total blindness. Since the macular area is responsible just for central vision, only this area is affected. However, a person afflicted with macular degeneration can feel very helpless and frustrated due to the loss of detail vision. The peripheral vision usually remains intact and therefore allows the person to function almost normally. This is especially true if only one eye is affected.

CONVENTIONAL TREATMENT

Lasers have been used in the treatment of the wet form of macular degeneration. In this procedure, the laser is used to coagulate (clot) the tiny blood vessels that have grown near the macula. Unfortunately, most forms of macular degeneration cannot yet be reliably treated either medically or surgically. In these cases, special low-vision aids can be of great help. These aids serve to magnify images so they are spread over a larger portion of the retina. For a description of some of these aids, see "Low Vision" on page 162.

Most doctors, when checking for macular degeneration, will administer a test called the Amsler Grid. For a sample grid and directions for using it, see "Cytomegalovirus Retinitis" on page 116. This test is valuable for following the course of the disease process, but certainly does nothing to resolve the condition.

SELF-TREATMENT

While you cannot change your age, your sex, or your family tree, there are some lifestyle changes that you can adopt to help protect your eyes. First, wear sunglasses or a brimmed hat whenever you are exposed to large amounts of UV light. Moderate amounts of UV light are good for the human body, but overexposure can cause damage to some parts of the eye. Even lightbulbs emit a modicum of UV light, and some people with macular degeneration have found that Chromolux Full Spectrum lightbulbs are easier on their eyes.

Anything that prevents clogging of your arteries may help to prevent macular degeneration (as well as the degeneration of the rest of your body). Therefore, watching your dietary fat and cholesterol, exercising regularly, not smoking, and watching your weight and blood pressure are wise moves. Limit your intake of alcohol to a maximum of six drinks per week if you are a man and three per week if you are a woman.

Finally, most doctors recommend that their older patients take antioxidant supplements to prevent or halt the progress of macular degeneration. Recent studies indicate that a well-rounded combination of antioxidants can slow macular-degenerative changes. Several research studies on ARMD are focusing on the role of a group of antioxidants called carotenoids. Two of these antioxidants, lutein and zeaxanthin, are the only pigments found in the macula. By contrast, beta-carotene is virtually absent from the eye (although its cousin, vitamin A, is plentiful in the retina). Lutein and zeaxanthin can be found in almost all fruits and vegetables, but are most likely to be present in dark green leafy vegetables such as spinach and collard greens. A study among male veterans showed that increasing the antioxidant intake can slow the progression of vision loss from dry ARMD.

NUTRITIONAL SUPPLEMENTS

Supplement	Directions for Use	Comments
Selenium	Take 400 mcg daily.	An antioxidant.
Shark cartilage (Benefin)	Take 1 gm for every 15 lbs of body weight daily.	Decreases the growth of new blood vessels In the macula area. *Note:* Be sure to use 100% pure, dried shark cartilage.
Vitamin A	Take 50,000–100,000 IU daily.	An antioxidant. *Note:* Use the emulsion form for easier assimilation and greater safety.
Vitamin C with bioflavonoids	Take 1,000–2,500 mg 4 times daily.	An antioxidant. *Note:* Use powdered buffered ascorbic acid.
Vitamin E	Take 600–800 IU daily.	An antioxidant and free-radical scavenger.
Zinc	Take 45–80 mg daily. *Caution:* Do not take more than 100 mg daily.	Deficiency has been linked to eye problems. *Note:* Use the zinc picolinate form.

HERBS AND HERBAL SUPPLEMENTS

Herb	Directions for Use	Comments
Bilberry	Take 160 mg daily.	Improves retinal function.
Blueberry	Drink 8–10 oz of tea daily.	Rich in flavonoids.
Ginkgo	Take as directed on the label.	The dry form stimulates blood flow in the capillaries.

HOMEOPATHIC REMEDIES		
Remedy	**Directions for Use**	**Comments**
Hamamelis virginiana 6c	Place 3–4 pellets under the tongue 3–4 times daily.	Alleviates venous congestion and vascular infiltration.
Lachesis 6c	Place 3–4 pellets under the tongue 3–4 times daily.	Good for macular degeneration with muscle fatigue.
Phosphorus 6c	Place 3–4 pellets under the tongue 3–4 times daily.	Good for many eye conditions. Improves tissue metabolism, and reduces vascular and blood degeneration.

RECOMMENDATIONS

■ While you can't stop the aging process, you can watch your diet. Eat a low-fat diet with lots of fresh vegetables and fruits, and a minimum of processed foods.

■ Increase your consumption of legumes; yellow vegetables; flavonoid-rich berries, such as blueberries, blackberries, and cherries; and foods rich in vitamins C and E, such as raw fruits and vegetables.

■ Avoid alcohol, cigarette smoke, all sugars, saturated fats, and foods containing fats and oils that were subjected to heat or exposed to the air, such as fried foods, hamburgers, luncheon meats, and roasted nuts.

■ Although there has been no study to show a direct correlation, shark cartilage is known to inhibit the growth of blood vessels, such as those that grow in wet macular degeneration.

Meibomian Cyst

See CHALAZION.

Migraine

See HEADACHE.

MS, Eye Problems Related to

See MULTIPLE SCLEROSIS.

Multiple Sclerosis

Multiple sclerosis (MS) is an inflammatory disease of the body's central nervous system. This disease—which may, it is now believed, originate with a viral infection—destroys the myelin sheaths, or coverings, of the body's nerves. Another theory is that MS is an autoimmune disease in which white blood cells attack the myelin sheaths as if they were foreign substances. The result is similar to what happens when you remove the insulation from wiring—the electrical impulses do not get to where they're going very well and also escape to the wrong places.

Multiple sclerosis can affect the optic nerve itself, causing poor vision ranging from mild symptoms to changes in color vision, blind spots, and blindness. It can also affect the nerves that control the muscles of the eyes, causing double vision from strabismus, poor binocular coordination, and an uncontrollable jerking of the eye muscles. Very often, these visual problems are the first symptoms of MS.

MS is usually diagnosed between the ages of twenty-five and forty. Women are affected nearly twice as often as men. MS is rarely diagnosed in children and in people over sixty years of age. Magnetic resonance imaging (MRI) may be used to diagnose MS. However, there is no single diagnostic test for the disease, and diagnosis must be done indirectly, by ruling out other possible causes of the symptoms.

CONVENTIONAL TREATMENT

Fortunately, most people with MS have periods of remission during which their symptoms improve or even disappear. Many years can go by before serious visual impairment occurs—and it doesn't occur at all in some patients. Systemic steroids and other medications are now used to improve the symptoms of multiple sclerosis, including the eye problems. If you have MS, you should see an ophthalmologist in addition to your regular doctor.

There is no known cure for MS, but the following supplement and dietary recommendations have been shown to be helpful. Long-term sufferers of MS may not benefit as much, but younger people who are just starting to exhibit symptoms may find that the correct supplements slow or even stop the progression of the disease.

SELF-TREATMENT

A strong immune system may help to prevent the development of multiple sclerosis by assisting the body in avoiding infection, which often precedes the onset of the disease. Once you have had MS confirmed as a diagnosis, start to educate yourself and your family about the disease, and seek out sources of emotional support. Contact the National Multiple Sclerosis Society. (For the address and telephone number, see "Resource Organizations" on page 255.) Watch your diet, take your supplements, and try to keep a positive attitude and a clean lifestyle.

NUTRITIONAL SUPPLEMENTS

Supplement	Directions for Use	Comments
Choline *and* inositol	Take as directed on the label.	Stimulate the central nervous system, and protect the myelin sheaths from damage.
Coenzyme Q$_{10}$	Take 90 mg daily.	Boosts the circulation, and improves tissue oxygenation. Strengthens the immune system.
Evening primrose oil, flaxseed oil, gamma linolenic acid (GLA), *or* omega-3 oils	Take as directed on the label 3 times daily with meals.	All of these are essential fatty acids that can help to control MS symptoms. Deficiency is common in MS.
Sulfur	Take 500 mg 2–3 times daily.	Protects against toxic substances.
Vitamin-B complex	Take 100 mg 3 times daily.	Aids immune function, and maintains healthy nerves.
Vitamin B$_6$	Take 50 mg 3 times daily.	Promotes red-blood-cell production, and aids nervous-system and immune function.
Vitamin B$_{12}$	Take 1,000 mcg twice daily.	Aids cellular longevity, and prevents nerve damage by maintaining the myelin sheaths. *Note:* Use the sublingual form.

HERBS AND HERBAL SUPPLEMENTS

Herb	Directions for Use	Comments
Alfalfa	Take as directed on the label.	A good source of vitamin K.
Burdock, dandelion, echinacea, goldenseal, red clover, St. John's wort, sarsaparilla, taheebo, *and* yarrow	Take as directed on the label.	All of these are excellent detoxifiers.
Garlic	Take 1,000 mg 3 times daily.	An excellent source of sulphur.
Lobelia, skullcap, *and* valerian	Take as directed on the label at bedtime.	Calm the nerves, and prevent insomnia.

HOMEOPATHIC REMEDIES

Remedy	Directions for Use	Comments
Aurum 6c	Place 3–4 pellets under the tongue 3–4 times daily.	Good for pain.
Gelsemium sempervirens 6c	Place 3–4 pellets under the tongue 3–4 times daily.	Good for headaches with fever.
Hyoscyamus 6c	Place 3–4 pellets under the tongue 3–4 times daily.	Relieves spasm.
Natrum muriaticum 6c	Place 3–4 pellets under the tongue 3–4 times daily.	Good for pain.
Nitricum acidum 6c	Place 3–4 pellets under the tongue 3–4 times daily.	Good for pain.

RECOMMENDATIONS

■ Eat only organically grown foods that have not been chemically treated and contain no chemical additives, including eggs, fresh fruits, gluten-free grains, raw nuts and seeds, fresh vegetables, and cold-pressed vegetable oils. The best diet for people with multiple sclerosis is vegetarian.

■ Eat plenty of raw sprouts and alfalfa, plus foods that contain lactic acid, such as sauerkraut and dill pickles. Also, green drinks, which contain plenty of chlorophyll, are good, as are dark green leafy vegetables. These are good sources of vitamin K.

■ Drink at least eight 8-ounce glasses of quality water each day to prevent toxic buildup in the muscles.

■ Do not consume any alcohol, barley, chocolate, coffee, dairy products, fried foods, highly seasoned foods, meat, oats, refined foods, rye, salt, spices, sugar, tobacco, wheat, and processed, canned, or frozen foods.

■ Take a fiber supplement. Fiber is necessary for avoiding constipation. Periodically take warm cleansing enemas. A clean colon is important for keeping toxic waste from interfering with muscle function.

■ Avoid stress and anxiety. Attacks of MS are often precipitated by a trauma or a period of emotional distress.

Myopia

See NEARSIGHTEDNESS.

Nearsightedness

Nearsightedness, also called myopia (my-OP-pee-ah), means having good near vision, but poor distance vision. For the myopic person, distance images (images at least twenty feet away) fall in front of the retina and look blurred. This misplacement of focus is the result of the eye being too long, positioning the retina farther back than normal; the cornea being too steeply curved; the eye's lens staying focused for near vision; or some combination of these and other factors. Myopia is the most common refractive error in humans, affecting over 32 percent of the population of the United States. It most often starts in childhood and continues to worsen until early adulthood, at which time, in the absence of other stress factors, it generally stabilizes.

It's been believed for a long time now that nearsightedness is inherited, and I don't deny that heredity may be a factor. Recent studies have shown that there is definitely a tendency for nearsightedness to develop more often in the children of nearsighted parents. But, this is probably not the whole story, because nearsightedness is much more prevalent in societies whose people do a lot of close work. Studies have found, for example, that nearsightedness is almost nonexistent in uneducated societies, and that it increases in proportion to the general level of education in the society. In other words, the more reading and near-point work a society does, the higher is its incidence of nearsightedness.

In a similar vein, studies have been conducted with Navy submariners, who are submerged for months at a time and spend their days in spaces where the maximum viewing distance is about eight feet. These studies showed an increase in nearsightedness during these extended periods of confinement. Dr. Francis Young of Washington University has done similar research with monkeys. Dr. Young kept rhesus monkeys in confined areas during various developmental periods of their early lives. The shorter the maximum viewing distance and the longer the confinement were, the more nearsighted the monkeys became.

So, what does this say about the way our eyes develop? The same as any biological system, our visual system changes in response to stress. When you read, you use near vision. Your eyes focus on a point only about fourteen to sixteen inches away. Your eyes accomplish this focusing through the process of accommodation. If you maintain a reading posture for long periods of time without taking breaks, your eyes will slowly adapt to the position in order to reduce the stress on the muscles controlling the lenses. Once adapted, the eyes can see more clearly up close with less effort. It's as if the muscles get comfortably "stuck" in the near-focus position. To make matters worse, when the eye muscles must work constantly to accommodate for near-point work, pressure builds up in the eye. Eventually, this pressure causes the eyeball to lengthen in an effort to relieve the pressure, moving the retina even farther back from the lens than it was originally. The result of all this? Nearsightedness. When a nearsighted eye relaxes in its attempts at accommodation and refocusing for distance vision, the images become blurred because they are too far forward of the retina. This relaxation doesn't happen just from reading steadily for a night or two. It's a gradual adaptation that your eyes make as they react to the strain of overwork.

In children, as you might expect, nearsightedness increases along with the amount of time spent focused for near-point activities. About 1.6 percent of children entering school in the United States have some degree of nearsightedness. That figure grows to 4.4 percent for seven- and eight-year-olds, 8.7 percent for nine- and ten-year-olds, 12.5 percent for eleven- and twelve-year-olds, and 14.3 percent for thirteen- and fourteen-year-olds. We used to say that the progression (worsening) of nearsightedness stabilizes at about twenty-one or twenty-two years of age. However, over the past fifteen years, eye doctors have seen more nearsightedness progressing well into the late twenties and even thirties. The reason? We're not quite sure, but computers are almost certainly one of the culprits. They require constant near-point focus, and more adults are spending more of their time in front of them.

CONVENTIONAL TREATMENT

For many centuries, the only treatment for nearsightedness was eyeglasses. The eyeglass lenses were (and still are) designed to weaken the focusing strength of the light entering the eye so that it falls further back toward the retina. The idea of using lenses that are in direct contact with the eye—that is, contact lenses—was actually conceived by Leonardo da Vinci. That idea became a reality in the mid-

1950s, and today there are many types of lenses in several materials. For a description of the different types of contact lenses currently available, see page 211.

There are several drawbacks to using eyeglasses or contact lenses to correct nearsightedness. Glasses have a limited ability to correct peripheral vision. In addition, the thickness of the lenses can be extreme and can cause perceptual distortions. Contact lenses can overcome these difficulties, but they have problems of their own. Since they are in direct contact with the eye tissue, they can accumulate debris and proteins from the tears and harbor bacteria, which can lead to infections. The eye can react to the lens material or to the debris on the lens, both of which can decrease your ability to wear the lenses successfully.

More recently, a third alternative, called refractive surgery, has emerged. Refractive surgery includes a number of procedures, but in general, all the procedures attempt to move the point of focus of the light entering the eye closer to the retina by surgically altering the shape of the cornea. Each of the surgical procedures has positive and negative aspects. For a discussion of the different types of refractive surgery being performed today, see page 228.

SELF-TREATMENT

There's probably no escape from activities that require near-point focus. Consider all the things we do with our eyes at the near point—reading, writing, drawing, typing, painting, sewing, crocheting, and even cooking and eating, to name just a few. And then there are those intermediate-distance tasks, such as playing the piano (and most musical instruments), shopping, working at computers, card playing, watching television, and enjoying a variety of hobbies. During the grade-school years, children read the equivalent of about 700 books. When this reading time is added to play time and computer time, it's not hard to see why so many people develop nearsightedness. Have you ever seen a lawyer, for example, who doesn't wear glasses? (If you have, he or she is probably wearing contacts!)

So, what can be done about all this? Well, you could stay away from near-point activities, but that's not too practical. Better is to first make an appointment for a complete vision examination with an optometrist or ophthalmologist who performs near-vision tests. Many doctors omit these tests because they take longer to do and evaluate than the simple tests for distance vision. Also, at home, make sure that you have enough light for your near-point activities, and do not do near-point work at a table or desk facing a wall. You want to be able to look up and focus for distance from time to time. Do about twenty to thirty minutes of near-point work, then take two minutes or so to look far away or close the eyes. Reading distance should be kept at fourteen to sixteen inches—no closer! If you are not able to read at this distance, something is wrong and a full examination is indicated. In short, give your eyes a chance to relax when doing a lot of close work, and schedule routine eye examinations to be sure everything is working properly.

If glasses are prescribed, they won't "cure" you, but they certainly will improve your distance vision. However, you might be advised to remove your glasses for reading and other near-point activities, since wearing them for those activities will only force your eyes to accommodate more and may hasten the progression of your nearsightedness. Or, you might be given bifocals, with each eyeglass lens including one clear section, for near vision, and one prescription section, for distance vision. With these kinds of biofocals, you don't have to keep taking your glasses off for near-point activities.

172

Vision therapy is another alternative for nearsightedness. However, it is more difficult to reverse nearsightedness than it is to prevent it. You must dedicate yourself to your vision-therapy program, and do all of the required techniques on a regular basis. Changing the way you see is a monumental task, but you may be able to do it if you commit to the process and follow through completely.

NUTRITIONAL SUPPLEMENTS

Supplement	Directions for Use	Comments
Calcium	Take 800 mg daily.	Important in collagen formation.
Chromium	Take 80–100 mg daily.	Deficiencies have been found in persons with nearsightedness.
Copper	Take 5 mg daily.	Important in collagen formation.
Vitamin A	Take 25,000 IU daily.	Good for all eye conditions.
Vitamin C	Take 2,500 mg daily.	Strengthens the collagen for stronger eyes.

HERBS AND HERBAL SUPPLEMENTS

Herb	Directions for Use	Comments
Eyebright	Take as directed on the label.	Good for the eye tissues.
Ming mu shang qing pian (Brion)	Take 4 pills twice daily.	Clarifies the vision. *Caution:* Do not use during pregnancy.

RECOMMENDATIONS

■ Have your eyes checked regularly. This is especially important for school-aged children. Make sure that your near vision is tested.

■ When doing a near-point activity, take regular breaks to give your eyes a rest.

■ Increase your intake of fiber, and reduce your intake of simple carbohydrates (sugar). Avoid most processed foods.

■ If you are sick with a fever, avoid near-point activities. High temperatures weaken and soften the collagen, which can easily become stretched with increased eye pressure.

Night Blindness

True night blindness is a relatively rare condition in the United States. The main symptom of this disorder is a decrease in visual acuity under nighttime viewing conditions. Most often, night blindness is caused by a nutritional deficiency—specifically, of vitamin A—and is common in underdeveloped countries. Vitamin A is necessary for the formation of visual purple, the pigment required by the retina to convert light energy to nerve energy. Other causes of night blindness are fatigue, emotional disturbances, and hereditary factors.

It is also very common for persons who are just beginning to become nearsighted to complain of difficulty seeing clearly at night. This, too, is different than true night blindness. The retina has a dual sensitivity—it is sharp in one area for daytime vision and in another for nighttime vision. The eyes generally become more nearsighted at night. In addition, our eyes are usually more fatigued after being used all day long in stressful situations, thus leading to a poorer focusing ability. When the light is dim, the pupil also dilates, causing the visual image to be distorted.

There are, however, some very serious eye conditions whose main symptom is night blindness. Most notable is retinitis pigmentosa, which is described in more detail beginning on page 194. If you notice that you are having difficulty reading those street signs at night, a complete eye examination is in order.

CONVENTIONAL TREATMENT

The treatment for night blindness depends on the cause of the problem. For the simple problem of nearsightedness, glasses are normally prescribed, often just for nighttime driving. Contact lenses may also be recommended, but most likely for full-time wear rather than just nighttime viewing. If your eyes are not permanently nearsighted but merely overstressed, you may be advised to use reading glasses for your daily near-point activities. These will allow the eyes to relax more during close work and therefore keep them from being stressed for nighttime viewing.

For the serious diseases such as retinitis pigmentosa, there are no conventional treatments available. However, new research is showing that nutritional supplementation might have a slowing effect on the progression of the disease.

SELF-TREATMENT

The best thing that you can do if you notice a problem with your nighttime distance vision is to make an appointment for a full eye examination. Ask your doctor what alternatives are available for your specific condition. In general, supplementing your diet with vitamin A will help to protect your eyes against night blindness. Also, vitamins B_1, B_2, and B_3, as well as zinc have been reported to relieve night blindness when vitamin A did not produce a response.

NUTRITIONAL SUPPLEMENTS		
Supplement	Directions for Use	Comments
Vitamin A	Take 50,000 IU daily.	Supports the retina.
Vitamin-B complex	Take 75–100 mg daily.	Good for nerve function.
Zinc	Take 15 mg daily.	Good in combination with vitamin A.

HERBS AND HERBAL SUPPLEMENTS		
Herb	Directions for Use	Comments
Eyebright	Take as directed on the label.	Good for all eye conditions
Qi ju di huang wan (Brion)	Take 8 pills 3 times daily or drink as a tea.	Aids liver function.

RECOMMENDATIONS

■ Have a complete eye examination once a year. Regular examinations can catch night blindness before it becomes disabling.

Night Vision, Decreased

See NIGHT BLINDNESS.

Nystagmus

Nystagmus (nis-TAG-mus) is characterized by involuntary movement of the eyes, which often seriously reduces vision. Many people with nystagmus are partially sighted, while some are legally blind. Few can drive a car; most encounter difficulties—both practical and social—in their everyday lives; and some even lose out on education and employment opportunities.

Depth perception is reduced by nystagmus, resulting in clumsiness and a proclivity to tripping. Coordination is adequate for most tasks, but not for those needing good hand-eye coordination, such as sports. Nystagmus affects about 1 in 1,000 people.

Nystagmus may be inherited or the result of a sensory problem. In a small number of cases, it occurs for no known reason. It can also develop later in life, sometimes as a result of an accident or illness, especially if the motor system has been affected. If you or a member of your family has nystagmus, consult an eye doctor. Nystagmus affects different people in different ways. While there are general patterns, good advice for one person may be inappropriate or even bad for another, especially if other eye problems are present.

CONVENTIONAL TREATMENT

Nystagmus cannot be corrected with eyeglasses. However, contact lenses, especially the gas-permeable type, occasionally are useful in reducing the magnitude of the jerkiness. Nystagmus often affects the nerves behind the eye rather than the eye itself. Sufferers are not simply nearsighted. Many can and do register as partially sighted or blind. Few people with nystagmus can see well enough to drive a car. Vision often varies throughout the day, and is likely to be affected by emotional and physical factors such as stress, fatigue, nervousness, and familiarity with surroundings.

There is no real treatment for nystagmus because it is simply a symptom of a more severe condition. It can be one of the first signs of multiple sclerosis. (For a discussion of multiple sclerosis, see page 168.) Since nystagmus most commonly begins at birth, the main goal of treatment is to minimize the visual disturbances caused by the condition.

SELF-TREATMENT

For persons with nystagmus, the angle of vision is important. Most sufferers have a null point, where eye movement is reduced and vision is improved. Those with such a null point often adopt a head posture that makes the best use of their vision. Sitting to one side of the computer monitor or blackboard often helps. Many can read very small print if they get close enough or use a visual aid. However, the option of using large-print material should be available, and all written matter should be clear. It is very hard for a person with nystagmus to share a book with someone else because the book will probably be too far away or at the wrong angle. In addition, the person's reading speed may be reduced because of the extra time needed to scan, but this should not be taken as a sign of poor reading ability.

Computers are used by many people with nystagmus, who find it helpful to be able to position the screen, adjust the brightness, customize the character sizes, and so on, to suit their own needs. However, some persons find it difficult to read computer screens.

Depending on the cause of the nystagmus, color therapy may be appropriate. (For a complete discussion of color therapy, see "Syntonics" on page 234.) Color therapy serves to stimulate the eyes to maximize the vision.

Following are some recommendations for the parents and teachers of students who have nystagmus:

1. Encourage the student to explain his or her visual needs. However, avoid continual and undue attention to these needs.

2. Allow the student to hold books and other objects close to the eyes, tilt the head, and adopt any other body posture that enhances vision.

3. Provide the student with personal books and worksheets. Sharing is impossible.

4. Enlarging materials often helps, although good contrast may suffice.

5. Place wall displays for reference at eye level and where the pupil can stand close to it (not above a filing cabinet or table, for example).

6. Allow the student to choose where he or she sits. Often, it is facing and near to the board, but it may also be off to one side. In addition, allow the student to sit close to demonstrations during activities.

7. Store visual aids so that the student can easily reach them when needed.

8. Allow the student to use prescribed tinted glasses, a cap, a hat, or eyeshades to reduce the effects of glare.

9. Read aloud when you write on the board, and describe any diagrams you draw.

10. Allow the student sufficient time to complete tasks, and to examine materials and objects.

11. Good (although not necessarily bright) lighting is essential. The light should be

behind the student and directed onto the object being viewed. Matte surfaces on walls, boards, and paper prevent light reflection and glare.

12. Use strong color contrast between letters, figures, and lines, and the background. Make sure to use good spacing.

13. To help the student keep track of his or her place while reading, encourage the use of a dark card or a finger. Keep on hand exercise books with matte paper, different colors, and ruled lines.

NUTRITIONAL SUPPLEMENTS

Supplement	Directions for Use	Comments
Vitamin-B complex	Take at least 100 mg daily.	Good for nerve function.

HOMEOPATHIC REMEDIES

Remedy	Directions for Use	Comments
Calacarea carbonica 6c	Place 3–4 pellets under the tongue 3–4 times daily.	Improves mineral absorption and utilization.
Magnesia phosphorica 6c	Place 3–4 pellets under the tongue 3–4 times daily.	Relieves spasm.

RECOMMENDATIONS

■ Good lighting is important, especially since some persons with nystagmus are also light sensitive. If necessary, hire a lighting specialist.

■ Ask your doctor about having an MRI. A brain scan will help to rule out disorders that may be contributing to the nystagmus.

Optic Atrophy

Optic atrophy (AT-roh-fee) was first described by the German eye specialist Theodore Leber in 1871, so it is often known as Leber's primary optic neuropathy. It consists of a slow decay, or dying, of the optic nerve. The illness usually occurs in males, although some females are affected. There is no warning of the onset of the condition.

Once a member of a family is diagnosed as having optic atrophy, other members of the family become potential sufferers or carriers. Only females can pass the problem on to their children, however; males are not known to transmit the disease. Fortunately, not every at-risk individual will become a sufferer. Unfortunately, there is no way of predicting who will develop the symptoms. If the symptoms do develop, both eyes are normally involved, even if to varying degrees. The eyesight can deteriorate over a period of hours to months. Very rarely, the eyesight may partially or completely improve again.

There is no proven cause of or cure for the disease. Genetic defects have been identified in some sufferers, but they do not yet help to predict future sufferers, as many people carry the defects, but do not lose their vision. Research has shown a deficiency of an enzyme called rhodanese, but the significance of this finding is also unknown. However, since one of the functions of rhodanese is to detoxify cyanide, doctors recommend that subjects at risk of developing optic neuropathy do not smoke and, when possible, avoid dietary cyanogens. Some of the early changes that occur in the eyes of sufferers, such as an increase in the number of minute blood vessels at the back of the eye and the loss of color vision prior to vision loss, may also be found in subjects at risk, but, as above, this does not help to predict which people will lose their sight.

CONVENTIONAL TREATMENT

Most sufferers of optic atrophy are registered as legally blind, although many retain enough usable eyesight to remain navigational—that is, they can move around fairly well in familiar surroundings, but cannot drive and cannot read without massive magnification. Typically, sufferers cannot recognize people in the street, although they may be able to discern moving shapes as they approach. Glasses and contact lenses are of no practical help. There is often no way of recognizing a sufferer in public because the defect is in the optic nerve. The eyes appear normal to the casual onlooker. During the acute phase of sight loss, however, cessation of physical exercise is recommended, as this helps to conserve energy at a time when the energy supply of the optic nerves may be failing.

SELF-TREATMENT

Optic atrophy is a severe condition that usually is not treatable. Some benefits may be derived from syntonics, a type of color therapy that can serve to stimulate and balance the nerves in the proper way. Maintaining a healthy lifestyle can help to overcome many disabilities.

NUTRITIONAL SUPPLEMENTS		
Supplement	Directions for Use	Comments
Vitamin A	Take 25,000–50,000 IU daily.	Good for all eye conditions.
Vitamin-B complex	Take 75–100 mg daily.	Maintains healthy nerves.

HOMEOPATHIC REMEDIES		
Remedy	Directions for Use	Comments
Nux vomica 6c	Place 3–4 pellets under the tongue 3–4 times daily.	Good for optic atrophy if the retina is atrophying. Reduces nerve and vascular irritability.
Phosphorus 6c	Place 3–4 pellets under the tongue 3–4 times daily.	Improves tissue metabolism, and supports nerve and vascular integrity.

RECOMMENDATIONS

■ Avoid smoking, smoke-filled rooms, and dietary cyanogens.

■ Consider treatment with hydroxycobalamin (vitamin B_{12}), which may be helpful.

■ Reduce your alcohol consumption, especially if you are in the process of losing your sight.

Optic Nerve, Decay of

See OPTIC ATROPHY.

Optic Nerve, Inflammation of

See OPTIC NEURITIS.

Optic Neuritis

Optic neuritis (nur-EYE-tis) is an inflammation of the optic nerve. It is also known as retrobulbar neuritis, since the nerve is behind (retro) the globe of the eye. Optic neuritis is generally experienced as an acute blurring, graying, or loss of vision, almost always in one eye, although occasionally in both eyes. The visual deficit usually reaches its maximum within a few days, and generally improves within eight to twelve weeks.

Optic neuritis typically presents with a triad of symptoms—loss of vision, disturbed color vision, and eye pain. The initial attack is in just one eye in 70 percent of adult patients and in both eyes in 30 percent. The mean age of onset of the disorder is the twenties, but it can develop anytime from birth through the sixties. The annual incidence of optic neuritis ranges from 1.4 to 6.4 new cases per 100,000 people. The associated visual symptoms include reduced perception of light intensity and visual deficit induced by exercise or increased body temperature.

The visual loss accompanying optic neuritis can be subtle or profound. In some cases, the vision may be 20/20 with the only symptom being blurring upon exertion. The rate of visual decline varies. The visual loss can occur over a period of hours (rarely) to days (most commonly). The peak visual loss most often is about one week after the onset of the disorder. The prognosis for visual recovery usually is good. The majority of patients (65 to 80 percent) recover a visual acuity of 20/30 or better. Most patients recover their visual acuity within a few months, although they often report some residual visual defects. These residual defects have included decreased contrast sensitivity, disturbed color vision, visual-field constriction, and light sensitivity.

It has been estimated that about 55 percent of patients with multiple sclerosis have an episode of optic neuritis. Frequently, optic neuritis is the first symptom of MS. While estimates of the subsequent development of MS in a person who presents with optic neuritis vary, studies with up to ten years of follow-up have demonstrated that approximately 50 to 60 percent of patients with isolated optic neuritis go on to develop MS. A more recent study reported that persons with optic neuritis who also had abnormalities in their spinal fluid were more likely to develop MS. Other studies have demonstrated that a majority of patients with optic neuritis have evidence of demyelination (wearing away of the nerve sheath) in the brain, as evidenced on MRI scanning. While other disease processes can cause optic neuritis, in a young, otherwise healthy person, MS is the most likely cause.

CONVENTIONAL TREATMENT

Recent studies suggest that a short course of intravenous steroids followed by a tapered course of oral steroids may be useful in helping to reverse and restore vision damaged by optic neuritis, although there is no definitive evidence that treatment with steroids effects a more complete recovery than no treatment at all.

SELF-TREATMENT

When a B-complex or B_1 deficiency is responsible for the optic neuritis, supplementing with these vitamins will result in recovery within three to four days. The B vitamins must be taken in adequate amounts even when a deficiency doesn't exist, however, since they are needed for the general health of nerve tissue.

A well-balanced diet is important for the maintenance and repair of the muscles and nerves. Whenever you have an infection, you should boost your protein, calorie, and fluid intakes.

NUTRITIONAL SUPPLEMENTS		
Supplement	Directions for Use	Comments
Essential fatty acids	Take as directed on the label.	Repair and rebuild the nerves.
Glutathione	Take 500–1,000 mg daily.	Supports the nerve and brain tissues.
Lecithin	Take 2 tbsp twice daily.	Protects and repairs the nerves. *Note:* Use the granular form.
Magnesium	Take 400 mg daily.	Helps the body to utilize the B-complex vitamins.
Protein	Take .5 gm for every 1 lb of body weight daily.	Important for the repair of body tissues.
Vitamin-B complex	Take at least 100 mg daily.	Good for nerve function.

HERBS AND HERBAL SUPPLEMENTS

Herb	Directions for Use	Comments
Bilberry	Take 60 mg daily.	An antioxidant.
Oats	Take as directed on the label.	Calms the nerves. Soothing for the mucous membranes.
Skullcap	Take as directed on the label.	Calms the nerves, and relieves spasm.
St. John's wort	Take as directed on the label.	An anti-inflammatory. Repairs and rebuilds the nerves.
Valerian	Take as directed on the label.	Calms the nerves, and relieves spasm.

HOMEOPATHIC REMEDIES

Remedy	Directions for Use	Comments
Aconite 6c	Place 3–4 pellets under the tongue 3–4 times daily.	Good for optic neuritis in the early stages. Good for pain and inflammation.
Apis mellifica 6c	Place 3–4 pellets under the tongue 3–4 times daily.	Good for inflammation.
Hypericum perforatum 6c	Place 3–4 pellets under the tongue 3–4 times daily.	Reduces nerve irritability.
Phosphorus 6c	Place 3–4 pellets under the tongue 3–4 times daily.	Good for many eye conditions.
Spigelia 6c	Place 3–4 pellets under the tongue 3–4 times daily.	Good for pain and nerve sensitivity.

RECOMMENDATIONS

■ Relaxation is a key component of the healing process. Reduce the stress level in all the areas of your life.

■ Avoid stimulants such as coffee, carbonated beverages, and cigarettes.

■ Increase your fluid intake.

■ Eat a diet of fresh fruits and vegetables, raw nuts and seeds, and whole grains.

Overconvergence of the Eyes

See CONVERGENCE EXCESS.

Photophobia

See LIGHT SENSITIVITY.

Pigment Deficiency

See ALBINISM.

Pimple on the Eyelid

See STYE.

Pinguecula

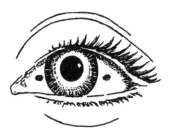

Pingueculae

The word "pinguecula" (pin-GWEK-yoo-lah) comes from the Latin word for "fatty." A pinguecula is a yellowish patch that forms in the white part of the eye, often at the three o'clock or nine o'clock position in relation to the cornea. There may be more than one pinguecula present in each eye. Pingueculae are completely different from jaundice, which causes a generalized yellowing of the entire sclera. Pingueculae are caused by exposure to excessive UV light, dust, or wind, and are common in farmers, gardeners, lifeguards, surfers, and construction workers. They do not need to be removed. Pingueculae do tend to swell when irritated, but they return to a stable condition once the irritant has been removed.

CONVENTIONAL TREATMENT

Currently, there is no medical treatment for pingueculae because they are not sight-threatening. They are cosmetically unappealing more than dangerous. However, the presence of pingueculae does indicate that the eye is under environmental stress, and that some action needs to be taken to remedy the situation. In general, the conventional treatment for pingueculae is to reduce the irritation to the eye.

SELF-TREATMENT

A soothing eyewash is the best remedy to quiet a pinguecula that is irritated. Use the herbal remedies below as eyewashes. *Do not* use eye drops that are intended to whiten the eye. Stay out of irritating environments, and wear sunglasses when outdoors for extended periods of time.

NUTRITIONAL SUPPLEMENTS		
Supplement	**Directions for Use**	**Comments**
Vitamin A	Take 25,000–50,000 IU daily.	Good for all eye conditions.
Vitamin C	Take 2,000–6,000 mg daily in divided doses.	Protects the eye, and aids tissue healing.
Zinc	Take 50 mg daily.	Enhances the immune response.

HERBS AND HERBAL SUPPLEMENTS		
Herb	**Directions for Use**	**Comments**
Chamomile	Apply as a hot compress or use as an eyewash.	Soothing for the eye tissues.
Eyebright and fennel	Apply as a hot compress or use as an eyewash.	Good for inflammation.

HOMEOPATHIC REMEDIES		
Remedy	**Directions for Use**	**Comments**
Apis mellifica 6c	Place 3–4 pellets under the tongue 3–4 times daily.	Relieves swelling around the eyes.
Pulsatilla 6c	Place 3–4 pellets under the tongue 3–4 times daily.	Good for eyelids that are stuck together.
Ruta graveolens 6c	Place 3–4 pellets under the tongue 3–4 times daily.	Good for hot, red eyes.
Sulphur 6c	Place 3–4 pellets under the tongue 3–4 times daily.	Good for red eyelids.

RECOMMENDATIONS

■ Watch your cholesterol level. Some experts feel that a pinguecula might indicate a high blood-cholesterol level. However, no research has as yet been conducted to explore this connection.

■ If you believe that you may have a pinguecula, see your eye doctor. A routine examination should confirm your self-diagnosis and allay any fears that your condition is more serious.

Pinkeye

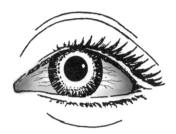

Pinkeye

Pinkeye, more properly known as conjunctivitis (con-junk-tiv-EYE-tis), refers to an inflammation of the conjunctiva (con-junk-TIE-vah). The conjunctiva is the mucous membrane that lines the eyelids and also covers the exposed surface of the sclera. Pinkeye can be caused by a bacterial, viral, or fungal infection; by an allergy; or by anything that has irritated the conjunctiva. When pinkeye is caused by an infection, it is highly contagious. It can be spread by sharing a towel, handkerchief, or makeup brush.

Bacterial conjunctivitis can be recognized by a discharge that contains pus and sticky, crusty eyelids that may have to be pried open in the morning. The area under the eyelids is beefy red, and the eyes feel sore. The white part of the eyes looks red, with large, twisted blood vessels. Bacterial conjunctivitis can strike people of all ages, but it's especially common in children, whose hand washing and other hygienic practices tend to be less than adequate. Children should be encouraged not to rub their eyes with dirty fingers. Bacterial conjunctivitis is usually self-limiting and generally responds to hot compresses, but if it doesn't resolve within a few days, you should see an eye doctor.

Viral conjunctivitis looks a little different from the bacterial type. The viral type is somewhat more common in adults than in children, although children also get it. This kind of infection may start in the eyes, or it may be a part of a systemic virus that is also causing a cold or sore throat. (When this happens, it just means that the virus has gotten into the conjunctiva along with other parts of the body.) The discharge from the eyes is usually more watery and less sticky than with a bacterial infection. The conjunctiva inside the eyelid is red and sometimes has raised spots that look like little cobblestones. The eyes hurt and look red. Antibiotics don't help viral conjunctivitis, but the infection usually clears up within a few days without any treatment.

Fungal infections of the conjunctiva can also occur, especially in people whose immune systems are not functioning properly, such as cancer and AIDS patients and people taking medications that suppress the immune system (for example, after an organ transplant). Fungal infections can be dangerous and require prompt treatment with special antifungal medications. It's hard to diagnose fungal conjunctivitis by yourself, but if you develop any kind of conjunctival infection while on medications that suppress your immunity or while being treated for AIDS or cancer, see your doctor immediately.

Allergic conjunctivitis is pinkeye caused by an allergy. An important feature that distinguishes allergic from infectious conjunctivitis is itching. Infections of the conjunctiva hurt; allergic reactions itch. Also, the eyelashes usually do not become matted with allergic conjunctivitis as they do with an infection, especially a bacterial one. The conjunctiva is usually swollen, and although the sclera may be red, the undersides of the eyelids are pale. There is a watery discharge. Allergic reactions involving the eyes frequently also involve sneezing, wheezing, and other symptoms of allergies to animals or plants. These reactions can be treated with antihistamines by mouth or with eye drops that block allergic reactions. It is also very helpful to wash out your eyes with an eyewash if you've been around something to which you're allergic.

In general, pinkeye can be a very trivial or a potentially serious problem. See your eye doctor if your pinkeye doesn't clear up within a couple of days.

CONVENTIONAL TREATMENT

The conventional treatment for pinkeye generally depends on the cause of the condition. Bacterial conjunctivitis is usually treated with antibiotics. Viral conjunctivitis can be treated with antivirals, but often it is left untreated because it may clear up as a result of the systemic viral treatment. Some doctors recommend the use of steroid ointments or eye drops to alleviate the inflammation in viral conjunctivitis, but this may be dangerous. If the infection happens to be caused by a herpes virus, the steroids can make it much worse. Sometimes it's best to just leave well enough alone. Fungal forms of conjunctivitis are treated with antifungals. Allergic conjunctivitis is treated symptomatically—that is, by reducing the itching and inflammation of the eye tissue along with treating the rest of the allergy symptoms.

SELF-TREATMENT

You can try to treat your pinkeye with a hot compress (very warm water on a washcloth) two or three times a day. Use this treatment specifically if your lids are sticking together in the morning. However, if the pinkeye doesn't resolve within a few days, see your doctor. If you suspect allergic conjunctivitis, use a cold compress to reduce the itching. In addition, be sure to clean your hands and face often, and splash your eyes with cold water. *Do not* use any over-the-counter preparations that promise to remove redness from the eyes. However, there are several herbal and homeopathic eye treatments that may help.

NUTRITIONAL SUPPLEMENTS		
Supplement	**Directions for Use**	**Comments**
Vitamin A	Take 25,000 IU daily.	Good for all eye conditions.
Vitamin C	Take 2,000–6,000 mg daily in divided doses.	Protects the eye, and aids tissue healing.
Zinc	Take 50 mg daily.	Enhances the immune response.

HERBS AND HERBAL SUPPLEMENTS		
Herb	**Directions for Use**	**Comments**
An mian pian (Brion)	Take 4 pills 3 times daily.	Purges "heat" from the liver.
Chamomile	Apply as a hot compress or use as an eyewash.	Soothing for the eye tissues.
Eyebright *and* fennel	Apply as a hot compress or use as an eyewash.	Boost the circulation.
Long dan xie gan wan (Brion)	Take 6 pills twice daily.	Purges "heat" from the liver and gallbladder.
Ming mu di huang wan (Brion)	Take 10 pills 3 times daily.	Good for red or itchy eyes.
Ming mu shang qing pian (Brion)	Take 4 pills twice daily.	Good for red, itchy, or burning eyes. *Caution:* Do not use during pregnancy.

Herb	Directions for Use	Comments
Nei zhang ming yan wan (Brion)	Take 8 pills 3 times daily.	Good for itchy, painful eyes. *Caution:* Contains aluminum, so limit its use.
Shi hu ye guang wan (Brion)	Take 1 pill twice daily.	Good for red or itchy eyes.
Xiao yao wan (Brion)	Take 8 pills 3 times daily.	Invigorates a congested liver.

HOMEOPATHIC REMEDIES

Remedy	Directions for Use	Comments
Aconite 6c	Place 3–4 pellets under the tongue 3–4 times daily.	Good for inflammation.
Allium cepa 6c	Place 3–4 pellets under the tongue 3–4 times daily.	Good for inflammation.
Anacardium 6c	Place 3–4 pellets under the tongue 3–4 times daily.	Alleviates swelling.
Apis mellifica 6c	Place 3–4 pellets under the tongue 3–4 times daily.	Good for pinkeye with swollen eyelids. Alleviates edema and inflammation.
Arnica montana 6c	Place 3–4 pellets under the tongue 3–4 times daily.	Good for inflammation.
Arsenicum album 6c	Place 3–4 pellets under the tongue 3–4 times daily.	Good for inflammation.
Belladonna 6c	Place 3–4 pellets under the tongue 3–4 times daily.	Good for inflammation.
Calcarea fluorica 6c	Place 3–4 pellets under the tongue 3–4 times daily.	Relieves discharge. Good for inflammation.
Calcarea sulfurica 6c	Place 3–4 pellets under the tongue 3–4 times daily.	Relieves discharge. Good for inflammation.
Causticum 6c	Place 3–4 pellets under the tongue 3–4 times daily.	Relieves discharge.
Euphrasia officinalis 6c	Place 3–4 pellets under the tongue 3–4 times daily.	Good for inflammation.
Mercurius corrosivus 6c	Place 3–4 pellets under the tongue 3–4 times daily.	Good for pinkeye with mucous discharge. An infection fighter.
Mercurius vivus 6c	Place 3–4 pellets under the tongue 3–4 times daily.	Relieves discharge. Good for inflammation.
Natrum muriaticum 6c	Place 3–4 pellets under the tongue 3–4 times daily.	Good for inflammation.
Pulsatilla 6c	Place 3–4 pellets under the tongue 3–4 times daily.	Relieves discharge. Good for inflammation. Good for allergic conjunctivitis.
Rhus toxicodendron 6c	Place 3–4 pellets under the tongue 3–4 times daily.	Good for inflammation. Alleviates swelling.
Ruta graveolens 6c	Place 3–4 pellets under the tongue 3–4 times daily.	Good for inflammation.
Sepia 6c	Place 3–4 pellets under the tongue 3–4 times daily.	Good for inflammation. Alleviates swelling.
Silicea 6c	Place 3–4 pellets under the tongue 3–4 times daily.	Good for inflammation.
Sulphur 6c	Place 3–4 pellets under the tongue 3–4 times daily.	Good for inflammation. Good for allergic conjunctivitis.

RECOMMENDATIONS

■ Pinkeye is one of the most contagious diseases currently known. Children seem to be more susceptible to it, probably due to their lack of proper hygiene. Teach your child to wash his or her hands properly and to keep the hands away from the eyes.

Pinkeye, Contact-Lens-Related

See GIANT PAPILLARY CONJUNCTIVITIS.

Presbyopia

During our first thirty to forty years of life, our eyes work busily to see everything they can, especially when we read and perform other near-point tasks. When our eyes are relaxed, they are, theoretically, in focus for distance vision. When we move closer to an object, we must actively increase the focal power of the lenses inside our eyes to keep the object clear. This is very easy to do when our eyes—and our bodies—are young. In fact, our focusing ability is at its maximum when we are five years old. As we grow older, however, our eyes' lenses become stiffer, and our maximum focusing ability—actually, the ability of our lenses to become rounded, as they must in order to do near-point work—diminishes. Eventually, we notice a blur at close range.

Although this process of the lenses becoming hardened is continuous throughout life, it isn't given a name until we are unable to clear the near (sixteen-inch) image comfortably. The condition is then called presbyopia (prez-bee-OH-pee-ah). The word comes from the Greek word *presbys*, which means "old", and *opia*, which refers to "vision."

Looking at this problem in perspective should help to give you a better idea of why it happens. Consider prehistoric man. In those early caveman days, the life expectancy was only about twenty-five to thirty years. The only near-point activities were cooking and making weapons, neither of which was extremely detailed work. Most of the visual requirements at that time were distance tasks, such as spotting that night's dinner and keeping from becoming someone else's dinner. So really, our eyes were made to focus for our entire lifetimes—except that we now outlive our eyes' focusing lifetimes.

CONVENTIONAL TREATMENT

One way to compensate for the deficiency in near vision is to use a prescription lens that helps the eye to focus. If you already wear glasses to see clearly at a distance, you'll need two different lens prescriptions—one for distance vision and one for near vision. One way to handle this double prescription is with bifocals, eyeglass lenses in which the top half of the lens is for distance vision and the lower half is for near vision. Do not use the kind of reading glasses that can be bought without a prescription. They are not likely to be the exact prescription you need, and the lenses will be of poor optical quality.

SELF-TREATMENT

There is a school of thought that says presbyopia is not an inevitable consequence of aging, but instead is the result of years of improper nutrition, stress, inadequate exercise, and faulty oxygenation of the body. Even if you do everything right, you cannot prevent the development of presbyopia entirely, but you may be able to postpone it or slow it down with good nutrition, aerobic exercise, and generally healthful living. Like any part of the body, the lens will stay younger longer with the aid of good overall health. In addition to general exercise and good nutrition, if you are reaching the "bifocal age," you should do the following simple technique several times a day. The technique consists of focusing from near to far (at least twenty feet away) and back to near again. This keeps the muscle that controls the lens in good working order. (For more techniques that may help, see "Vision Therapy" on page 235.)

NUTRITIONAL SUPPLEMENTS		
Supplement	Directions for Use	Comments
Glutathione	Take as directed on the label.	Maintains the clarity of the lens.
Vitamin B$_2$	Take 50 mg daily.	Alleviates eye fatigue.
Vitamin C	Take 5,000–6,000 mg daily in divided doses.	Maintains the flexibility of the lens.
Vitamin E	Take 200 IU daily.	Alleviates eyestrain.

HOMEOPATHIC REMEDIES		
Remedy	Directions for Use	Comments
Calcarea fluorica 6c	Place 3–4 pellets under the tongue 3–4 times daily.	Supports the connective tissue.

RECOMMENDATIONS

■ Presbyopia is a gradual process, though you may wake up one day and discover that reading is suddenly difficult. Maintaining your focusing ability is much easier than trying to regain a lost ability. Watch what you eat, get enough exercise, and try to keep your stress level down. In addition, as you approach your fortieth birthday, practice the focusing technique described in "Self-Treatment," above.

Pterygium

A pterygium (ter-IDJ-ee-um) has some similarity to a pinguecula, but is shaped differently, is located in a different spot in the eye, and has more blood vessels. A pinguecula is a yellowish patch on the white part of the eye. (For a complete discussion of pingueculae, see page 182.) A pterygium is a triangular-shaped white area containing a lot of blood vessels. In fact, the word "pterygium" comes from the Greek word for "wing." While a pinguecula does not interfere with vision and therefore does not need to be removed, a pterygium grows onto the cornea, where it can obscure vision, and therefore should be removed. To determine if what you have is a pinguecula or a pterygium, look in the mirror. If the patch is starting to cover a part of your iris, you have a pterygium. There is usually only one pterygium in each eye, and it is most often located on the side of the eye nearest the nose. No exact cause for pterygiums is known, but the condition does occur more frequently in hot, dusty climates, and it is often seen among surfers, who spend hours in the windy ocean spray and sun.

Pterygium

CONVENTIONAL TREATMENT

Most eye doctors prefer to leave pterygiums alone until they begin to encroach on the line of sight, where they can interfere with vision. Previously, pterygiums tended to grow back after being removed. However, the newer laser procedures are more effective at removing them, and regrowth is now rare.

SELF-TREATMENT

Once a pterygium has started to grow, the best thing you can do is to reduce the environmental assault on it. Stay out of windy, dusty, sunny, and smoky environments. In addition, keep your eyes lubricated and moist.

NUTRITIONAL SUPPLEMENTS

Supplement	Directions for Use	Comments
Vitamin A	Take 25,000–50,000 IU daily.	Good for all eye conditions.
Vitamin C	Take 2,000–6,000 mg daily in divided doses.	Protects the eye, and aids tissue healing.
Zinc	Take 50 mg daily.	Enhances the immune response.

HERBS AND HERBAL SUPPLEMENTS

Herb	Directions for Use	Comments
Chamomile	Apply as a hot compress or use as an eyewash.	Soothing for the eye tissues.
Eyebright *and* fennel	Apply as a hot compress or use as an eyewash.	Boost the circulation.

HOMEOPATHIC REMEDIES		
Remedy	Directions for Use	Comments
Apis mellifica 6c	Place 3–4 pellets under the tongue 3–4 times daily.	Relieves swelling around the eyes.
Ruta graveolens 6c	Place 3–4 pellets under the tongue 3–4 time daily.	Good for hot, red eyes.
Sulphur 6c	Place 3–4 pellets under the tongue 3–4 times daily.	Good for red eyelids.

Ptosis

See DROOPING EYELIDS.

Pupils, Different-Sized

See ANISOCORIA.

Recurrent Corneal Erosion

Recurrent corneal erosion is a condition in which the outermost cells of the cornea fail to adhere to their basement membrane. It usually follows a corneal abrasion, and most often happens in dry-eye conditions.

The outermost cells of the cornea are about five rows deep and are anchored to the membrane located behind them. When you scratch your cornea, these cells are scraped away, leaving very sensitive nerves exposed. Normally, the cells grow back rapidly, in as quickly as twenty-four hours. However, if the scrape is unusually deep, you may have lost all five layers of cells and exposed the bare membrane. In this situation, it will take longer for the cells to grow back because of the extent of the damage. In addition, while your eye heals, you may try to function as normal, and may irritate the area and stall the healing process. The new cells may be brushed off before they have had a chance to adhere firmly to the basement membrane.

CONVENTIONAL TREATMENT

The mildest approach to treating this disorder is to use artificial tears or a temporary antibiotic. This often includes the use of a lubricating ointment at bedtime to prevent the eyelids from sticking to the loose corneal cells. If this approach is not successful, a bandage contact lens may be used to protect the cornea from physical contact with the eyelids. This bandage contact lens will likely be in the form of a disposable soft contact. If the scratch is deep, a pressure bandage may be required.

If these mild treatments are not effective, a more radical approach will be necessary. This radical approach is called anterior stromal puncture (ASP), in which about forty to sixty micropunctures are made into the front part of the cornea. These micropunctures allow the cells to adhere better to the basement membrane. Though somewhat painful, ASP is effective in severe cases of recurrent corneal erosion.

SELF-TREATMENT

If your doctor diagnoses recurrent corneal erosion, prepare yourself for a long healing process. It will take anywhere from a week to a month or more, and will depend mostly on your environment. Use the lubricants prescribed by your doctor as often as necessary. Even more important are the ointments prescribed for application at bedtime. Use warm compresses to relax your eyes before you open them in the morning. (Obviously, you will need help preparing them.) Finally, stay out of dry or smoky environments.

NUTRITIONAL SUPPLEMENTS

Supplement	Directions for Use	Comments
Vitamin A (Viva-Drops)	Take 1–2 drops 3–4 times daily for 2 days.	Supports the corneal tissue as it heals.
Vitamin C	Take 500 mg twice daily for 2 days.	Builds collagen tissue.

HERBS AND HERBAL SUPPLEMENTS

Herb	Directions for Use	Comments
Bayberry, eyebright, *and* goldenseal	Use as an eyewash twice daily.	Good for all eye conditions. *Caution:* Do not take goldenseal internally for more than 1 week. Do not use goldenseal during pregnancy.
Comfrey	Use as an eyewash.	Promotes healing.
White willow bark	Take 400 mg as needed.	Good for pain.

HOMEOPATHIC REMEDIES

Remedy	Directions for Use	Comments
Aconite 6c	Place 3–4 pellets under the tongue every 3–4 hours, or put 2 drops in 1 cup of water and use as an eyewash.	Good for pain. Good for inflammation.
Hypericum perforatum 6c	Place 3–4 pellets under the tongue every 3–4 hours, or put 2 drops in 1 cup of water and use as an eyewash.	Reduces the effects of a nerve injury.

RECOMMENDATIONS

■ Keep your eyes well lubricated at all times. Even during sleep, the lids may creep apart, allowing the eye to dry out to some degree. If necessary, use surgical tape to keep the lids closed while sleeping.

■ Avoid sunny, windy, dusty, and other drying environments.

Red Eyes

See BLOODSHOT EYES.

Refractive Errors, Differing

See ANISOMETROPIA.

Retina, Peeling

See RETINAL DETACHMENT.

Retinal Bleeding

See DIABETIC RETINOPATHY.

Retinal Detachment

Retinal detachment is the peeling away of the retina from the back of the eye, the way you might imagine wallpaper peeling away from a curved surface. A healthy retina is securely attached to the choroid layer of the eye. In retinal detachment, a hole or tear in the retina allows fluid to collect between the retina and the choroid, leading to separation.

Retinal detachment can occur for many reasons, not all of them injuries, although a blunt or penetrating injury to the eye is a common cause of the condition. Nearsighted eyes and protruding eyes are more prone to retinal detachment than normal eyes and farsighted eyes, probably because the retinas are more tautly stretched. Recent cataract surgery is another risk factor.

Everyone should know the symptoms of retinal detachment because failure to seek treatment in time can result in blindness in the affected eye. A developing retinal detachment is heralded by flashes of light that look like sparks or flickers, a large number of floaters in the field of vision, and a shadow or curtain that spreads from the edge of the visual field to the central vision. You may also notice a shimmering effect, such as what you see when you look through gelatin. However, you will not feel pain from the retina, since the retina does not contain pain receptors. (You may, of course, feel pain from elsewhere in the eye if an injury caused the detachment.)

FIRST AID FOR RETINAL DETACHMENT

✚ Stabilize your eye—lie down and keep your eyes very still, preferably closed.

✚ Have someone take you to the eye doctor or emergency room quickly, but carefully.

CONVENTIONAL TREATMENT

A detached retina can be reattached by an ophthalmologist if it is caught in time. If there is only a small hole, a laser may be used to seal it. If there is a large tear and the retina is actually peeling away from the eye, a freezing probe will be used to make the retina adhere to the choroid again. Many times, a strap called a scleral buckle is attached around the eyeball to compress it slightly and allow the retina to contact the choroid once again.

In extreme cases, an air bubble is injected into the vitreous portion of the eye. Air bubbles always rise, so the patient is put on a tilted table and rotated to the position that will allow the rising bubble to push the retina back into place.

SELF-TREATMENT

There isn't much that you can do for yourself to reattach a detached retina. Getting prompt attention is your first priority; seconds count! The only thing to do is to lie down very quietly and stay in this position. This occasionally allows the retina to fall back into place. Do not make any sudden moves—either with your head or your eyes—and stay quiet and relaxed until you can see an ophthalmologist.

NUTRITIONAL SUPPLEMENTS		
Supplement	Directions for Use	Comments
Vitamin A	Take 25,000–50,000 IU daily.	Supports the retina.
Vitamin-B complex	Take at least 100 mg daily.	Good for nerve function.

Retinal Holes or Tears

See LATTICE DEGENERATION.

Retinitis Pigmentosa

Retinitis pigmentosa (ret-in-EYE-tis pig-ment-OH-sah) is an inherited disease that affects approximately 1 out of every 3,700 people. Retinitis pigmentosa (RP) causes deterioration of the retina with progressive loss of sight starting at about the age of ten. The first symptoms are increasing night blindness and difficulty seeing in dim light. Then, the peripheral vision gradually decreases, until the person feels as if he or she is looking through a tunnel (tunnel vision), with only a small "island" of central vision. Fortunately, this island may last until the person is well along in years. However, the loss of peripheral vision will eventually make it impossible for the person to drive or do many mobile tasks.

CONVENTIONAL TREATMENT

The medical community has no treatment for RP. Traditional medical practitioners recommend getting in touch with a low-vision clinic and using the best low-vision aids you can obtain.

However, a recent breakthrough in tackling retinitis pigmentosa was made by a team of molecular geneticists in New Zealand. The researchers found defects in two genes in the retinal epithelium, a layer of cells at the back of the eye. They discovered that a number of retinal diseases are caused by genetic mutations in the epithelium. The two defective genes give instructions to two proteins that play a vital role in transporting vitamin A to the eye's light-detecting cells, which need a continuous supply of the nutrient to function. These researchers believe certain RP cases can be cured by supplementation with raised levels of vitamin A, something that has been suspected for many years, but could not be proved. The ancient Egyptians treated blindness with ground-up roasted ox liver, a high source of vitamin A. One of the New Zealand researchers conducted much of his practical research in India, in communities where intermarriage and large families are common. This researcher said that it may take generations to prove vitamin A is a preventive cure. But for some known sufferers, vitamin-A treatment could be as dramatic as insulin treatment is for diabetics.

For persons with RP who do not respond to vitamin A, another treatment possibility is transplantion of the epithelial layer. This technology, which is already within grasp, may offer a cure to up to one-third of RP sufferers.

NUTRITIONAL SUPPLEMENTS		
Supplement	Directions for Use	Comments
Vitamin A	Take 75,000 IU daily.	Good for all retinal conditions. *Note:* Use the emulsion form for easier assimilation and greater safety.

194

HOMEOPATHIC REMEDIES		
Remedy	Directions for Use	Comments
Nux vomica 6c	Place 3–4 pellets under the tongue 3–4 times daily.	Good for nerve inflammation.
Phosphorus 6c	Place 3–4 pellets under the tongue 3–4 times daily.	Supports nerve and vascular integrity.

RECOMMENDATIONS

■ For more information on RP, contact the Retinitis Pigmentosa Foundation. For the address and phone number, see "Resource Organizations" on page 255.

Retrobulbar Neuritis

See OPTIC NEURITIS.

Scratched Cornea

See CORNEAL ABRASION.

Spots Before the Eyes

See FLOATERS.

Strabismus

"Strabismus" (stra-BIZ-muss) is the technical term for crossed eyes. Actually, "crossed" is somewhat of a misnomer, because in strabismus, an eye can be turned upward, downward, inward, or outward. Crossed eyes is just one form of strabismus. When an eye is turned toward the nose—toward the nasal side—it's usually called cross-eyed. When an eye is turned toward the ear—toward the temporal

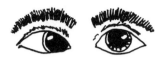

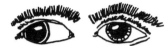

Strabismus

In the top pair of eyes, the eye on the left is cross-eyed. In the bottom pair of eyes, the eye on the left is wall-eyed.

side—it's called wall-eyed. In children, strabismus usually involves an eye that is turned nasally. About half of the people who have strabismus were born with it. Somewhere along the line, the eye-brain hookup became incorrectly "wired." Some authorities believe that strabismus is hereditary. It may be, since it often occurs in the same family.

What is the cause of strabismus? Believe it or not, we don't really know for sure in many cases. Strabismus may be induced by a poor visual environment—for example, by isolating an infant in a dark room or by keeping an infant positioned with the same eye closer to the mattress. The eyes are intended to receive light; they function best in light. The more they are used, the better they develop. The more visual stimulation a child is given, the more visual experience the child has, and the better is his or her visual development. If a child's visual stimulation is deficient or limited to one side, the child's visual system will not develop symmetrically.

The eyes are directly connected to the brain and are controlled from there. So are the six sets of eye muscles attached to the eyeballs. (For an illustration of the eye muscles, see below.) These muscles control where the eyes are aimed. Years ago, doctors thought that the incorrect turning of an eye was a purely mechanical error, caused by an eye muscle that was too long or too short. They believed that all they had to do to straighten out the eye was to surgically shorten or move a muscle. Sound logical? Well, maybe. But consider this: An eye muscle is a hundred times stronger than it needs to be to turn an eyeball. Why, then, can't it just pull the eye in the correct direction without the benefit of surgery?

The answer turns out to be that strabismus is usually a problem of eye-brain coordination, not just of muscles being too short or too long. When the eye muscles of a child with strabismus are tested, they are usually found to be in perfect working order—even though the child can't aim both of the eyes in the same direction.

CONVENTIONAL TREATMENT

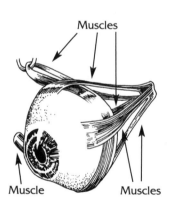

The muscles that control the eye.

Some ophthalmologists still routinely recommend eye surgery to correct strabismus. I usually advise against surgery for strabismus, although it does help in some extreme cases. Most of the time, I find that surgery doesn't really correct the problem; it only makes the eyes appear to be aimed at the same point. If you have been given a recommendation to have this type of surgery, first consult an ophthalmologist who specializes in the procedure, as well as an optometrist who uses nonsurgical therapeutic techniques to teach the eyes to work together. (For a discussion of nonsurgical therapeutic techniques, see "Vision Therapy" on page 235.)

Surgical treatment for strabismus, however, is beneficial in some cases. For children, pediatric ophthalmologists sometimes choose to operate on the muscles of both eyes, even though only one eye may be turned. They move the muscles on both eyes further back, thus loosening the tension on the muscles. They operate on both eyes because they have found that when only one eye is operated on, the other eye may end up "following" the first eye. For example, if a nasally-turned eye is operated on and pulled temporally, the other eye may turn nasally. Therefore, the operation that is often performed to straighten a nasally-turned eye will weaken the power of the muscles on the nasal side of both eyes.

Another surgical procedure for strabismus involves only the turned eye. If the eye is turned nasally, the muscle on the nasal side is moved back, as in the other operation, to reduce the tension on that side. In addition, the muscle on the temporal side is shortened to increase the tension on that side and turn the eye toward the temporal side. To turn an eye toward the nasal side, the muscle on the temporal side is moved back, with the muscle on the nasal side shortened.

SELF-TREATMENT

There are several ways to treat strabismus without surgery. One way is to force the child to use the turned eye by covering the good eye for prescribed periods of time. This is called occluding the vision in the good eye. The good eye can be covered with a patch or with an opaque lens in a pair of eyeglasses. The vision in the good eye can also be occluded with the use of eye drops that cause blurring. However, you have to be careful not to obscure the vision in the good eye for too many hours of the day or you may risk losing it. Futhermore, because strabismus is a binocular problem, simply using one eye is not the final answer. It is simply a first step in assuring that each eye works to its maximum ability. Your eye doctor should be able to guide you to the best nonsurgical therapy.

Another way to treat strabismus without surgery is to use eyeglasses. Sometimes, childhood strabismus is caused by farsightedness. The child tries to compensate for the farsightedness by overconverging the eyes—that is, making both of the eyes turn inward too much. This kind of strabismus should be treated with glasses that correct the farsightedness.

There are also a number of techniques and activities that can be done to prevent or treat strabismus in an infant or child:

■ Place your infant on his or her back. Standing directly in front of the child, gently grasp both of the child's wrists and slowly pull him or her up. Repeat this technique a few times as if it were a game, being careful not to tire the child. This technique will help the child's neck muscles to develop properly. Good control of the neck muscles aids in the development of binocular vision.

■ Hold your infant in the air and attract his or her attention to your face. Gradually bring the child closer to you, causing the child's eyes to converge. Bring the child all the way to your face and make a funny sound when your noses touch, then lift the child away again. Repeat this technique a few times as if it were a game, being careful not to tire the child. This technique will develop the child's ability to converge the eyes effectively.

■ Drape a piece of material with bold black and white stripes over the edge of your child's crib. The stripes will stimulate the child's visual development.

■ Place your child in an infant seat or high chair, and line up four or five squeaky toys just out of his or her reach. Sitting across from your child, squeeze the farthest toy on your left. As soon as your child looks at that toy and attempts to grasp it, squeeze the farthest toy on your right. When your child reaches for this second toy, squeeze a toy on your left again. Continue squeezing different toys only as long as the child feels it's a game; stop if the child becomes frustrated or irritable. This technique will stimulate the child's eyes to move in both directions.

■ Have your child look through a stereoscopic viewer, such as a View-Master, at three-dimensional slides. Stereoscopic slides are available with cartoon characters, animals, and other things that children enjoy. Ask the child whether the character or animal looks as if it's "sticking out" (three dimensional). The child will see a three-dimensional image only if he or she uses binocular vision.

For older children, try the techniques recommended for coordination on page 23.

NUTRITIONAL SUPPLEMENTS

Supplement	Directions for Use	Comments
Manganese	Take 4 mg daily.	Stimulates the nerve-muscle connection.
Vitamin A	Take 25,000 IU daily.	Good for all eye conditions.
Vitamin-B complex	Take 100 mg daily.	Good for proper nerve growth.

HOMEOPATHIC REMEDIES

Remedy	Directions for Use	Comments
Aluminum 6c	Place 3–4 pellets under the tongue 3–4 times daily.	Good for strabismus affecting the right eye. Improves coordination.
Calcarea carbonica 6c	Place 3–4 pellets under the tongue 3–4 times daily.	Good for strabismus affecting the left eye. Relieves spasm.
Phosphorus 6c	Place 3–4 pellets under the tongue 3–4 times daily.	Good for many eye conditions.

RECOMMENDATIONS

■ Always get a second opinion if your doctor recommends surgery for strabismus. Once the muscles are cut from the eyeball, their signals to move the eye are never the same.

■ Therapists very often recommend gross-motor techniques, such as ball bouncing, hopping, jumping, and crawling, to help the body acclimate to bilateral stimulation. Play games with your child that incorporate these movements, such as basketball, hopscotch, and jumping rope.

Stye

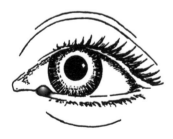

Stye

A stye, technically called a hordeolum (hord-ee-OH-lum), is a common problem caused by a bacterial infection in one of the small glands on the edges of the eyelids or just under the eyelids. Children frequently get styes from rubbing their eyes with dirty hands, but adults also get them from time to time, and sometimes it's hard to say how the infection got started.

A stye looks and feels like a pimple on the eyelid—because that's what it really is. It is often somewhat painful. You can differentiate a stye from a chalazion, a similar infection, by tugging slightly at the eyelid skin. If the pimple or swollen area moves *with* the skin, it's probably a stye. If the skin slides *over* the mass, it's likely a chalazion. Chalazia are most often painless. (For a complete discussion of chalazia, see page 101.)

CONVENTIONAL TREATMENT

Most styes go away within a week or so, but a stubborn one can be incised and drained by a doctor. Topical antibiotics are also sometimes used.

SELF-TREATMENT

A stye can be brought to a head by steam bathing. One way to do this is to cover a wooden spoon with gauze, dip the spoon in boiling water, and then hold the spoon so that it *does not touch the eye*, but the steam rises to the eye. Repeat the procedure when the spoon cools. You can also use a washcloth soaked in warm water or one of the herb teas listed below.

There are some over-the-counter remedies for styes that contain a compound called mercuric oxide. These remedies may work, but the mercury in these preparations can be very irritating to the eye. Mercury causes itching, stinging, and redness in many people. For this reason, I don't recommend these products.

FIRST AID FOR A STYE

✚ Apply a warm wet washcloth as a hot compress to the affected eye three to four times a day.

✚ *Do not* squeeze the stye, even if it comes to a "head."

NUTRITIONAL SUPPLEMENTS		
Supplement	**Directions for Use**	**Comments**
Vitamin A	Take 25,000–50,000 IU daily.	Good for all eye conditions. Especially beneficial if styes are a frequent problem.

HERBS AND HERBAL SUPPLEMENTS		
Herb	**Directions for Use**	**Comments**
Eyebright	Apply as a compress or use as an eyewash.	Good for all eye conditions.
Raspberry	Apply as a compress or use as an eyewash.	Alleviates redness and irritation.

HOMEOPATHIC REMEDIES		
Remedy	**Directions for Use**	**Comments**
Apis mellifica 6c	Place 3–4 pellets under the tongue 3–4 times daily.	Alleviates swelling.
Graphites 6c	Place 3–4 pellets under the tongue 3–4 times daily.	Good for styes accompanied by severe discharge.
Lycopodium 6c	Place 3–4 pellets under the tongue 3–4 times daily.	Good for styes accompanied by severe discharge.
Pulsatilla 6c	Place 3–4 pellets under the tongue 3–4 times daily.	Good for styes accompanied by mucous discharge. Especially good for styes in the upper eyelids of children. Good for inflammation.

Remedy	Directions for Use	Comments
Sepia 6c	Place 3–4 pellets under the tongue 3–4 times daily.	Good for styes accompanied by watery discharge.
Staphysagria 6c	Place 3–4 pellets under the tongue 3–4 times daily.	Good for lumps in the eyelids. Especially good for recurrent styes. Supports the connective tissue. Good for inflammation.
Sulphur 6c	Place 3–4 pellets under the tongue 3–4 times daily.	Good for recurrent styes. Good for inflammation.

RECOMMENDATIONS

■ Do not attempt to drain the head of a mature stye. Doing this can lead to more serious problems. Instead, contact your doctor for proper treatment.

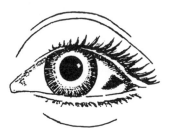

Subconjunctival Hemorrhage

Subconjuntival Hemorrhage

A subconjunctival (SUB-con-junk-TIE-val) hemorrhage is bleeding from broken blood vessels under the conjunctiva of the eye, between the conjunctiva and the sclera. It is a problem that looks much more serious than it is. A subconjunctival hemorrhage can result from a jarring injury, such as a blow to the head from a basketball, or from anything that increases the pressure in the delicate blood vessels of the conjunctiva, such as intense coughing, sneezing, vomiting, or pushing during childbirth. The area where the bleeding occurs appears as a bright red patch on the white sclera. There is no pain, and vision is not affected. Of course, if you're having any symptoms that concern you, such as pain or visual disturbances, see your eye doctor.

CONVENTIONAL TREATMENT

Since the blood will be absorbed and the eye will return to normal within one to three weeks, a subconjunctival hemorrhage does not need to be treated. In fact, no real treatment exists for this particular problem. However, since subconjunctival hemorrhages are often caused by trauma to the eye, it is important to have a professional evaluation performed to assure that all of the structures of the eye are intact and functioning normally.

SELF-TREATMENT

If you notice a subconjunctival hemorrhage and know when you received it, apply cold compresses to your closed eyelid for the first day or two. This will slow any bleeding. For the next day or two, do nothing, then begin to apply warm compresses. This treatment will help the pooled blood to break down more quickly and the condition to resolve. In any case, a subconjunctival hemorrhage will usually disappear on its own in a short time.

TREATMENT FOR SUBCONJUNCTIVAL HEMORRHAGE

✚ Apply a cold wet washcloth as a compress to the affected eye when you first notice a subconjunctival hemorrhage. Repeat several times during the first twenty-four hours.

✚ No treatment other than the cold compresses on the first day is necessary during the first forty-eight hours.

✚ On the fourth day, begin applying warm compresses to the affected eye. The warm compresses will hasten the breakdown of the visible blood.

NUTRITIONAL SUPPLEMENTS

Supplement	Directions for Use	Comments
Calcium *and* magnesium	Take 1,000–1,500 mg of a combination supplement daily.	Essential for blood clotting.
Vitamin A	Take 25,000–50,000 IU daily.	Good for all eye conditions.
Vitamin C	Take 3,000 mg daily.	Important for blood clotting.

HERBS AND HERBAL SUPPLEMENTS

Herb	Directions for Use	Comments
Alfalfa	Take as directed on the label.	A good source of vitamin K.

HOMEOPATHIC REMEDIES

Remedy	Directions for Use	Comments
Arnica montana 6c	Place 3–4 pellets under the tongue 3–4 times daily.	Good for subconjunctival hemorrhage caused by injury. Reduces hemorrhaging and venous congestion.
Sanguinaria 6c	Place 3–4 pellets under the tongue 3–4 times daily.	Improves vaso-motor activity, and reduces congestion.

RECOMMENDATIONS

■ If you experience subconjunctival hemorrhages frequently, especially without apparent causes, you should consult your internist.

Suppression

As discussed in "The Eyes and the Visual System" on page 5, your two eyes receive images that must be fused together in the brain to form one picture. If this fusion isn't accomplished with efficiency, you will experience two pictures, or "see double." Since double vision is a most unwanted condition, the brain will probably turn off one of the two images it perceives. This is called suppression.

Fortunately for your brain and visual system, you can experience double vision without ever knowing it. Unfortunately, there may be no clues that let you know you need to seek help. The suppression of images therefore can go on for years with no indication of a problem, especially if the problem begins early in life. Most children think that all people see the same way. Whether their vision is good or bad, they have no concept of clear vision.

Studies have found that children who are efficient at suppression are actually good readers and learners. This may sound contradictory, but it really isn't. If there is a severe conflict between the two eyes and the brain has a very difficult time fusing the two images, it makes it very easy for the brain to suppress one image and see fine with the one eye that it chooses to use. However, if there is a very subtle difference between the two eyes and the brain occasionally suppresses one image, or if the two eyes constantly battle for fusion, there will be a conflict and the symptoms of poor reading and decreased learning will become apparent.

CONVENTIONAL TREATMENT

The treatment for suppression depends, unfortunately, on the doctor you see for your eye examination. Since suppression in some people is subtle and occasional, it takes a special, in-depth type of examination of the visual system to be detected. If your doctor is more interested in just making sure your eyes are healthy and seeing 20/20, your suppression problem will likely be missed.

Since suppression problems affect children and their learning abilities the most, it is critical that an examiniation for this condition be included in all their vision exams. An optometrist who specializes in functional, or behavioral, vision will give the most appropriate evaluation. If found early, suppression usually can be treated with a program of vision therapy. (For a discussion of vision therapy, see page 000.)

SELF-TREATMENT

Since the visual system follows the path of least resistance to seeing, there may not be much that you can do to force your brain not to suppress your vision. However, a good vision-therapy program should include techniques that you can perform at home on a regular basis. These techniques should allow you to use both eyes efficiently and effectively. Check with your doctor to see what kind of vision therapy would be best for your particular condition.

RECOMMENDATIONS

■ Vision therapy is not a quick fix, so be patient (no pun intended!). However, you also need to be aggressive in taking control of your vision.

Tunnel Vision

See RETINITIS PIGMENTOSA.

Underconvergence of the Eyes

See CONVERGENCE INSUFFICIENCY.

Vision, Distorted

See ASTIGMATISM.

Vision Suppressed in One Eye

See SUPPRESSION.

Wall Eyes

See STRABISMUS.

White Patch on the Cornea

See PTERYGIUM.

Yellow Patch on the Sclera

See PINGUECULA.

Part Three
Eye-Care Techniques and Procedures

Introduction

There are several techniques and procedures used by eye-care specialists that help to serve your visual needs. Included are a variety of procedures and materials to produce appliances to enhance eyesight, as well as a number of surgical procedures to save eyesight. In Part Three, we will review these techniques and procedures concerned with preserving and improving vision. We will examine such "extreme" methods as acupressure and color therapy, as well as more common ones such as eyeglasses and contact lenses. We will also delve into such interesting techniques as cataract surgery, corneal transplant, ortho-keratology, refractive surgery, and vision therapy. Hopefully, you will gain enough of an understanding of each of these techniques and procedures to enable you to discuss them with your eye doctor if you ever need to decide which is the most appropriate method for resolving your particular condition.

Acupuncture and Acupressure

The basis of traditional Chinese medicine is acupuncture, a technique for treating certain conditions and for producing anesthesia by passing long thin needles through the skin to specific points that affect the nerve-transmission signals. Although acupuncture has been practiced for about 5,000 years, and textbooks on the subject go back about 2,000 years, the practice is only now becoming accepted in the West.

The technique known as acupressure is a modification of acupuncture. It is a safe, simple, and inexpensive treatment. Acupressure is a method of achieving relaxation and inducing healthy tissue changes (such as increased blood flow) by massaging the same points that the Chinese penetrate with needles. Although both acupressure and acupuncture have been promoted as pain-reducing procedures, they also increase energy to the points in the body, as well as achieve a number of specialized results.

Some of the points used in both acupuncture and acupressure are shown in the illustrations below. The points on the faces and hands in these illustrations are used by Chinese acupuncturists to treat conditions such as nearsightedness and other refractive errors, excessive tearing, eyelid twitching, sinusitis, and strabismus. You can use these points to give your eyes and head area a healthful, relaxing massage. To give yourself an acupressure massage, refer to the illustrations as you read the following instructions:

1. Locate the point on your hand called *hoku*. To do this, move the thumb of the hand you wish to massage up next to the forefinger of the same hand. Notice the hump that results in the muscle within the *V* formed by the bones of the thumb and forefinger. (See Figure 3.1, below.) The peak of that hump is the *hoku* point.

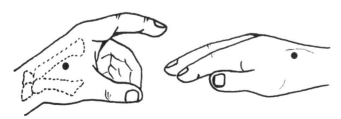

Figure 3.1. The *hoku* point.

Press the *hoku* point while relaxing the other muscles in that hand. Repeat with your other hand. Massaging the *hoku* point is believed to increase the circulation and nerve energy to the head region.

2. Using the thumb and forefinger of one hand, massage the two points on either side of the bridge of your nose at the level of your eyes. (See Figure 3.2, below.) These points are called *jing ming*, and massaging them is believed to fight eye disease and facial payalysis.

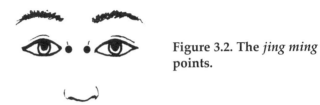

Figure 3.2. The *jing ming* points.

3. Press the forefingers and middle fingers of each hand together, then place the pairs of fingers on your cheeks next to your nose near the nostrils. Anchor your thumbs under your lower jawbone, then remove your middle fingers and massage your cheeks with your forefingers. These points on your cheeks are called *si bai*, and massaging them is believed to combat eye disease, headache, and eyelid twitching. (See Figure 3.3, below.)

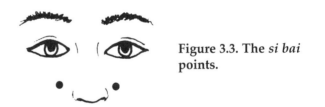

Figure 3.3. The *si bai* points.

4. Using the outsides of your forefingers, rub along the bony ridges above and below your eyes. (See Figure 3.4 on page 210.) Keep your other fingers curled under, and anchor your thumbs on each side of your forehead. By rubbing along the bony ridges, you will massage four points around each eye—*zan zhu* (point 1 in the illustration), located above the inside corner of the eye; *yang bai* (point 2 in the illustration), located over the eye; *tong zi liao* (point 3 in the illustration), located at the outside corner of the eye; and *cheng qi* (point 4 in the illustration), located below the eye. Massaging the *zan zhu* point is believed to fight headaches. Massaging the *yang*

bai point is believed to help night blindness and glaucoma. Massaging the *tong zi liao* point is believed to combat the headaches accompanying eye diseases. And massaging the *cheng qi* point is believed to improve conjunctivitis, nearsightedness, and optic atrophy.

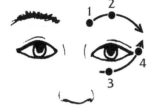

Figure 3.4. Massaging the *zan zhu* (point 1), *yang bai* (point 2), *tong zi liao* (point 3), and *cheng gi* (point 4) acupressure points.

To massage an acupressure point, apply threshold pressure to the point with your finger or thumb. Threshold pressure is firm pressure, pressure on the "threshold" of becoming painful. The idea behind acupressure is to stimulate the point, but not cause the muscles to tighten from pain. The pressure should be firm but gentle. Apply threshold pressure to a point for ten seconds, then release for ten seconds. Repeat the pressure-release cycle eight times. Another method is to apply continuous pressure for one to five minutes.

Cataract Surgery

A cataract is a clouding of the lens within the eye. As discussed in "Cataracts" on page 96, the clouding can be partial or complete. Therefore, the interference to vision that cataracts cause runs the gamut from slight to severe. However, a cataract that causes a slight problem today may develop into a disabling condition. This is because the type of cataract that occurs with advancing age is generally progressive. Luckily, not all cataracts reach the point where they obscure vision.

When your cataract does interfere significantly with your vision and your lifestyle, your doctor will most likely recommend surgery. Consider that cataract surgery is the most common surgical procedure done in the United States today, with about 1.5 million operations performed annually. Most surgeons will ask you how well you feel you are functioning in your daily life with your cataract. Your answer will be a determining factor in the decision on whether or not to operate. A few different surgical techniques are currently in common use, and you and your surgeon can decide which one is best for you. Sometimes, cataract surgery can be done as an outpatient procedure.

TYPES OF CATARACT SURGERY

The two types of surgery most commonly used for cataracts are extracapsular cataract extraction and intracapsular cataract extraction.

The lens of the eye is surrounded by a capsule that helps to keep it in place. In extracapsular cataract extraction, a bit of this capsule is removed, with the cataract-covered lens either taken out or washed out of the remaining capsule. The main advantage of this procedure is that most of the capsule is left intact to continue performing its function of dividing the front and back parts of the eye. In addition, it can support an artificial lens implanted in your eye as a replacement for the extracted lens. (For a further discussion of this, see "How You See After Cataract Removal," on page 211.) Extracapsular cataract extraction is now used in about 65 percent of cataract operations.

Another way to remove a cataract is to remove the cataract-covered lens while it is still in its capsule—that is, both the lens and lens capsule are removed. This procedure is called intracapsular cataract extraction. These days, the lens and capsule usually are frozen first to make extraction easier and to minimize bleeding. The main advantage of this method is that every bit of lens tissue and capsule tissue is removed so that no cataract or cloudiness can form in the future. When the capsule is left in the eye, it may itself become opaque, or remnants of the old lens may grow over it and make it cloudy. These problems are known as secondary cataracts, or aftercataracts. The main disadvantage of intracapsular cataract extraction is that, once the lens capsule has been removed, the vitreous humor no longer has a dam to prevent its oozing into the front part of the eye, where it doesn't belong and can cause some trouble. Another problem is that the capsule is no longer present to support an artificial lens implant.

A technique that can be used during an extracapsular extraction is phacoemulsification (fake-oh-ee-MUL-si-fi-KAY-shun). With this technique, the cataract is emulsified (broken up) using ultrasonic energy. Once emulsified, it is aspirated (sucked out). Phacoemulsification has the advantages of a smaller incision and faster postsurgical wound healing than other methods of extraction.

Contrary to what many people believe, lasers are not normally used in cataract surgery. Lasers burn holes in tissue, and a lens with a hole isn't any better than a lens with a cataract. However, lasers are usually used to get rid of secondary cataracts.

New and better procedures are now being developed to remove cataracts. The new procedures involve smaller incisions and have fewer complications.

HOW YOU SEE AFTER CATARACT REMOVAL

By now, you may be wondering: "But if my lens is removed, how will I be able to see?" Without a lens, you will have very poor visual acuity. Fortunately, there are ways to get around this problem. You may have heard of cataract glasses or may have even seen people wearing them. Years ago, these heavy, thick glasses had to be worn after cataract surgery. They were not only unsightly, but also left something to be desired in terms of optical correction. Nowadays, people who have a lens removed have it replaced with either a contact lens worn on the cornea or with a plastic lens inserted in the eye right where their own lens used to be. The latter type of lens, called an artificial intraocular lens, is put into place immediately, during the cataract surgery. Today, almost 100 percent of persons who have a cataract extracted have an intraocular lens implanted within the eye.

Both the lens worn on the cornea and the artificial intraocular lens work only for distance vision, however. No artificial lens is yet available that can change the shape of the eyeball to change the focus, although some are currently in the early stages of research and development. There are some trial studies being done in which an artificial intraocular lens is ground into the optical correction of a bifocal, therefore allowing the person to see both distance and near objects clearly. This device is still experimental, though, and doesn't always work effectively. For most people to do near-point work such as reading, glasses are still necessary—but most people old enough to have a cataract need reading glasses anyway!

Contact Lenses

Contact lenses are an optical device made to fit over the cornea of the eye to change its refractive characteristics and improve vision. Many people ask me how I feel about contact lenses. Well, I feel fine about contacts, but I don't have to wear them. Contact lenses are a highly individual experience. Some people love their contacts, and others simply can't wear them no matter what kinds they try. About 27 million Americans now wear contact lenses, and many additional people give them a trial run every year.

If you can move past the idea of putting something in your eye, you will find that contacts do offer some advantages over glasses. Perhaps the most obvious one is that the majority of people prefer the way they look without glasses. In addition, you can now go one step beyond just removing your glasses—you can actually change your eye color through the use of tinted contacts. However, appearance is not the only reason to wear contact lenses. If you're very nearsighted, for example, your eyeglass lenses will be concave in shape. When you look straight ahead through the centers of the lenses, you will find that your prescriptions are exactly what you need, but as you get away from the centers and move out toward the peripheries of the lenses, you will experience a lot of distortion. The lenses, out of necessity, are thicker around the peripheries, so they don't correct your vision very well when you look through that part. Nor do you have any correction beyond the edges of the frame. With contacts, the lenses stay right on the corneas and move with your eyes, so you are always looking through their optical centers, where there is virtually no visual distortion.

Until the 1970s, contact lenses caused a lot of problems. They were made of hard, impermeable materials—glass until the late 1930s, and a hard plastic until the 1970s. In addition, until the 1950s, they covered the entire front of the eye, not just the cornea, as they do now. The cornea needs to take in oxygen and get rid of carbon dioxide, and it must stay wet. The early contacts didn't permit oxygen and carbon dioxide to permeate, thus causing the cornea to swell. In the 1970s, new materials became available, and lenses that are gas-permeable and hydrophilic (water-loving) were developed. Today, lenses are also available in soft and rigid materials.

Let's take a look at some of the different kinds of contacts, and how to wear them and care for them.

TYPES OF CONTACT LENSES

Modern contact lenses have been around since the 1950s, but they've come a long way since then in terms of the materials from which they're made, their comfort and wearability, and the kinds of conditions they can correct. In general, today's contacts are much more comfortable than those of the past, but not everyone can wear them. Among those who have difficulty with contact lenses are people with chronically dry eyes because of a medical condition or medication (antihistamines are a problem); people with allergies that make their eyes itch and swell; and people with extremely sensitive eyes who can't tolerate the thought of having something resting on their eyeballs. But with the variety of materials and designs available today, most people do find something that fits their needs.

Hard Contacts—The Originals

The earliest contact lenses were developed in Germany in 1927. They were made of glass and covered the entire visible sclera. In 1937, an early type of plastic was developed for use in contact lenses, but the lenses still covered the whole visible sclera. These newer lenses were introduced in the United States in 1938.

In 1940, a plastic called polymethylmethacrylate (PMMA) came into use for contacts, which were still made to cover the whole front of the eye. In 1950, the first patent was granted for lenses made of PMMA that covered only the cornea. These smaller plastic lenses were routinely fitted during the 1950s. They were somewhat flexible, but they still earned the name "hard lenses." The plastic could be molded inexpensively, polished to a smooth optical surface, and modified with relative ease. (A minor prescription change was an office procedure.) The lenses maintained a good optical transparency that did not fade with time, they didn't crack too easily, they didn't sustain bacterial growth (which could cause infection), and they could be tinted slightly to make them easier to see when dropped.

These lenses, however, also had a downside. The material had no ability to transmit oxygen or carbon dioxide, which made them unhealthy for the cornea, and solutions had to be used to help water or tears adhere to the surface. It took some determination to wear these lenses because they were so uncomfortable. However, a certain number of brave souls were able to tolerate them, and they were a definite improvement for those with very high prescriptions. The lenses, if not lost, could sometimes last for as long as ten or fifteen years (though no contact lens should be used for that long).

Today, hard contact lenses are obsolete. The newer materials have all but displaced them from optometrists' inventories. If you're still wearing a hard lens material, ask your eye doctor about the newer types of lenses. They're more comfortable and healthier for your eyes.

Soft Contacts for Daily Wear

In the 1960s, a Czechoslovakian chemist named Dr. Otto Wichterle developed a new type of plastic that he thought could be utilized to make artificial blood vessels and organs until he used a child's erector set to experiment with using it for contact lenses. Called hydroxyethylmethacrylate, or HEMA, this material changed the world of eye care forever.

These soft contacts—now referred to as daily-wear soft lenses—were introduced to the public in 1971 by the Bausch & Lomb Company of Rochester, New York, and marked the beginning of a whole new era in contact-lens technology. The material was 38-percent water, and was called hydrophilic because it also absorbed water. The lenses were more permeable to oxygen and carbon dioxide than hard lenses, and their comfort level was incredible compared to that of the hard lenses. However, the vision through the soft lenses was not quite as sharp as that through the hard lenses, and these early lenses could not correct for astigmatism. Also, in addition to absorbing water, these lenses had an affinity for infection-causing bacteria. The care of the lenses was therefore complicated, often calling for disinfection by heat unit every night. Even so, the incidence of eye infections in soft-lens wearers remained higher than that in hard-lens wearers. The lenses tended to yellow with age, could rip rather easily, and lasted for only a year or two despite their substantial price. But for persons who were nearsighted, did not have astigmatism, and were reliable enough to disinfect the lenses every night and replace them every year or two, these lenses were wonderful.

In 1976, soft contact lenses became available for people with astigmatism. These lenses, called toric lenses (*torus* is Latin for "bulge"), were manufactured using a computerized lathe that could cut different curves into different areas of one lens in much the same way that eyeglass lenses are made. These lenses also had some limitations, however, and were unable to correct for large amounts of astigmatism, but they worked very well for many people. The first astigmatism lenses were slightly uncomfortable because they had a bulge on the lower edge to keep them positioned properly over the cornea. This thickness was noticeable, but the lenses were still more comfortable than hard lenses. They were made of the same material as daily-wear soft contacts, so their care was the same, and so were their other problems. The current astigmatism lenses have thinner edges and are also available in other materials.

Today, soft contacts for daily wear are still popular and can be chemically disinfected instead of needing to be sterilized with heat.

Rigid Gas-Permeable Contacts for Daily Wear

Patented in 1974 and introduced to the public in 1979, rigid gas-permeable lenses were the next advancement in technology for hard lenses. They looked and acted like hard lenses, but they could absorb small amounts of fluid and were able to transmit oxygen and carbon dioxide to and from the eye. This was due to the addition of silicone to the plastic material. The silicone made the lenses more comfortable and adaptable than the original hard lenses. Because these new lenses were not as hard as the original lenses, they were called "rigid" rather than "hard." Many people who wore the hard lens but had some discomfort were now able to upgrade to the newer material with almost no change in their vision or care regimen. The only drawback to the updated plastic material was that, although the silicone aided in gas transmission, it made the surface difficult to wet. Therefore, some people experienced a drying of the eyes toward the end of a day of wearing the lenses. Luckily, this was more of a discomfort than a danger. Today, there is a newer generation of gas-permeable lenses that can be comfortably worn by most people. These lenses are a good alternative for those patients who can't get good visual correction with soft lenses or who don't want the risk of infection that soft lenses pose.

Soft Contacts for Extended Wear

Probably the biggest explosion in the contact-lens field was the advent of contact lenses that could actually be worn overnight for days at a time. The only problem seemed to be that the lenses were extremely fragile, although that drawback has been significantly improved since the early days.

In 1981, the FDA approved extended-wear soft con-

tacts designed to be worn for thirty days at a time without cleaning or disinfecting. Unfortunately, this proved to be too long a wearing period and earned the lenses some bad press—not entirely undeserved. In September 1989, the *New England Journal of Medicine* published an article based on a study sponsored by the Contact Lens Institute, a group of contact-lens manufacturers. The study noted that the risk of corneal ulcers, which can occur with infections of the cornea, was five times greater in extended-wear-lens users than in daily-wear-lens users, although the problem still occurred in only 0.2 percent (2 out of every 1,000) of all extended-wear-lens users. All of a sudden, everyone was afraid to sleep in contact lenses. Many medical practitioners called for no overnight wear of lenses, even though the study did note that the risk of infection increased proportionally with the wearing time.

The members of the Contact Lens Institute now recommend that extended-wear lenses not be worn for more than seven days and nights by the average patient. They also recommend that certain patients not wear their lenses overnight at all or do so only occasionally. People who have a high level of protein in their tears, have chronically dry eyes, have eyes that do not close completely due to surgery on the eyelids, or work in exceptionally dirty environments are advised to remove, clean, and disinfect their lenses every night.

Many patients remove their lenses every night that they're home, but leave them in occasionally over the weekend or during a camping trip, for example. This practice has been called "flexible wear," and it is in fact a term that some manufacturers are now using to describe these lenses in an attempt to get away from the controversy associated with the term "extended wear." Today's extended-wear soft lenses are less fragile than their predecessors, and can stand up to being handled daily as well as being left in the eye for a few days.

Rigid Gas-Permeable Contacts for Extended Wear

In early 1987, the FDA approved rigid gas-permeable contact lenses that could be worn overnight for up to seven days. These lenses were made of a material specifically designed for extended wear, and had the optical and handling advantages of hard lenses combined with a wearability closer to that of soft lenses. The key difference was the addition of fluorine to the silicone material during the manufacturing process.

This allowed the best combination of gas transmission and moisture maintenance of any lenses yet developed. Rigid gas-permeable lenses for extended wear have been available for some time now, with several manufacturers elaborating on the basic concept. The lenses offer many advantages in the areas of lens life and visual clarity. The material allows for a flexible wearing schedule similar to that of extended-wear soft lenses. It is durable enough to be handled daily, yet apparently is safe enough to be left in the eye for several days. The Contact Lens Institute study on extended-wear problems did not include any rigid gas-permeable lenses. More research needs to be done to determine the safety of this kind of extended-wear lenses. However, these lenses seem to have great potential for capturing the hearts of millions of contact-lens wearers.

Disposable Contacts

In 1987, Johnson & Johnson's contact-lens subsidiary, Vistakon, released the first disposable contact lenses, called Acuvue. Acuvue lenses were the same as extended-wear soft lenses, but were made in an entirely new way. In fact, the new process enabled the lenses to be produced and sold so cheaply that they could be discarded after being worn for just one or two weeks.

I have my patients wear their disposables for up to two weeks, and I tell them to use a disinfecting solution on the lens between wearings. (Some patients take their lenses out before going to bed, for example.) Some doctors feel, however, that disposable lenses should be worn only once; once a lens is out of the eye, it should be discarded, even if it was in the eye only for an hour. There is some controversy about this, so I recommend that you follow your doctor's instructions, which should be based on the condition of your eyes.

A small number of eye doctors have some reservations about disposable lenses and whether or not patients use them correctly, but the patients I fit with them simply love them. Most contact-lens companies make disposables, and almost all doctors fit them. If you choose to have these, just be sure that you complete the follow-up care. Wearers of disposable lenses should visit their optometrists for a vision examination every three months, as compared to every six to twelve months for the wearers of other types of lenses. Simply ordering lenses by mail is asking for trouble.

Vistakon has kept pace with the changes in contact lenses by introducing daily-wear disposable lenses, called Surevue. Surevue lenses are essentially the same as Acuvue lenses except they are thicker and easier to handle. They are designed to be removed daily, cleaned regularly, and disposed of every two weeks. In 1994, Vistakon also released One-Day Acuvue lenses. These are daily-wear disposables—they are inserted in the morning and thrown away at night. One-Day Acuvue lenses are much more expensive than the other types of lenses, especially since you need 720 lenses a year, but they do have some applications.

You can also get disposable contacts that are clear but block up to 90 percent of UV light. I don't routinely recommend contacts as a substitute for a good pair of UV-blocking sunglasses, but people concerned about UV exposure to the eye may find them very useful.

Frequent-Replacement Contacts

Since disposable soft contact lenses were first developed, the trend has been toward more frequent replacement of contacts. The traditional daily-wear soft lenses are gradually becoming obsolete, with frequent-replacement contacts becoming the preferred lenses. Frequent-replacement lenses, though not really disposable, are replaced every one to three months, depending on your particular program.

Doctors are very enthusiastic about frequent-replacement lenses because they stay cleaner due to being replaced more often. This is especially true since the publication of the studies showing that lenses which are worn longer are more likely to cause infections. Most patients also appreciate the convenience of frequent-replacement lenses. The lenses are comfortable, and the cost is becoming more comparable to that of daily-wear lenses when the solution costs are factored in. Lenses replaced monthly do not require an enzyme cleaner, the cost of which is a major expense.

Bifocal Contacts

Even back in the 1970s, bifocal contacts were available. However, the original bifocal contacts had all the drawbacks of hard lenses and weren't tolerated very well by a large number of patients.

Nowadays, bifocal contacts are available in rigid gas-permeable and soft materials. The rigid types have a success rate for vision correction of about 70 percent, and people who are already used to this material seem to have little trouble adapting to the bifocal version.

The first bifocal soft contact lenses became available in 1985. The theory of how they should work was well-developed, yet in practice the lenses did not perform as expected. Since then, there have been several different forms of bifocal soft contacts, each using a different technique to achieve clarity for near as well as distance vision. Unfortunately, none has proven to be the ultimate lens design. Current success rates for vision correction are running at about 40 to 50 percent at best.

But presbyopes, take heart. Since most contact-lens wearers are baby boomers who are now reaching their early fifties, many contact-lens manufacturers are putting big money and effort into the research and development of a successful and comfortable bifocal contact lens. New designs are being developed constantly, so it should be only a short time before the next generation of lenses hits the market. There is even a bifocal disposable lens that was recently introduced.

Until a bifocal contact lens that works for a larger percentage of the population is developed, many doctors are using a technique called monovision for bifocal patients who want contacts. In the monovision technique, one eye is fitted with a near-vision prescription lens, and the other eye is fitted with a distance-vision prescription lens. Then, because of suppression, the brain shuts off the image from the distance lens when you look at something close up, and it shuts off the image from the near lens when you focus for distance. You don't develop lazy eye because each eye is used some of the time. This way of seeing takes the brain about two weeks to learn, but it works surprisingly well (although not perfectly). If you don't want to wear glasses but need bifocals, you might want to give monovision a try.

Tinted Contacts

For many years, hard and rigid contact lenses have been available with a slight tint, called a handling tint, that is not really visible on the eye, but just dark enough to allow the lenses to be found if accidentally dropped. Manufacturers haven't, and probably won't, try to make these lenses able to change a person's eye color because both these types of lenses are slightly smaller than soft lenses and don't quite cover the iris.

If you had brown eyes and wore a pair of these lenses tinted blue, for example, you'd have a blue lens ringed by a brown iris, which might look interesting, but isn't likely to become popular.

Beginning in about 1984, however, a process of tinting lenses enough to change eye color was developed for soft lenses. These tinted soft lenses caught on and gave lens wearers an additional choice. The first tinted lenses only changed the color of light blue or green eyes. Then, in 1986, Wesley-Jessen, Inc. of Chicago introduced lenses with an opaque tint that would actually make a brown eye appear blue, green, or aquamarine. The contact-lens industry boomed again. About a third of the new tinted lenses that were sold had no prescription, but were purchased for cosmetic purposes only. Today, these lenses are available in colors with names such as baby blue, sapphire, and misty gray, and many optometrists offer free trials to see what difference they can make in your appearance. Theoretically, there's nothing wrong with wearing contact lenses to change your eye color, but it's important to remember that these lenses are made of the same material as prescription daily-wear and extended-wear soft lenses, and need to be given the same care. They are still medical devices, not makeup.

ADAPTING TO CONTACT LENSES

Although the contact-lens experience is a very individual one, there are a few common symptoms and signs of which you should be aware.

When you first start wearing contact lenses, your eyes will go through a period of physiological adaptation; they will actually learn to ignore the contact lenses. (In fact, you could adapt to and ignore an eyelash stuck in your eye if it were present long enough.) Adaptation to rigid lenses can take up to a week or two; to soft lenses, up to a few days. Contacts (unlike eyelashes) are designed to be on your eyes, and most people will adapt to them. By the way, calluses do not build up on the insides of the eyelids when you wear contacts, as some people believe.

You will be put on a wearing schedule when you first get your lenses. Be sure to stick to the wearing times, even if the lenses feel great. Sometimes a problem may exist that you can't feel until the lens is removed. An average wearing schedule for adapting to soft lenses and rigid gas permeables is four hours the first day, five hours the second day, and so on, adding progressively more hours until you can wear your lenses all your waking hours by the seventh day. Follow your doctor's advice about adapting to your lenses.

Some of the sensations you may notice with rigid gas-permeable lenses include an increased sensitivity to the sun and wind, awareness of the lenses, frequent blinking, fluctuating tear flow, and transient blurred vision. If any of these symptoms persists for more than seven days, tell your doctor when you return for your follow-up exam.

Soft-lens adaptation is much more subtle. The lens sensation usually disappears within the first thirty to ninety minutes of wearing time. Although these lenses are very comfortable, your vision may occasionally blur, and you may experience some drying of the lenses and of your eyes. Again, let your doctor know what you experience.

WEARING AND CARING FOR CONTACTS

Rigid gas-permeable and soft contacts require slightly different kinds of care. Following is what I tell my patients about wearing and caring for their contact lenses. Your doctor may have other do's and don'ts to add to this list.

For all types of contact lenses:

■ Wash your hands with a non-creamy, non-oily soap before handling your lenses. Most pump soaps contain creams. Use Ivory or a clear soap such as Neutrogena.

■ Keep your fingernails manicured and short.

■ Check your lenses often for nicks and other damage. If a lens has a defect, you can still wear it if it's comfortable, but be especially careful about how you handle it. Order a replacement lens as soon as possible.

■ Never use saliva to wet your contact lenses. Saliva is full of bacteria. It's not the same as tears, which are free of bacteria unless you have an eye infection. You can cause a very serious infection by inserting saliva-coated lenses into your eyes. In fact, it's better to put rigid gas-permeable lenses on dry than to wet them with saliva. If necessary, you can wet rigid lenses with bottled, distilled, or filtered tap water. Wet your soft lenses only with a wetting solution; do not use water. Unfiltered tap water is not clean enough, and any kind of water, including bottled and distilled, will be absorbed by the lenses and may cause distortions.

Soft-lens wearers should always have some wetting solution on hand to use in an emergency.

■ Close the drain when you insert or remove your lenses over a sink.

■ Never insert lenses if your eyes are red or irritated. Wait twenty-four hours, and if the symptoms persist, call your doctor.

■ Insert your lenses before applying makeup, but after using hair spray.

■ Use cream (not powdered) eye shadow and water-soluble makeup. Oils and face creams can cause a film to build up on the lenses.

■ Do not rub your eyes intensely while the lenses are in place.

■ Avoid anything that may cause dry eyes, such as smoke, wind, and dust.

■ Do not swim with your lenses inserted unless you wear goggles. Wait at least one hour after swimming in chlorinated water to reinsert the lenses.

■ Wear sunglasses to help reduce any light sensitivity caused by your lenses.

■ Remove a lens immediately if a foreign body becomes lodged in your eye. Rinse your eye and the lens thoroughly before re-inserting the contact. Do not wear the lens if the discomfort continues.

■ Establish a routine of always removing the same lens first to avoid accidentally interchanging your lenses.

■ Clean your lenses, rinse them thoroughly, and disinfect them daily as directed. In addition, change the storing solution daily. How well you do this has a profound effect on how long your lenses will last.

■ Use the cleaning and storing solutions that your doctor recommends. There are hundreds of different solutions on the market today, so be careful what you buy if you switch brands. Do not switch solutions without your doctor's approval.

■ Clean your lens case periodically by boiling a pot of water, removing it from the heat, and soaking your empty case for at least twenty minutes. A dirty case can contaminate clean lenses.

■ Do not wear lenses when using eye medications or when you have an eye infection. Do not use commercial eye-whitening drops.

■ Call your doctor if you have a question about wearing your lenses while using a systemic medication.

■ Do not sleep with your lenses without your doctor's approval.

■ Keep a backup pair of glasses on hand, even if you wear your lenses all the time. There may be a time when you are unable to wear your contacts, because of either an infection or a lost lens.

■ Have your ocular health, visual acuity, and lens performance evaluated at least once a year.

For soft contacts:

■ Handle your lenses as little as possible and then only with your fingertips. Never handle your lenses with your fingernails. Do not crease your lenses.

■ Check your lenses before inserting them to make sure they are not inside out. If a lens is inside out, it may pop out of your eye when you blink or cause irritation, discomfort, or blurred vision.

■ Keep your lenses wet when they're not in your eyes. Should a lens dry out, carefully place it in your storing solution or saline for at least four hours. If it is intact, feels comfortable in your eye, and does not negatively affect your vision, it can be safely worn. However, once a lens has dried, it is weakened and may tear more easily.

■ Use only the disinfecting method prescribed by your doctor. Chemical disinfecting systems, including hydrogen peroxide, cannot be interchanged with heat disinfecting systems. Do not change methods without your doctor's approval.

■ Ask your doctor about ultrasonic cleaning, which is highly effective in slowing down the buildup on lenses when performed regularly. (Soft lenses cannot be polished.)

For a listing of the different characteristics of hard, soft, rigid gas-permeable, and disposable lenses, see the table below.

Most vision problems today can be at least partially corrected with contact lenses. Much of the success of contacts, however, still depends on motivation. In my practice, I prefer to start a patient with soft lenses because of the comfort factor, and then move to rigid lenses if the soft lenses aren't satisfactory. Other optometrists like to start with rigid gas-permeable lenses, then go to soft lenses if the rigid ones don't work out. However, some cases call for a gas-permeable fit right away. If you've been wearing hard lenses without much discomfort, you should probably go to rigid gas-permeable rather than soft lenses because the visual acuity is somewhat better with the rigid lenses, and the required care and handling will be closer to what you're used to.

If you're interested in wearing contacts, ask your eye doctor for the latest information on the lenses that are appropriate for your eye problem.

LENS CHARACTERISTICS OF THE DIFFERENT KINDS OF CONTACTS

Characteristic	Hard Lenses	Soft Lenses	Rigid Gas-Permeable Lenses	Disposable Lenses
Visual acuity	Excellent	Good	Excellent	Good
Resistance to deposits	Excellent	Poor	Good	Poor
Comfort during first 1–2 weeks	Poor	Excellent	Fair	Excellent
Comfort after first 1–2 weeks	Good	Excellent	Good	Fair
Gas permeability	Poor	Good	Good to excellent*	Good
Durability	Excellent	Fair	Good	Poor
Ability to remain moist	Excellent	Excellent	Good to excellent	Good
Ease of care	Excellent	Fair	Excellent	Excellent
Ease of customizing fit	Excellent	Fair	Excellent	Fair
Flexibility in wearing time	Poor	Good	Good to excellent	Fair
Tintability	Good	Excellent	Good	Good

* Rigid gas-permeable lenses vary in their exact formulation depending on the manufacturer, so it's harder to generalize about their characteristics than about those of the other types of lenses.

Corneal Transplant

There are times when the cornea becomes deformed or defective. One of the more common versions of this is keratoconus. (For a complete discussion of keratoconus, see page 155.) Whatever the cause of the corneal deformity or defect, there is a procedure in which the damaged cornea can be removed and replaced with a donor cornea. Eye banks in major cities collect healthy corneas from recently deceased individuals who had indicated they wished to donate their organs, and fulfill requests from eye surgeons for these corneas. (This is the only use for donated eyes.) This is a highly organized and sophisticated system, and corneal transplants are quite common operations and very successful. The probability of rejection is less than that for any other transplanted organ simply because the cornea has no blood supply. The rejection of other organs is usually due to incompatibility between the donor and the recipient, and is mediated by blood cells.

While corneal transplantation has a 95-percent rate of success, this procedure, the same as all operations, involves potentially serious risks. In cases where the first transplant is not successful, a second can be undertaken with success. However, permanent loss of vision, though extremely rare, can also occur. Corneal transplantation is considered only in those cases in which contact lenses cannot be worn or provide inadequate vision correction.

While the surgical transplantation of a new cornea resolves the basic problem of corneal-surface irregularity, eyeglasses or contact lenses are usually still needed for vision correction. In many cases, rigid gas-permeable contact lenses are required to correct the large amount of visual distortion that is associated with transplants.

Corneal-transplant surgery is the most successful of all the transplant procedures, and the techniques are being improved constantly. Either general or local anesthesia can be used in this surgery, and you may need to spend a night or two in the hospital. You will need someone to drive you home, and once there, you will have to rest and relax for several days.

Corneal-transplant surgery involves the use of a high-tech instrument called a trephine, which is used like a cookie cutter first to remove your distorted cornea and then to cut a similar "button" from the donor cornea. The donor cornea button is placed in the round hole of your cornea and stitched in place. This is all done by a surgeon looking through a surgical microscope. The suture (thread) that is used is much finer than a human hair and is easily overlooked by the naked eye.

Most people experience surprisingly little pain and discomfort following a corneal transplant. The time taken off from work varies with the individual and the kind of work the individual does. Generally, if you have a sedentary job, you will be back to work in a week or two. Your bandages may likely be removed in one to two weeks after the surgery, but you will not be able to see clearly yet. It will probably be several months before your vision stabilizes, but your doctor may prescribe eyeglasses or contact lenses. Keep in mind that individual cases vary a great deal, so the time frames mentioned should be considered very general.

Eyeglasses and Lenses

Most people who wear eyeglasses don't think about them very much. But the fact is that millions of us wouldn't be able to function without them. It's worth taking a look at how eyeglasses work, how they're made, and how to find a pair that's both attractive and durable.

EYEGLASS LENSES

There are two basic types of lenses prescribed for vision correction—lenses for nearsightedness and lenses for farsightedness. These two basic types of lenses can also be combined into one lens that corrects for both near and distance problems, as well as one lens that corrects for near, distance, and intermediate problems. Furthermore, these combination lens can be crafted to meet the specific requirements of a certain work situation or hobby. In this section, we will discuss the two basic types of lenses and the variations that are in popular use today.

Minus Lenses and Plus Lenses

The two basic types of lenses prescribed for vision correction are the minus lens, which corrects for nearsightedness, and the plus lens, which corrects for farsightedness. The minus lens is concave in shape—thinner in the center than at the edges. Because of this shape, the minus lens weakens the focusing power of light before it enters the eye, so that the image of the object the eye is observing falls farther back, on the retina. (See Figure 3.5, below.) The minus lens is needed for the nearsighted eye to see clearly at a distance.

The plus lens is convex in shape, much like the shape of the lens in the eye. It is thicker in the center than at the edges, and increases the focusing power of light before it enters the eye. Because of this, images fall farther forward in relation to the retina. (See Figure 3.6, above right.) This increase in focusing power is needed for the farsighted eye to see clearly.

A plus lens is also used to correct for presbyopia. (For a complete discussion of presbyopia, see page 187.) In presbyopia, which is a normal part of aging, the eye's own lens has hardened and can no longer accommodate to see things up close. A lens that moves images farther forward to fall on the retina (in other words, a lens that corrects for farsightedness) can compensate for an eye that cannot accommodate for near vision.

The lens used for astigmatism is usually a combination of plus and minus lenses, to fit the particular curvatures of the astigmatic eye. This type of lens does not not look like either a minus or plus lens because of the way lenses are now manufactured, but the principle on which it is based is the same.

Your eye doctor will prescribe exactly the lens power you need. Your doctor also will measure the distance between the pupils of your eyes when they are aligned for distance and then again for near

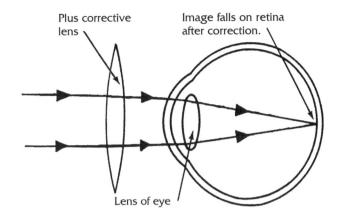

Figure 3.6. The plus lens is convex in shape. It is thicker in the center than at the edges, and increases the focusing power of light. The makes images fall farther forward—on the retina in cases of farsightedness and presbyopia.

vision, and will make sure the lenses' optical centers (the parts you look through when you look straight ahead) correspond to those distances.

Beware of the do-it-yourself reading glasses available at pharmacies and discount stores. These glasses are not of high optical quality, and, needless to say, they were not made with your exact prescription in mind. The optical centers of pharmacy glasses will probably be different from those of your eyes, which can cause a lot of eyestrain. Also, do-it-yourself lenses cannot compensate for astigmatism.

Bifocals

Minus lenses correct for nearsightedness, and plus lenses correct for farsightedness and presbyopia. But what do you do if you're already nearsighted and then become presbyopic as you get older (a common situation)? You'll still need your distance prescription to see the television and the road when you're driving, but you'll also need some correction for very close work such as reading. In other words, you now have a problem with both near and distance vision, and have only a narrow range in between at which you can see without correction. You could keep wearing your distance glasses for getting around in the world, and get a pair of reading glasses for near work. Some people do this. Or, you could enter the world of bifocals.

Bifocals, as their name implies, are lenses that have two focal corrections, one for near and one for dis-

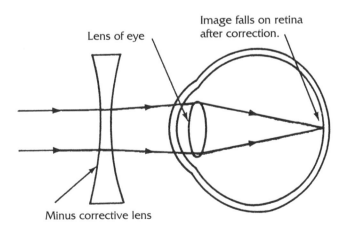

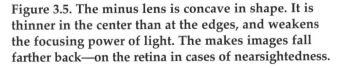

Figure 3.5. The minus lens is concave in shape. It is thinner in the center than at the edges, and weakens the focusing power of light. The makes images fall farther back—on the retina in cases of nearsightedness.

tance. If your examination reveals that you need bifocals, take heart—you aren't the first, and you won't be the last. Let's take a look at bifocals, and see where they came from and where they're going. You might be surprised.

The first bifocal was developed by Benjamin Franklin in the late 1700s. He took his distance glasses and cut them in half, took his reading glasses and cut them in half, and then glued the two halves together so that the distance lens was on top of the near lens. This primitive but functional solution kept Franklin from having to switch back and forth between two pairs of glasses.

In 1908, John Borsch, Jr., created the first fused bifocal by cutting a segment out of the lower portion of a distance lens, inserting a portion of a near lens in the hole, and then heating the two sections to melt them together. The lines between the two lens pieces were not as obvious as that in the Franklin bifocal, but the optics were not as sharp either.

The first good one-piece bifocal came along in 1910, when technology had advanced enough to allow the production of a single glass lens with two different curves, one curve for each focal point. The reading segment of this bifocal was large, but the line between the segments was obvious and the glass lenses were heavy. However, this is the same type of lens as today's executive bifocal, which has a line going all the way across. The executive bifocal is available in either glass or plastic. Its major drawbacks are the prominent line between the segments and the "jump" in image as the eye passes from the distance segment to the near segment.

After the first good one-piece bifocal came the flat-top bifocal, the most popular type of bifocal in recent times. The flat-top is similar to the fused lens invented by Borsch, but the top portion of the reading segment is made of the same material as the distance lens so that, when the lenses are fused, the material "disappears" and leaves a crescent-shaped reading segment. This lens has some significant optical advantages, as well as a very thin, hardly noticeable line. Many of today's bifocals are made this way.

In 1946, a bifocal was developed that was similar again to the Borsch lens, but the distance and near segments were blended together at their junction to reveal no noticeable line. This was cosmetically appealing because the lens did not look like a bifocal. However, when the wearer changed focus, his vision blurred significantly in the transition zone between the two seg-

ments. This was unacceptable to most wearers, so the flat-top remains the bifocal of choice today.

Trifocals

Bifocals are adequate for the majority of people with a need for both distance and near corrections. Most people's eyes can focus for intermediate activities—such as computer work, card playing, music reading, seeing prices on grocery shelves, and working at a large desk—by using either the distance-lens or near-lens segment of their glasses. But there are some people whose eyes need a special lens for this intermediate, arm's-length distance. The answer for these people is—you guessed it—trifocals. Trifocals correct vision at three different focal distances.

The first trifocals were developed in the 1940s and were similar in design to the flat-top bifocals. The only difference was that the trifocals had a third lens segment, for intermediate vision, inserted between the near and distance segments. The fitting of these lenses was extremely difficult. The intermediate segment needed to be low enough so that the wearer could look comfortably through the distance segment while driving, but it also needed to be high enough so the wearer could look comfortably through the reading segment at, for example, groceries on a supermarket shelf while keeping the head in a normal position. It was no surprise that few people adapted well to the first trifocals.

The next evolution in trifocals came in France in the early 1950s, when Bernard Maitenaz developed a single lens that incorporated the distance, intermediate, and near prescriptions without any visible lines. This lens was called a progressive addition lens (PAL) because the power change from distance to near was gradual and uninterrupted, similar to the power change normally accomplished by the eye itself. Many people today mistakenly call this lens a "no-line bifocal," but it is more accurately termed a "multi-focal" lens. Unfortunately, Maitenaz's first-generation design caused severe distortions at the edges of the lens that created a swimming effect when walking.

These days, technological advances in optics have not only overcome most of the problems in Maitenaz's lens, but also improved the lens enough so that it is now the correction of choice in many situations. Currently, more than twenty companies make about sixty types of PALs, and the latest versions seem to be easy to adapt to and comfortable to wear.

The topmost part of the lens corrects for distance viewing; the central part corrects for intermediate viewing; and the bottom part corrects for near viewing. The head positions required, although still a consideration, are not nearly as much of a complicating factor because of the gradual transition in lens power.

Occupational Lenses

Many people, as they perform their jobs, find that conventional lenses just don't allow clear or comfortable vision. This can be due to unusual working distances or angles. For example, computer users must be able to clearly see their monitors, often positioned straight ahead at an intermediate distance. In addition, they also need to clearly see the keyboard, as well as papers on their desk. There are now lenses, called occupational lenses, available that are specifically designed to solve unusual on-the-job problems.

Since your job may have a variety of visual requirements, discuss your needs with your doctor to see if there is a lens appropriate for you. There are a number of computer lenses available, as well as other types of unusual designs for different working conditions. It is important to have accurate measurements of all your working distances and angles so that your doctor can make the proper recommendations.

UNDERSTANDING AN EYEGLASS PRESCRIPTION

If you have ever had a prescription for eyeglasses, you may have noticed that it looked rather confusing. Whatever happened to 20/20? As you may remember from our discussion about 20/20 in "The Eyes and the Visual System," a prescription for glasses cannot be derived from reading letters on a chart. Look at Figures 3.7 and 3.8, right, and I'll explain how to read a prescription so that you can judge for yourself how your eyes are doing.

The basic prescription is broken down into two general categories—distance vision and near vision. In the illustrations, you see the abbreviations "OD" and "OS." These, respectively, stand for *oculus dexter*, the Latin term for "right eye," and *oculus sinister*, the Latin term for "left eye." Some prescription forms simply say "right" and "left," or "R" and "L."

The first blank column on the left, labeled "Sphere," is for indicating the basic power of the lens-

es. If the numbers in this column are preceded by minus signs, the prescription is for minus lenses, which correct for nearsightedness. If the numbers are preceded by plus signs, the prescription is for plus lenses, which correct for farsightedness. (It is possible to be farsighted in one eye and nearsighted in the other, although this is uncommon.) The unit of measurement is the diopter, which gives the refractive power of the lens. The larger the number is, the greater is the requested correction. A typical prescription for a mildly nearsighted patient would be about -.25 to -1.50 diopters; -1.75 to -3.00 diopters would be a moderate prescription; -3.25 to -6.00 diopters would be for a significant correction; and over -6.00 diopters would be a severe prescription. For farsightedness, up to about +1.50 diopters would be considered a mild prescription; +1.50 to +2.50 diopters would be a moderate prescription; and over +2.50 diopters would correct for significant farsightedness.

In the nearsighted prescription illustrated in Figure

FOR MR. JOHN DOE		EXAM DATE			
R	SPHERE	CYLINDER	AXIS	PRISM	BASE
DIST. OD	-1.00	-0.75	180	—	—
DIST. OS	-2.25	-1.25	15	—	—
NEAR OD					
NEAR OS					

PD 64/60 SPECIAL INSTRUCTIONS _____

_____ O.D.

Figure 3.7. Eyeglass prescription to correct nearsightedness.

FOR MS. JANE DOE		EXAM DATE			
R	SPHERE	CYLINDER	AXIS	PRISM	BASE
DIST. OD	+1.50	—	—	—	—
DIST. OS	+0.50	-0.50	90	—	—
NEAR OD					
NEAR OS					

PD 64/60 SPECIAL INSTRUCTIONS _____

_____ O.D.

Figure 3.8. Eyeglass prescription to correct farsightedness.

3.7, the patient needs a distance correction of -1.00 diopters in his right eye and -2.25 diopters in his left. (Pop quiz: Which of this patient's eyes is worse—the left or the right? Would his right eye be considered mildly, moderately, or significantly nearsighted? What about his left eye?)

In the prescription illustrated in Figure 3.8, the patient is farsighted. Her right eye needs a distance correction of +1.50 diopters, and her left eye needs a correction of +0.50 diopters. (Is she mildly, moderately, or significantly farsighted in her right eye? What about in her left eye?) A similar prescription might be written for a presbyopic patient.

The second and third blank columns on both prescriptions are labeled "Cylinder" and "Axis." They are for indicating the amount and the direction of any astigmatism. Picture the cornea of a normal eye as being shaped like a basketball (a sphere) and that of an astigmatic eye as more like a football (a squashed sphere). The "Cylinder" column gives the amount of correction the astigmatic eye needs. It is expressed in diopters with a plus or minus sign. The "Axis" column gives the direction of the astigmatism—that is, which way the "football" is turned. This is expressed in degrees between 1 and 180. The prescription illustrated for the nearsighted patient shows astigmatism in both eyes. The farsighted patient needs correction for astigmatism only in the left eye. Changes in the degree of nearsightedness and farsightedness are common over time. Astigmatism normally remains about the same in adulthood, although minor changes may occur after the age of sixty.

The fourth blank column on both prescriptions is headed "Prism." A prism correction bends light and may be prescribed for special problems. It isn't a common prescription. The final blank column, entitled "Base," refers to whether the base of the prism in the lens should point up, down, in, or out.

The "PD" at the bottom of the form is short for "pupillary distance," the distance between the patient's pupils. It is usually written using two numbers, as in the illustrations. These figures express the distance between the pupils when looking at a distant object and when looking at a near object. These distances are measured in millimeters and don't change during adulthood.

In most states, eyeglass prescriptions expire after one year, although in some, they remain good for two years. You should have your eyes checked at least once a year anyway!

LENS MATERIALS

Up until the late 1950s, all eyeglass lenses were made of glass (which is why they weren't called "eyeplastics"!). Since then, however, the advent of an optical plastic called CR-39 has revolutionized lenses. This material was originally developed during World War II, and since then, it has been further refined to improve its optical properties. CR-39 plastic is now used in about 80 percent of American lens prescriptions. Its main advantage over glass is that it is light in weight—about 50 percent of the weight of a glass lens per diopter of power. This makes it much more comfortable to wear, especially for people with a higher prescription, either for nearsightedness or farsightedness. Plastic also offers much more protection to the eyes. A plastic lens can still break, but it takes a much greater force to break one than it does to break a glass lens. In addition, plastic doesn't splinter into tiny slivers the way glass does. Plastic lenses can easily be tinted different colors, and the color can be changed if desired. (Glass cannot be so easily tinted, although it can be done.) Plastic lenses can be treated to block out ultraviolet light, which makes it as good a material for sunglasses as glass. (Glass lenses block most UV light without being treated.) If you like rimless frames, plastic is the lens material you should choose because it won't chip at the exposed edge nearly as easily as glass does.

In 1985, a new kind of plastic lens, called a polycarbonate lens, entered the market, and it has some advantages over the CR-39 lens. The bending ability of this plastic allows it to be formed into lenses that are much thinner than the lenses made of CR-39 plastic and yet achieve equal optical power. Polycarbonate lenses are also 50-percent lighter than conventional plastic lenses, have inherent UV protection, and can be treated to be scratch-resistant. One of the most impressive properties of polycarbonate plastic is that it is practically unbreakable. A twelve-gauge shotgun fired at a polycarbonate lens at close range only dented it! This is obviously the ideal material to use for protective eyewear. The only drawback is that the usable optical zone (the part through which you see) of polycarbonate lenses is slightly narrower than that of conventional plastic lenses, so distortions can occur in the peripheral vision, which bothers some people with a higher prescription.

Adding to the choices now is a higher-density plastic, called high-index plastic. This plastic is similar to

CR-39 plastic, except it is more dense, allowing lenses to be made thinner and lighter, even lighter than polycarbonate lenses.

The chief disadvantage of CR-39, polycarbonate, and high-index plastics is that they scratch more easily than glass. However, a scratch-resistant coating can be applied to plastic lenses to reduce their susceptibility. Scratch-resistant coatings are very effective, but they do not approximate the hardness of glass.

Glass lenses are still available and do have certain advantages. If you have a mild prescription and a frame that is not very large, the weight of the lenses may not be a problem. They are more scratch-resistant than plastic, and they have an inherent ability to block out UV light. There is also a new version of glass that simulates some of the properties of high-index plastic, forming thinner, lighter glass lenses that are scratch-resistant.

Glass lenses are available as photochromic lenses, which react to light and automatically darken as the surrounding light gets brighter, such as when you move from indoors to a sunny outdoor environment. Plastic lenses that react to light are now also available and are called Transitions lenses. Transitions lenses can change, but do not get as dark as glass photochromic lenses. Ordinary tinting does not work as well in glass as in plastic lenses. It can't be changed if you change your mind about the color, and it isn't as uniform in glass in the higher prescriptions as it is in plastic. Polycarbonate lenses are not tinted as darkly as the other plastics.

The main problem with glass lenses, in addition to their weight, is that they can splinter when broken and seriously injure your eyes. Today's glass lenses are tempered (required by Federal law) to minimize splintering, but they are still not as safe as plastic lenses. I do not recommend glass lenses when playing sports.

So, which is the best lens for you? If you just need to wear glasses occasionally for reading and you have a tendency to toss them around carelessly, glass is the best way to go. If you wear glasses on a full-time basis, but your prescription is not very high, CR-39 plastic will do nicely. If your prescription is very high or you're in a high-risk environment for breakage, polycarbonate or high-index plastic is for you. For kids, who are always tough on glasses, polycarbonate is recommended, since it's the safest way to go. Glass will certainly last longer and not become as badly scratched, but polycarbonate is much safer. For a quick comparison of glass, CR-39, polycarbonate, and high-index lenses, see the table below.

LENS COATINGS

Have you ever noticed how in photographs of people wearing glasses, you can see their glasses, but not their eyes? That's because of the reflection of the room lights or sunlight off the front surface of the glasses. This occurs because only 92 percent of light passes through a lens; 8 percent bounces off the surface. An anti-reflective lens coating was recently developed to take care of this problem. The coating has some distinct advantages. With an anti-reflective coating on the lens, over

COMPARISON OF DIFFERENT LENS MATERIALS

Lens Characteristic	Glass	CR-39 Plastic	Polycarbonate Plastic	High-Index Plastic
Weight	Heavy	Light	Very light	Very light
Impact resistance	Fair	Good	Excellent	Good
Tintability	Fair	Excellent	Good	Good
UV protection	Excellent (inherent ability)	Poor (can be treated)	Excellent (inherent ability)	Poor (can be treated)
Scratch resistance	Excellent	Fair	Fair	Fair
Thickness per diopter	Thick	Thicker	Very thin	Thinnest
Available as photochromic lens?	Yes	Yes	Yes	Yes
Suitable for rimless frames?	No	Yes, in lower prescriptions No, in highter prescriptions	Yes	Yes

99 percent of the light can pass through, with less than 1 percent deflected. Other people can see the wearer's eyes through the lenses and sometimes not perceive at all that glasses are being worn. Some people consider this a major cosmetic advantage, especially if they wear one of the higher prescriptions, which occasionally cause rings of reflected light to be visible in the lens. People who drive at night appreciate the coating because it eliminates the glare from oncoming headlights. It has one disadvantage, however—it tends to smudge and needs special cleaning and handling, although newer technology is making it better.

Lenses can also be treated with coatings that block UV light, coatings for scratch resistance, and tinted coatings. Sunglasses can be treated with a mirror coating. The photochromic process is not a coating. Having your lenses coated may add $50 to $75 to the price of your glasses. Discuss the different lens materials and coatings with your optometrist or optician. Find out what's available and which products best suit your needs.

FRAME MATERIALS

Most eyeglass frames are made of some version of either plastic, metal, or nylon. However, researchers are hard at work trying to come up with new materials for frames.

Plastic Frames

The traditional plastic frame is made from a material called zyl (ZILE). Zyl has the unique property of being easily bent into a particular shape when heated and holding that shape when cooled. This is critical when trying to adjust frames to fit thousands of different faces. Zyl is also available in a variety of translucent and opaque colors.

The 1960s saw the advent of a new type of material, called optyl (ahp-TEEL). Optyl weighs 30-percent less than zyl. It can also take on translucent colors. The only problem with optyl is that it tends to lose its shape when repeatedly exposed to heat (for example, by being left in a hot car too often). This material has lost some of its popularity.

Carbon fiber is made by adding carbon powder to plastic, which gives the material the strength of metal and the weight of plastic. Carbon-fiber frames are very durable and hold their shape very well. The color choices are numerous, but are all opaque (not translucent).

Cellulose proprionate is an inexpensive plastic that is usually used for cheap sunglass frames. It is highly breakable, difficult to adjust, and difficult to color completely.

Plastics are still popular for fashionable frames. Each type of plastic has its advantages, and can be used to enhance your appearance.

Metal Frames

Although many metal frames are gold colored, it is rare to find real gold in eyeglass frames today. Up until the "gold rush" of the early 1980s, most metal frames were gold-filled. However, when the price of gold shot out of reach for most of the eyewear manufacturers, a process called electroplating came into use. With electroplating, a gold-colored surface is put on a less expensive metal. Most of today's frames are still made using this process.

Aluminum offers a high strength-to-weight ratio—it is light in weight, yet strong. It is resistant to corrosion, and can be treated to take on a variety of colors. Since it cannot be soldered or welded easily, the design possibilities are limited, and screws and rivets must be used to connect the frame sections.

Beryllium is a metal that was developed by the National Aeronautics and Space Administration (NASA). It is strong, lightweight, and resilient. Because of its high cost, however, it is often combined with other metals, such as copper, to make frames.

Stainless steel is actually 67-percent iron and 18-percent chrome. It is very resistant to corrosion, and frames can be made thin because of its springiness. However, it does not hold adjustments well, or allow for easy soldering repair. In addition, it is slightly brittle.

Titanium is a metal that has a high tensile strength, is ultralight in weight, has impressive durability even when thin, and has excellent corrosion resistance. It is easy to adjust. It is, however, difficult to weld or solder, and is extremely expensive. Titanium-composite frames have the amazing ability to return to their original shape regardless of how much they are bent out of shape. These composite frames are becoming much more popular.

Metal frames have excellent qualities and offer a high-class look. However, beware of metals that are too inexpensive, since they usually lack durability.

Nylon Frames

Nylon is used mostly for sports and safety glasses, the most popular example being Vuarnet sunglasses. The frames are unbreakable when new, but lose moisture and become brittle with age.

Polyamide is a blend of nylons and features durability, reduced weight, flexibility, scratch resistance, a non-irritating surface, and the ability to hold translucent colors. It does, however, lose its adjustment if heated.

Rimless and Nearly Rimless Frames

Back in the 1960s, granny glasses were all the rage. These were frames that were barely there. They had only two temples (the part that goes from the lens to your ear) and a nosepiece bridge, which were held to the lenses with a few screws. Any shape lenses could be used, though the small round ones were the most popular. Granny glasses are harder to come by these days, but can still be found. Their main disadvantage is that holes must be drilled into the lenses, and the screws used to attach the frame pieces to the lenses often loosen. Drilling a hole in a lens can cause it to crack. If you have rimless glasses such as granny glasses, be careful when handling them, especially when putting them on, taking them off, and cleaning them.

Frames that have an upper portion but just thin nylon cords to support the bottoms of the lenses are called rimlon frames. The cords are positioned in grooves cut into the edges of the lenses. Rimlon frames have many advantages. They are light in weight, are not very noticeable on the face, and yet are durable if they are of good quality. They also have disadvantages, though. The nylon cords stretch with time, so the lenses can pop out (replacing the cord is easy, however); the edges of the lenses are exposed and can chip; and the higher prescriptions look very obvious. Using polycarbonate or high-index lenses in these frames reduces the thickness of the lenses' edges.

CHOOSING A FRAME

Have you ever heard the saying: "Boys don't make passes at girls who wear glasses"? This saying is so out of date now that you may not ever have heard it. Eyeglass frames have gotten much more attractive over the past twenty years, and today are even con-

sidered an enhancement, much like makeup and jewelry. To choose a frame for your glasses, go to a reputable optical shop and plan to spend some time there. Look for quality and style, not just price.

Quality

Selecting quality eyewear is like picking out fine jewelry. Unless you know what you're looking for and how to judge it, you may be fooled into paying for something you're not getting. Certainly not all frames are alike.

Fashion designers have created quite a stir in the eyeglass-frame world in the past few years. The optical industry is suddenly a part of the fashion scene. Most designers have some knowledge of what goes into a product that bears their name. However, some just sell their name, handing total control over to the manufacturer, who is then free to use the least expensive manufacturing methods. It's best to examine a frame carefully and to ask the optician to tell you about its durability and other characteristics.

The quality of a frame is evident in the material used, the workmanship, the attention to detail, and the integrity of the hinges and nose pads. Examine a frame as you would a piece of jewelry to see if the quality stands out. You may want to compare a few different frames to get a sense of what represents quality workmanship. Also, check any warranties that come with the frame. Good frames are warrantied for at least a year or two. In general, expect to pay about $75 to $100 for a high-quality plastic frame, and $175 to $225 or more for a metal frame. Rimless frames usually run a bit more. A frame that won't crack, chip, peel, tarnish, or corrode is valuable and a pleasure to own.

Style

Styles change in frames as they do in clothes, cars, makeup, and just about anything else we use to adorn ourselves. There are basic styles that have been around for years and will be here for years to come. And there are styles that make a statement, albeit for a short period of time. Picking the right frame for your face shape, skin tone, hair color, makeup, clothing, and lifestyle takes some expertise. Try to find a trustworthy optician who has experience, knowledge, and taste in eyewear. Word-of-mouth referrals are a good source. If you see someone who has good-looking glasses, find out where he or she got them.

Here are some tips to help you select the right frame for you. First, determine your face shape. To do this, pull your hair away from your face, look in a mirror, and outline your face on the mirror with lipstick. (This is a bit messy, but it works.) Once you know the shape of your face, you can choose the general shape of your eyeglasses. The general rule is that your eyewear shape should contrast with your face shape. "Choosing a Frame for Your Face" on page 227 gives specific advice for the seven different face shapes. Some additional fashion tips to consider are:

■ If you have a long nose or wide-set eyes, look for a thick, darkly colored bridge that rests low on the nose.

■ If you have close-set eyes, look for a high, thin, lightly colored bridge or a thin frame shape.

■ If you have a short face or a wide face, look for a highly placed temple.

■ If you have a full hairstyle around your face, look for a thin, light frame.

■ If you have minimal or sleek hair around your face, look for a bold frame.

Take some time to choose the right frame for you. Don't limit yourself to ten minutes to find a frame that you might wear for two years. Remember that people will see your eyeglass frame before they see your face, so think about the image you want to project. Consider this: Most people have at least six pairs of shoes and only one pair of glasses, but how often do other people look at your shoes?

CHOOSING FRAMES FOR CHILDREN

Choosing frames for children takes special effort and care. Try to make it fun, not frustrating. Approach the process in a way that makes your child want to wear and enjoy the glasses.

Children's frames need to be durable. The glasses will probably be on and off a dozen times a day, and should be able to withstand the wear and tear. Many kids' frames have spring hinges on the temples. When the temples are bent outward, they just spring back to the proper position. (These hinges are becoming popular for adults, too.) To make staying on the child's face easier, many frames have cable temples, which wrap around the ears. Glasses with cable temples are especially good for smaller children.

For infants and toddlers, patience is the key to fitting glasses. Let the baby play with the glasses first so that he or she can become familiar with them and want to keep them. Have the baby put the glasses on, and don't worry if they're upside down. Make a game out of it—on and off, on and off a few times. Let the baby enjoy the experience.

Older kids want frames that are "cool," and those frames are often the same ones that adults have. Smaller versions of the more popular adult frames are big sellers for kids. Many are adapted to children's sizes by building up the nosepiece bridge to fit the smaller face. Brighter colors are used because children's clothes are brighter.

Treat your older child with respect, and discuss the different features of each frame and whether the frame is good for his or her needs. Your optician should be able to advise you here. The optician should make sure that the bridge of the frame fits the child's nose correctly, since children's skin is softer and more sensitive to pressure. The temples should be adjusted so that there is no excessive pressure behind the ears. Comfort is a function of the weight and tension of the glasses being distributed as evenly as possible. Expect a growing child's frame to fit for about a year. Don't buy a frame that is too big and expect the child to grow into it.

When you and your child pick up the finished glasses, have your child first look at the glasses. Let your child put the glasses on himself or herself, and look through them. (If your child is an infant or toddler, you will probably need to play the on-and-off game again.) At this point, the optician can advise your child and make adjustments to the frame. The optician should also explain how to clean and care for the glasses, and give your child a glasses case, stressing the importance of keeping the glasses in the case when they are not being worn. Bring your child back in a week or two for an adjustment. Your child can then tell the optician about wearing the glasses, and the optician can reinforce how well the child is doing.

The prices of children's frames shouldn't be as high as the prices of adult frames, but don't skimp on quality to save a few dollars. In general, children's frames should sell for about $80 to $100. The keys to a successful frame for children are function, fit, and, comfort. And don't forget: Children who wear corrective lenses should have their vision checked every year.

Choosing a Frame for Your Face

OVAL FACE

Description: An oval face is considered to be a "well-balanced" face. The top half balances the bottom half.

Frame: An oval face can wear just about anything, as long as the frame is in proportion to the face.

ROUND FACE

Description: A round face has a large, curved forehead with a rounded chin. The face looks "full," with very few angles.

Frame: Angular or geometric frames give better contours to a round face.

HEART-SHAPED FACE

Description: The forehead is the widest part of the heart-shaped face. Then the face narrows, and the chin is slightly pointed.

Frame: Try a frame with straight top lines and rounded sides, such as "aviator" or "butterfly" shapes.

RECTANGULAR FACE

Description: The rectangular face is long and narrow with a squarish chin.

Frame: Frames with a strong top bar and round bottom lines are a good choice.

TRIANGULAR FACE

Description: The triangular face has a narrow forehead, but is full around the cheeks and chin.

Frame: A heart-shaped frame is best. Square frames, aviator frames with a straight top or wire frames that are rimless on the bottom can also work well.

SQUARE FACE

Description: The square face has a wide forehead and a wide cheek and chin area. The jaw is angular.

Frame: Oval or round frames add soft lines to a square face.

DIAMOND-SHAPED FACE

Description: The diamond-shaped face has a small forehead, a wide temple area, and a small chin area.

Frame: A butterfly-shaped frame is best. You can also try a square frame.

Chart courtesy of You! Are Something Beautiful, La Habra, CA.

TAKING CARE OF GLASSES

Taking care of glasses doesn't take much time or effort, but a little care can go a long way. When you first get your glasses, make sure that they are adjusted by someone who knows what he or she is doing.

There is nothing more annoying than having your glasses hurt behind your ears or slip down your nose while you're reading.

To check the fit of your glasses, look down at the floor with the glasses on and and shake your head firmly. The glasses shouldn't slip at all. Sometimes it's a few days before glasses that are too tight start hurting. Don't get discouraged if it takes two or three return visits to the optician to get a proper fit.

Many opticians and pharmacies sell little eyeglass-repair kits. These kits are okay, but be careful. The screwdrivers are small, and it doesn't take much to strip the head of a tiny screw or to "inject" yourself with the tiny screwdriver. The best thing to do is to take your glasses back to your optician every three months or so for a tightening and "tune-up." If you take them back to the shop where you bought them, you should not be charged for this service.

You should always wet plastic lenses before wiping them. If you don't, the dirt on the lens may scratch the surface. I recommend using a one-to-one mixture of glass cleaner and water. Dry the lenses with a soft cotton cloth, not with paper tissues. Lenses with an anti-reflective coating must be cleaned with a special cleaning agent, which you most likely can buy from your optician. To clean your frames, soak the glasses in detergent overnight. Even with good care, lenses generally need to be replaced about every one to two years, and frames about every two years. Take good care of your glasses, and they'll take good care of your vision.

Orthokeratology

When hard contact lenses were first being worn, doctors discovered that they caused a slight change in the shape of the cornea. They also noted that this flattening of the cornea caused a reduction in the degree of nearsightedness.

In the early 1970s, a group of optometrists started to discuss what they believed was happening to the corneas of contact-lens wearers. They called the process orthokeratology (or-tho-care-ah-TOL-oh-gee), from the Greek words *orthos*, which means "straight," and *kerato*, which pertains to the cornea. They saw this process of "straightening" the cornea with special contact lenses as similar to straightening the teeth with dental braces. More research has since been done, and now there are documented cases of contact lenses actually reducing nearsightedness to the point of complete correction. This process used to take anywhere from twelve to eighteen months, depending on the degree of nearsightedness. With the new lens designs and materials, however, it now can take as lit-

tle as four to six weeks to achieve the same effect. It all seems too good to be true—well, maybe.

The lenses now used for orthokeratology are made of the same material as the rigid gas-permeable lenses used for standard vision correction, but they are constructed with a curvature on the back that works to flatten the curvature of the cornea. They can cost up to four times more than standard rigid gas-permeable lenses because the program requires several visits to the optometrist—about eight or more visits over the course of four to five months—as well as multiple lens changes. After the corneas have flattened, "retainer" lenses must be worn to keep them that way.

Because of the variety of materials and techniques currently available, the retainer time varies for different people. Some people need to wear their retainer lenses a few hours a day to maintain their clear vision. Others use them every other day. In some cases, a person can insert the lenses before going to bed, sleeping with them in place and then removing them in the morning. Your final wearing schedule will depend on how well you respond to the program.

If orthokeratology sounds interesting to you, contact the International Orthokeratology Society for help in locating a doctor in your area who specializes in the procedure. For the address and phone number of the society, see "Resource Organizations" on page 255.

Refractive Surgery

Refraction is the changing of the path of light, which, in the optical arts, results in the light entering the eye coming to a focus on the retina. Light starts to refract toward the retina as soon as it enters the eye. In nearsightedness, however, the light refracts in a way that causes it to focus in front of the retina when looking at a distant image. In farsightedness, the light is focused in back of the retina. In astigmatism, because the cornea is shaped like a barrel instead of a sphere, the light is focused in two different points, which cannot be reconciled. Since about 80 percent of the eye's refractive power comes from the front part of the cornea, refractive surgery consists of altering the shape of the cornea to cause the light rays to refract properly and focus directly on the retina. When successful, it can dramatically reduce or eliminate your need for glasses or contact lenses. However, the same as all surgery, it is not something you should jump into without complete information. Here's the scoop on the latest in refractive surgery.

TYPES OF REFRACTIVE SURGERY

Four of the more popular types of refractive surgery are radial keratotomy, photorefractive keratectomy, lamellar keratoplasty, and laser-assisted intrastromal keratomileusis. A fifth type, the intracorneal ring, is currently being put to the test in clinical trials. All of the procedures involve changing the shape of the cornea so that light entering the eye comes to a focus more accurately. For a quick comparison of the four most popular procedures, see the table below.

Radial Keratotomy

Modern radial keratotomy (RK) was introduced in the 1970s by a Russian surgeon named Svyatoslav Fyodorov. It has been performed in the United States since around 1980. In RK, a tiny diamond blade is used to make four to sixteen incisions around the center of the cornea like the spokes of a bicycle wheel. As the cornea heals, it flattens in the center. This flattening has the effect of changing the refraction of the

light rays entering the eye. A different incision pattern but a similar technique are used to treat astigmatism.

According to the National Eye Institute, about 250,000 RK procedures are done each year in the United States, up from 30,000 in 1990. To date, more than 1,000,000 people have had RK. Currently, however, even though RK is constantly being improved due to new technologies, it is suffering a decline in popularity, most likely because of the advances in the laser techniques that have been gaining in popularity.

Photorefractive Keratectomy

Photorefractive keratectomy (PRK) is a computer-assisted surgical technique that uses an excimer laser to correct refractive errors. In October 1995, the FDA approved the first excimer-laser system for use in this procedure. In PRK, the cornea is reshaped using the energy from the light emitted by the laser. Specifically, the laser produces an ultraviolet beam of light and emits it in pulses. Each pulse delicately removes microscopic layers of tissue from the cornea. The laser is controlled by a computer that is preset to your particular correction needs.

After the procedure, healing may take several weeks.

COMPARISON OF THE FOUR MOST POPULAR TYPES OF REFRACTIVE SURGERY

Characteristic	Radial Keratotomy (RK)	Photorefractive Keratectomy (PRK)	Lamellar Keratoplasty (LK) and Automated Lamellar Keratoplasty (ALK)	Laser-assisted Intrastromal Keratomileusis (LASIK)
Range of correction	-1.00 to -8.00 D	-1.00 to -20.00 D	+1.00 to +5.00 D -10.00 to -15.00 D and up	-3.00 to -10.00 D
Accuracy of prediction of final prescription	-1.00 to -6.00 D	-1.00 to -9.00 D	-6.00 and up	-9.00 D and up
Length of procedure	5 minutes	5 minutes	20 minutes	20 minutes
Risk of complications	Low	Low	Low	Low
Physical recovery time (back to work)	As little as 1 day	3 days	As little as 1 day	As little as 1 day
Visual recovery time (visual acuity)	Less than 1 week	Several weeks or more	Up to several weeks	Up to several weeks
Side effects immediately after surgery	Watering and mild discomfort	Irritation, watering, and sometimes burning	Scratchy sensation	Scratchy sensation
When second eye can be treated	In less than 1 week	In several weeks or more	In less than 1 week or at same time as first eye	In less than 1 week or at same time as first eye

D = diopters.

For the first few days, a contact lens is used to bandage the eye. Drops are used for several weeks to help reduce the inflammation. To date, more than 1,000,000 people in forty countries have had PRK.

Lamellar Keratoplasty

In lamellar keratoplasty (LK), the cornea of the eye is reshaped using an instrument called a microkeratome. This instrument, which is designed to function much like a carpenter's plane, is used to create a corneal flap, revealing the inner corneal tissue. To correct for nearsightedness, a thin wedge of inner tissue is removed, and the flap is closed. Removing this wedge of tissue changes the shape of the cornea, which alters the way light entering the eye is refracted. LK is used to correct high degrees of nearsightedness and low degrees of farsightedness.

Since a farsighted eye is too short and its cornea must be made steeper, the LK procedure used is a little different. Only one pass is made across the cornea with the microkeratome, but a thicker flap is created. The normal inner pressure of the eye then assists, pushing against the cornea and making it steeper. The flap is repositioned, and the farsightedness should be reduced or eliminated.

Automated lamellar keratoplasty (ALK) was developed in the late 1980s after the introduction of the automated microkeratome. Manual LK has been in use for almost fifty years. Tens of thousands of patients to date have had LK or ALK.

Laser-Assisted Intrastromal Keratomileusis

Laser-assisted intrastromal keratomileusis (LASIK) is a procedure that combines the use of the excimer laser from PRK with the creation of a corneal flap from LK. Instead of using a microkeratome to cut out a wedge of tissue, an excimer laser is used to reshape the inner corneal tissue or, in some cases, the flap itself.

LASIK may be more successful than PRK for patients with severe or extreme cases of nearsightedness or astigmatism. It may be an alternative for patients ineligible for PRK, such as people with lupus, rheumatoid arthritis, or severely dry eyes.

LASIK has been in use since the late 1980s, just about the same number of years as ALK. To date, the procedure has been performed on several thousand patients in the United States and thousands more worldwide. LASIK is quickly becoming the procedure preferred by eye surgeons around the world. ALK and PRK, the two procedures that make up LASIK, have been approved by the FDA.

Intracorneal Ring

The intracorneal ring (ICR) is yet another type of refractive surgery. In this method, two bands of surgical plastic are inserted into the central portion of the cornea. The bands are angled in a way that makes them stretch the cornea to flatten the curvature, thus creating the same effect as the other types of surgery. The good news is that the bands can be removed, so the procedure is reversible. Thus far, there have been very few side effects or drawbacks to this procedure, which is designed mostly for nearsightedness.

IS REFRACTIVE SURGERY RIGHT FOR YOU?

Only your doctor can determine whether refractive surgery is an option for you, and can counsel you about which treatment may produce the best result. Many doctors, for example, believe that RK is best for patients with low myopia and shouldn't be performed on people with vision weaker than about 20/500. (A person with 20/500 vision typically cannot see the big *E* on the eye chart.) In addition, age, sex, and internal eye pressure may also be determining factors.

WHAT TO EXPECT DURING AND AFTER REFRACTIVE SURGERY

Refractive surgery is typically performed on an outpatient basis with a topical (eye-drop) anesthetic. Immediately after the surgery, you can expect the following:

■ *RK.* For the first few days following your RK procedure, you will probably experience mild discomfort, and your vision will be cloudy. However, most patients are able to return to work in a few days and to resume driving within a week.

■ *PRK.* The postoperative discomfort of PRK is generally more significant than what follows RK, so your doctor may prescribe a soft contact lens that functions as a bandage and eases the discomfort, as well as eye drops that reduce the inflammation. Infection is also a risk during the first two to three days following the procedure, but you will be given antibiotic eye drops and told which activities to avoid to minimize this risk. Most doctors recommend that you stay home from work for a few days, but after that, you can resume your normal activities.

■ *LK and ALK.* The discomfort and disruption following LK and ALK are minimal compared to what accompanies RK and PRK. Some patients feel a scratchy sensation, but the discomfort is generally minor. You most likely will be able to return to work as early as the next day.

■ *LASIK.* The risk of postoperative pain for LASIK surgery is somewhat lower than it is for PRK. You may just feel a scratchy sensation, as with LK and ALK. Your visual recovery may be faster than it is with PRK. In fact, again as with LK and ALK, you may be able to return to work as early as the day after surgery.

Refractive surgery is usually performed on one eye at a time so that your healing can be better monitored. However, bilateral surgery (surgery on both eyes at the same time) may be considered possible for some patients.

THE RESULTS TO EXPECT FROM REFRACTIVE SURGERY

The amount of time it takes the vision to stabilize after refractive surgery varies from days to months, since the healing process differs from patient to patient. However, in general, most people can expect the following results:

■ *RK.* If you have a moderate degree of nearsightedness, you should expect good results from RK. In fact, the less nearsighted you are, the better your results will likely be. While everyone will not see 20/20 without glasses or contacts after this procedure, your vision should be improved. Studies have shown that the vision of over 90 percent of RK patients is 20/40 (driver's license vision) without corrective lenses after surgery.

■ *PRK.* If you have mild to moderate nearsightedness, the chances are excellent that you will end up with 20/40 vision or better from PRK. However, the jury is still out as far as results are concerned in cases of severe nearsightedness.

■ *LK and ALK.* If you are severely nearsighted (-10.00 diopters or more), LK and ALK have been found to be the most effective types of refractive surgery. They

have also been used to correct up to +5.00 diopters of farsightedness.

■ *LASIK.* If you have a case of severe nearsightedness or astigmatism, you will be better off with LASIK, which has been found to have more predictable results than PRK for this disorder, as well as a decreased probability of regression. However, LASIK has not been studied for as long as PRK.

These expectations are general guidelines, and your experience may be different. Be sure to fully discuss the expected results with your doctor before the procedure.

THE SIDE EFFECTS OF REFRACTIVE SURGERY

Minor side effects, most of which are temporary, are relatively common after refractive surgery, especially while the cornea heals. Depending upon the procedure performed, here's what you should expect:

■ *RK.* The side effects of RK include glare sensitivity, halos around lights, flashing lights, astigmatism, light sensitivity, fluctuations in vision, and, initially, the inability to wear contact lenses. Often, these side effects improve with time. The cornea is weakened by RK, increasing the risk of eye rupture from physical trauma. According to the American Academy of Ophthalmology, however, there have been reports of severe eye trauma without damage to the incision wounds. The report also says that potentially blinding complications, such as corneal infection or perforation, are rare.

■ *PRK.* The most common complaints after undergoing PRK are a hazy sensation and halos around lights. For some patients, it may take from weeks to months to reach optimal vision after PRK, often depending on the initial lens prescription. Several newer medications have reduced this time significantly.

■ *LK, ALK and LASIK.* If you have either LK, ALK, or LASIK, you may experience halos around lights and glare sensitivity, both of which sensations that may be similar to what you experienced while wearing your contacts before the surgery. These side effects usually fade during the weeks and months following the surgery.

Other complications, although rare, include infections and a reduction in the best visual acuity (that is, your vision may be slightly less sharp than it was before surgery). If you are undercorrected or overcorrected, or if your vision regresses over time, your doctor may suggest further surgery to improve the result. However, many patients require only a single procedure.

THE FIRST STEP

If you decide that refractive surgery may be a good idea for you, the first steps you should take are to get a complete eye examination and to discuss the possibilities with your doctor. Besides determining your refractive error, your doctor will also check that you have no disease or corneal irregularity that could complicate a refractive-surgery procedure. The doctor will also ask you questions about your lifestyle and occupation, and discuss your needs and wishes. This is when you should ask your doctor any questions you may have, for example:

■ Am I a good candidate for refractive surgery?

■ Which procedure would be best for me?

■ What are the risks of the surgery?

■ What are the side effects?

■ How long will the side effects last?

■ How long will it take my eyes to fully heal?

■ If the results are less than I had hoped for, what can be done?

■ How long do I have to wait after my first eye is done to do my second eye?

Both optometrists and ophthalmologists are qualified to discuss refractive surgery and the different procedures currently being used. They also should be able to answer all your questions. Many optometrists work with a particular ophthalmologist, and this team may work on your case together.

Refractive surgery is an individual decision. Your particular refractive problem, as well as your goals, the expected outcome of surgery, your tolerance for discomfort and side effects, and even your lifestyle and occupation, are among the factors that you and your doctor should take into consideration when discussing the possibility of surgery for you. Refractive surgery is not for everyone—but it just might be a good solution for you.

Sunglasses

Sunglasses are a specific type of eyewear for a specific purpose. They should be chosen carefully because they alter the light that reaches your eyes. In this chapter, we'll take a look at the different properties of sunglasses and what you should look for in a quality pair.

SUNGLASSES FOR PROTECTION

Sunglasses have traditionally been worn for comfort in bright sunlight and for style. Now, research has added protection from harmful light rays to the list. Any eyeglass prescription can be made in a tinted lens for use in sunlight. If you don't wear glasses, you should get a pair of quality nonprescription sunglasses.

Protection From Ultraviolet Light

Ultraviolet light—also called ultraviolet radiation—is light that is not visible to the human eye because it is below the visible spectrum in wavelength. However, it is above the visible spectrum in wave frequency, another way of measuring light, which is why it is called ultraviolet, meaning "beyond violet." UV light rays come from the sun, and some of them reach the earth and our eyes. They are responsible for sunburn, skin cancer, and snow blindness, and may contribute to the formation of cataracts. UV light may also have a hand in the formation of pingueculae, yellowish spots on the front of the eye. (For a discussion of pingueculae, see page 182.) Although pingueculae are not a serious condition, an irritated spot can be uncomfortable, and is easily inflamed by excessive wind, dust, sun, or smoke.

Commercial, "off-the-rack" sunglasses of the type for sale in pharmacies and dime stores offer no UV protection. In fact, the lenses in these kinds of sunglasses may actually cause your eyes to absorb more UV light than normal. This is because your pupils dilate when you wear sunglasses. If the sunglasses don't filter out UV light, more UV light will enter your eyes than it would if you weren't wearing sunglasses at all and your pupils were constricted just the usual amount! But even if a manufacturer claims that a pair of sunglasses offers "100-percent UV protection," the optical quality of off-the-rack sunglasses is poor.

Glass lenses block about 98 percent of UV light, and CR-39 and high-index lenses can be treated to also offer good UV protection. The new polycarbonate lenses offer 100-percent protection against UV light. (For a complete discussion of all these types of lenses, see "Eyeglasses and Lenses" on page 218.)

Protection From Blue Light

Blue light has a wavelength of between 400 and 500 nanometers, and is perceivable by the eye. It is considered less dangerous than ultraviolet light, but, according to recent evidence, it may be responsible for damage to the eye's retina. Most UV light is absorbed by the lens of the eye, where it may eventually cause a cataract to develop, while blue light goes through the lens and is absorbed by the retina.

Blue light also causes glare on sunny days, so blue-blocker sunglasses have been around for a while. Amber and brown sunglass lenses block blue light, improving the contrast in your vision and reducing the glare, as well as protecting your retina from long-term exposure to blue light. However, as just mentioned, protection and optical quality are two different properties in sunglasses and should both be present for the best results. So, if you're paying only $10 for a pair of sunglasses, you're definitely *not* getting a quality product.

Protection From Infrared Light

Infrared light, with a wavelength of more than 700 nanometers, is not visible to the human eye. Its wavelength is longer than what we can perceive. However, its wave frequency is less than what we can perceive, so it is called infrared, which means "less than red." Infrared light passes through the cornea and is absorbed mostly by the lens. It produces heat, and is more intense at high altitudes and around bodies of water. It is also produced by the kind of flame used in glass blowing and welding. Therefore, high-altitude skiers, boaters, and some glass blowers and welders are at risk for infrared damage, which can cause cataracts after repeated exposure over a number of years. Some high-quality sunglasses block infrared light, but most sunglasses do not.

RATING SUNGLASSES

UV light has a wavelength of between 286 and 400 nanometers. It can be further divided into subsections—UVC light has a wavelength of less than 286 nanometers;

UVB light has a wavelength of between 286 and 320 nanometers; and UVA light has a wavelength of between 320 and 400 nanometers. UVC light is not normally considered a threat because much of it is blocked out by the earth's atmosphere before it reaches us.

The FDA has approved a voluntary labeling system to assist consumers in judging the UV protection offered by sunglasses. The FDA has adopted three categories of lenses:

1. Cosmetic lenses are "just for looks," or fashion accessories. They block out 70 percent of UVB light, 20 percent of UVA light, and 60 percent of visible light.

2. General-purpose lenses are for activities such as boating and hiking. They block out 95 percent of UVB light, 60 percent of UVA light, and 60 to 92 percent of visible light.

3. Special-purpose lenses are for activities such as skiing and sunning. They block out 99 percent of UVB light, 60 percent of UVA light, and 97 percent of visible light.

Look for the UV-light rating on your next pair of sunglasses. Many optical shops can measure the amount of UV transmission through a lens with a special meter. However, keep in mind that even the best UV-light protection is no guarantee of good optical quality in a sunglass lens.

POLARIZING LENSES

People who spend time around water know the value of polarizing lenses. These lenses polarize light—that is, they prevent it from scattering and causing glare. Polarizing lenses are made from crystals that are aligned in such a way that they change the orientation of light rays.

The best polarizing lenses are made of glass, but some good-quality plastic polarizing lenses are also available. Polarizing sunglasses are not necessarily more expensive than other sunglasses, but having the lenses of your prescription sunglasses polarized will add to their total cost.

LENS COLORS

The color that you choose for the lenses of your sunglasses is a matter of personal preference. However, most experts agree that gray, green, brown, and amber are the lens colors that reduce glare the best. Gray lenses are neutral, transmitting all the colors evenly, so you see all the colors as they are. Green lenses resemble your natural color sensitivity and allow a maximum amount of useful light to reach your eyes. (The human eye is more sensitive to the colors in the green part of the spectrum than in the other parts, so it "tunes in" better to those colors.) Brown and amber lenses have the advantage of blocking out blue light.

Photochromic lenses such as Corning's Photogray have been around for about thirty years now and continue to be very popular. These lenses automatically darken to a gray or brown color when the surrounding light becomes brighter, and lighten as it becomes darker. The color change takes about a minute to complete. Photochromic lenses will not become completely dark while you're driving because the windshield of the car will block out some of the UV light. The original photochromic process could be used only with glass lenses, but Transitions lenses, which are plastic, are becoming quite popular. Transitions lenses do become lighter indoors than photochromic glass lenses do, but they do not become quite as dark outdoors. Both glass and plastic photochromic lenses are of excellent quality, and the color-change process never wears out. Prescription-eyeglass wearers like these lenses a lot because they can wear them all the time rather than having to switch to sunglasses when they go out into the sun.

SUNGLASS QUALITY

Many people choose their sunglasses based on how well the frame fits and how the glasses look, rather than on the quality of the lenses.

Off-the-rack sunglasses are likely to have lenses made of a type of plastic called cellulose acetate. This plastic is usually stamped out into a lens shape and inserted into a frame. The lenses often warp and distort the light passing through them, which can cause headaches. With their low-cost materials and low labor costs, these "fun glasses" sell for between $5 and $15. This low price has led to the unfortunate notion that sunglasses should be cheap and easily replaced when lost or broken. I often hear people say they want cheap sunglasses because they're "just for the beach"—but the beach is where sunglasses are needed the most for protection.

Quality sunglasses are a different story. They are made of optically ground plastic, usually CR-39, or glass. Lenses that are optically ground have true curves, substantial "body" that helps to maintain their shape, and clear optics. Plastic lenses can be tinted any color, as well as bleached of color if you change your mind later and want to use them as regular glasses. Glass lenses can be tinted, but not bleached.

Glass lenses are almost always optically ground, so they work well as sunglasses. Many of the more popular brands of sunglasses are glass. Good sunglasses are made in one of two ways—the color can be incorporated directly in the lens, or a tinted coating can be applied to the front, back, or both surfaces of the lens. The only disadvantage of the coating method is that the coating can be scratched off accidentally. With proper care, however, either type of tinted lens works well.

While the lenses are the most important part of a pair of sunglasses, you also need to pay attention to the frame. The frames of off-the-rack sunglasses usually can't be tightened or properly adjusted. The frames used for good sunglasses are of the same quality as those used for prescription glasses. They can be adjusted to fit properly, and will hold their adjustment.

Don't let price be your primary consideration when choosing sunglasses. Evaluate your specific sunglass needs. For example, do you need them for the beach, bike riding, or driving a car? Choose a store that is convenient so that you can go in for adjustments or repairs periodically. Make sure that someone in the store can adjust glasses. In addition, try on several styles, and check for fair pricing. As with most things, you do get what you pay for in sunglasses.

Syntonics

Syntonics (sin-TAHN-iks), also known as optometric phototherapy, has been used clinically for over sixty years in the field of optometry. It is the branch of ocular science dealing with the application of selected visible-light frequencies through the eyes. It has been utilized with continued success in the treatment of visual dysfunctions such as strabismus, lazy eye, accommodative insufficiency, convergence insufficiency, and vision-related learning disorders, as well as for the visual consequences of traumatic brain injury.

Through most of history, the role of light in human

function has been limited chiefly to the process of seeing. Early pioneers found that color, applied to the skin, could have a non-intrusive curative effect on bodily ailments. At the turn of the century, it first became known that light entering the eyes not only serves vision, but also travels to other important brain regions. It was believed that applying certain frequencies of light by way of the eyes could restore balance within the body's regulatory centers, thereby directly affecting the source of visual dysfunctions. This balance is referred to as syntony.

A phototherapy-treatment plan may span a period of one to two months and require three to five sessions per week. A series of twenty phototherapy sessions of twenty minutes each may be prescribed to begin a vision-therapy program, or phototherapy may be implemented concurrently with other vision-therapy techniques. Although syntonics is rarely used in isolation from other procedures, in some cases, along with a lens prescription, it may be enough to solve the visual complaint.

As so often happens, positive clinical experience with syntonics has preceded any validating research, so many doctors feel that this therapy is not "accepted." Researchers and other professionals are still a step away from understanding the clinical methods and practice of light stimulation, which syntonists has used with positive results for over half a century. However, the interest in phototherapy has increased in recent years. Research showing that color changes the interaction and timing in the visual-processing system may be one of the reasons. Another may be the use of approaches such as the Irlen method, which uses color overlays and tinted eyeglass lenses to help improve reading. (For a complete discussion of the Irlen method, see "Irlen Lenses" on page 21.)

One other development that supports the validity of phototherapy is the discovery of a condition now known as seasonal affective disorder (SAD). This is a condition of psychological depression that usually occurs during the winter months, when the daylight hours are short. Between 1992 and 1994, more than 5,000 articles were published in the medical literature describing light's effect on physiology. Roughly 1,100 studies used color, and nearly 800 dealt with experimental phototherapy. It is now widely accepted that the natural light of the sun is more beneficial to the human system than artificial light. In addition, it is now common to find full-spectrum lighting in indoor environments, especially classrooms.

The College of Syntonic Optometry was established in 1933 and is dedicated to research on the therapeutic application of light to the visual system. For help with finding a professional trained in syntonics, contact the College of Syntonic Optometry. (See "Resource Organizations" on page 255 for the address and phone number.)

Vision Therapy

Some people just want to go to an eye doctor—or any doctor, for that matter—and get a prescription and be on their way. However, a growing number of people want to play a more active role in their health care, and are interested in learning how to take care of themselves. For these people, a program of vision therapy is the perfect prescription.

Could your eyes benefit from vision therapy? Answer the following questions to help you decide:

■ Is your vision, near or distance, ever blurry, even for a few seconds?

■ Do you ever see double?

■ Do you lose your place while reading?

■ Do your eyes feel tired if you read for an hour or more?

■ Do you get a headache toward the end of the day, especially around your forehead or temples?

■ Do your friends see things before you can bring them into focus?

■ Do you do a lot of close work on the job, and then go home and use a computer?

■ Does squinting improve your eyesight?

■ Do you need stronger glasses every year or two?

If you answered "yes" to any of these questions, you may find vision therapy to be of help to you.

Tomorrow morning, take a good look at your eyes in the bathroom mirror immediately after you get up. Try to describe how your eyes look, and then try to describe how your body feels. After you eat breakfast and take a shower, but before you leave for work, take another close look at your eyes. Do you see any difference? How does the rest of your body feel? After work, look at your eyes once again and see if they had a "hard day at the office," too.

Your eyes do a lot of work in an average day and can get stressed just like any other body part. Thinking about the above questions and taking a close look at your eyes from time to time can help you to get to know your eyes better. Techniques to relax the eyes and improve the vision can help your eyes to work better.

Vision therapy is a program of techniques and other activities designed to reduce stress, guide the development of the visual system, improve the visual skills, and enhance visual performance. The idea of vision therapy dates back at least as far as the 1920s, although today's vision therapy—which is sometimes called optometric vision therapy—is quite different from the programs of the past.

THE BATES METHOD

In the 1920s, a New York ophthalmologist named William H. Bates developed a theory that stress and eyestrain are the primary causes of all vision problems. He reasoned—though not entirely scientifically by today's standards—that reducing stress on the eyes would reduce refractive errors, and he developed a program of relaxation techniques in line with his theory. Dr. Bates advised his patients never to stare or look directly *at* objects, but rather to look *through* them. He advised against prolonged fixation of the eyes in one position, and recommended doing techniques such as "swinging," which consisted of shifting your weight from foot to foot while scanning a room, and "sunning," which involved closing your eyes, turning toward the sun, and rolling your head back and forth.

Dr. Bates appreciated the connection between the mind, brain, and eyes, and said that memory and visual perception are also linked. He wasn't entirely wrong. Stress certainly does influence vision, and there is a close connection between the eyes and the brain. His techniques probably did help people to relax their eyes, but his explorations didn't go far enough and didn't effectively treat most vision problems. Today, optometric vision therapists still use some of Dr. Bates's ideas. In fact, the palming and head rolling techniques presented on page 241, are based on Dr. Bates's techniques.

MODERN OPTOMETRIC VISION THERAPY

Modern vision therapy was first practiced in the 1930s by A.M. Skeffington, an American optometrist, and is still being refined. Today, it is practiced primarily by optometrists who specialize in vision therapy. Optometric vision therapy combines a series of office visits with exercises done at home. "Exercise," in this case, does not refer to aerobic exercise or strength training, but rather to activities designed to improve binocular coordination and eye-brain coordination. When you practice vision exercises, or techniques, you won't strengthen your eye muscles (they're already strong enough), but you will improve the efficiency and smoothness of the muscles that control your eye movements and the focusing of your eyes' lenses. You'll also improve the connections between your eyes and your brain, and between your two eyes.

The office visits for vision therapy, which normally takes several months, are generally thirty to sixty minutes in length and held two to three times a week. In the office, lenses, prisms, and techniques involving light and pictures are used to encourage the eyes to work differently from the way in which they have been working. Some optometrists also try to improve vision by stimulating the visual system with different flashes of color. (See "Syntonics" on page 234.) The homework consists of techniques intended to improve vision, but without much equipment.

True optometric vision therapy is more than just a group of techniques. It is an individualized program of progressively arranged conditions of learning for the development of a more efficient and effective visual system. It can be used to improve nearsightedness, farsightedness, presbyopia, visual discomfort, learning difficulties, strabismus, lazy eye, slow reading, poor reading comprehension, poor visual perception, poor sports performance, and job-related visual disabilities. Some of the visual skills that optometric vision therapy seeks to improve are:

■ Tracking—the ability to follow a moving object, such as a ball in flight or vehicles in traffic, smoothly and accurately with both eyes.

■ Fixation—the ability to quickly and accurately locate and inspect with both eyes a series of stationary objects, one after another, such as the words in a sentence while reading.

■ Accommodation—the ability to look quickly from far to near and vice versa, such as from the dashboard to the cars on the street, or from the chalkboard to a book, without blurriness.

■ Depth perception—the ability to judge the relative distances of objects, and to see and move accurately within a three-dimensional space, such as when parking a car.

■ Peripheral vision—the ability to monitor and interpret what is happening around you while attending to a specific task with your central vision; the ability to use visual information perceived from a large area.

■ Binocular coordination—the ability to use both eyes together, smoothly, equally, simultaneously, and accurately. This includes the ability to converge the eyes, aiming them toward each other to look at a near object; and to relax the convergence, moving the eyes away from each other to refocus on a distant object.

■ Hand-eye coordination—the ability to use the hands and eyes together in a synchronized manner so that a task such as hitting a ball can be performed with efficiency.

■ Attention maintenance—the ability to continue doing a particular skill or activity with ease and without interfering with the performance of other skills.

■ Near-vision acuity—the ability to clearly see, inspect, identify, and interpret objects at near distances (within twenty feet of the eyes).

■ Distance-vision acuity—the ability to clearly see, inspect, identify, and interpret objects at a distance (more than twenty feet away from the eyes).

■ Visualization—the ability to form mental images in the "mind's eye" and retain them for future recall or for synthesis into new mental images beyond the current or past experiences.

■ Relaxation—the ability to relax the eyes and the visual system. This is important for preventing and treating eyestrain.

Even in the absence of a complete vision-therapy program, vision-therapy techniques can help to improve these visual skills.

VISION-THERAPY TECHNIQUES

Vision-therapy techniques are designed to be used to improve the skills just mentioned. Following are some techniques you can do at home. It's usually best to do these techniques early in the day, before your eyes are too tired. Don't try to do all of the techniques every day. Instead, spread them over the course of a few days. See which of the techniques are the most difficult for you, then concentrate on those particular ones for several weeks, and see what improvements you can make in your vision.

Accommodative Rock

The accommodative rock helps to improve the eyes' ability to change focus and see clearly at near and at distance. Accommodation is the process by which the eyes change focus, and is probably the most important and most often performed function of the eyes. The ability to focus decreases with age, but adequate focusing ability can be maintained for longer periods of time with techniques such as this one. To do the accommodative rock:

1. Fasten some large letters, such as a banner newspaper headline, to a wall, and stand back twenty feet. If necessary, use your glasses to see the letters clearly.

2. Take some small letters, such as the body of a newspaper article, and hold them in one hand.

3. Cover one of your eyes with your free hand, keeping the eye itself open, and bring the small print as close to your face as you can while still being able to see it clearly. Stop.

4. Look at the large letters on the wall again. Are they clear?

5. Continuing to hold the small print at the same distance, look at it again. Is it clear?

6. Repeat steps 4 and 5 for a few minutes until you can see both the the distance and near letters easily. The accommodation should take only a second. Try the technique with the other eye, then repeat it with the small letters held one-inch closer.

Do this technique for five minutes with each eye at least twice a day. Preferably, finish both sessions before evening tiredness sets in. You can also try this technique throughout the day, whenever you find yourself with a near and a distant object on which to focus—for example, a wall clock and your wristwatch.

Rotations

Rotations increase the eyes' tracking ability and help your ability to pay attention to an activity. Smooth eye movements are basic to good vision. You'll need an empty pie pan and a marble for this technique. To do rotations:

1. Put the marble in the pie pan, and hold the pie pan about sixteen inches from your eyes.

2. Tilt the pie tin so that the marble rolls around the edge at a steady pace. Follow the marble with your eyes only; do not move your head.

3. Repeat step 2, rolling the marble around the edge of the pie pan in the opposite direction.

Do this technique for two minutes in each direction once a day. (You'll become dizzy if you keep the marble going in the same direction for more than two minutes). If possible, have a friend watch your eyes to see how smoothly they move.

Alphabet Fixations

Alphabet fixations improve the ability to center the eyes—that is, to fixate them—on an object in an instant. Fixation is one of the skills used in reading. This technique also helps with near-vision acuity. To do alphabet fixations:

1. Cut two strips of paper. Type or clearly print the alphabet in a vertical direction on each strip.

2. Hold the strips about eighteen inches from your face and a bit farther apart than shoulder width.

3. Call out the letters in alphabetical order, making sure to read each letter off a strip before calling out its name. Alternate between the strips, reading the "a" from one strip, the "b" from the second, the "c" from the first strip again, and so on. Keep your head absolutely still as you do this.

4. Spell words using the strips, again reading the letters before calling them out and alternating between the two strips as in step 3. For example, spell the word "boy" by taking the "b" from the left-hand strip, the "o" from the right-hand strip, and the "y" from the left-hand strip again. Your speed should increase with practice.

Do this technique for five minutes once a day.

Monocular Fixations

The monocular (one-eyed) fixation technique en-

hances the ability to fixate with one eye at a time. This particular technique is also designed to improve hand-eye coordination. You'll need a string, a small ring (such as a wedding band or a key ring), and a knitting needle or long pencil. To do monocular fixations:

1. Tie the string to the ring and hang the string (from a doorway, for example) so that the ring is at eye level. Stand about two feet away from the ring.

2. Hold the knitting needle or pencil in your right hand, cover your left eye, step forward on your right foot, and try to put the knitting needle or pencil through the ring without touching it. Try this several times.

3. Move the knitting needle or pencil to your left hand, cover your right eye, step forward on your left foot, and try to put the knitting needle or pencil through the ring again without touching it.

4. After mastering the technique using a stationary ring, repeat steps 2 and 3 with a swinging ring. This is great practice for many sports.

Do this technique for five minutes with each eye once a day.

Wall Fixations

Wall fixations improve your ability to fixate and your peripheral vision at the same time. You'll need eight white three-by-five-inch index cards, a felt-tipped marker, a blank wall, a book, and maybe some gentle music. To do wall fixations:

1. Number the index cards from one to eight, one number per card. Using the felt-tipped marker and a bold stroke, position each number in the center of the card and make it two inches tall. Fasten the cards in a haphazard order to a blank wall in an eight-foot square shape. (See Figure 3.9 on page 239.)

2. Stand about six feet from the wall, facing the center of the card pattern. Put a book on your head to keep your head steady, and cover one eye.

3. Starting with the "1" card, shift your eyes from card to card in numerical order. Keep your head very still and look directly at each number, being aware of the other numbers in your peripheral vision. If you wish, do this technique to gentle music to help keep your eye movements smooth and steady.

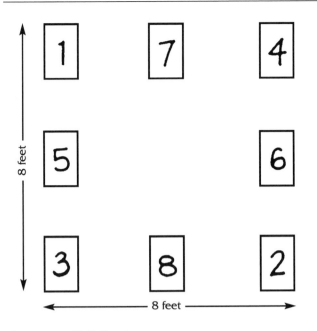

Figure 3.9. Wall fixations.

4. When you become adept at shifting your eyes from card to card, move closer to the wall. Continue to move closer as your skill improves. As you move closer to the wall, your eye movements will need to become more extreme.

5. Repeat steps 3 and 4 first with the other eye, then with both eyes together.

Do this technique for two minutes with each eye, then for two minutes with both eyes, once a day.

Marsden Ball

The Marsden ball technique is a great activity for improving tracking and fixation, as well as hand-eye coordination and attention maintenance. You'll need a rubber ball about four inches in diameter, some strong thread or string, and a ballpoint pen. To do the Marsden ball:

1. Write letters randomly all over the ball with the ballpoint pen. Attach the thread or string to the ball, and suspend the ball (from a doorway, for example) so that it can swing freely.

2. Cover one of your eyes, give the ball a slight push, and try to touch one letter at a time, calling out the letter at you do so. Keep your head as still as possible.

3. Repeat step 2 with the other eye.

Do this technique for two minutes with each eye once a day.

Deep Blink

The deep blink is designed to improve your ability to accommodate and the acuity of your distance vision. It's also a relaxation technique. Note that if you feel dizzy or faint at any time while performing the technique, stop and rest. You'll need a blank wall, a chair, and some large letters, such as a banner newspaper headline. To do the deep blink:

1. Fasten the large letters to the wall, and remove your glasses or contacts. Stand a few feet from the letters and gradually move back until the letters start to blur. Position the chair at that point.

2. Sit in the chair in a relaxed posture. Take a deep breath, and let it out slowly. Repeat this a few times until you feel relaxed.

3. Take a deep breath and hold it. With your breath held, close your eyes, clench your fists, and tighten the muscles in your whole body—legs, arms, stomach, chest, neck, face, head, and eyes. Keep your muscles tightened for about five seconds.

4. At the end of the five seconds, snap your hands and eyes open, exhale quickly through your mouth, and relax your entire body. Breathe slowly, and look at the letters, blinking gently as necessary. Stay very relaxed and try to look *through*, rather than *at*, the letters. After a second or two, the letters should become clear. (If you feel dizzy or faint after tightening and relaxing your muscles, omit this part. Just take slow, deep breaths, and practice looking through the letters on the wall.)

5. If the letters remained clear, push your chair about a foot back from the wall, and repeat steps 3 and 4. Continue moving your chair back to see how far away you can sit from the letters and still keep them clear. You may be amazed to find that after a few weeks, you can sit quite a few feet further back from where you started and still see those letters.

Do this technique at least once a day.

Brock String Technique

The Brock string technique helps to improve depth perception, peripheral vision, and binocular coordination. You'll need a piece of string four feet in length. To do the Brock string technique:

1. Tie a knot in the middle of the string. Attach one end of the string to any object that is at your eye level. (You can sit or stand for this technique.) Hold the string between your thumb and forefinger, stretch it taut, and hold it up against your nose.

2. Look at the far end of the string. You should see an *A* without the crossbar. You should see the knot in the middle of the string as two knots, one on each side of the *A*. (See Figure 3.10, below.)

3. Look at the knot in the string. It may take a few seconds, but you should be able to see an *X* pattern with one knot in the middle.

4. Shift your gaze back and forth from the *A* to the *X* pattern until the movement is smooth and requires little effort.

5. Move your gaze up the string toward your nose. As you do this, you should find the center of the *X* moving up toward your nose, too. When your gaze gets very close to your nose, the *X* should become a *V*, and the knot in the middle of the string should appear to be two knots, one on each side of the *V*, in your peripheral vision.

6. Shift your gaze from the *A* to the *X* to the *V* pattern until the movement is smooth and requires little effort. Continue shifting your gaze, shortening the string, but keeping the knot centered.

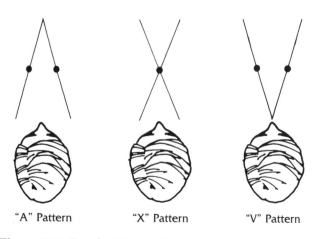

"A" Pattern   "X" Pattern   "V" Pattern

Figure 3.10. Brock string technique.

Do this technique for five minutes once a day.

Convergence Stimulation

Convergence is the aiming of the eyes toward one another as you look at near objects. This skill is critical for all near-point activities, such as reading. Convergence stimulation helps to develop binocular coordination, of which convergence is one aspect, and good depth perception. It also improves attention maintenance. You'll need Figure 3.11 on page 241 and a pencil. To do convergence stimulation:

1. Hold the illustration at your normal reading distance and focus your eyes on it. If necessary, wear your glasses or contact lenses. You should see two sets of concentric circles.

2. Position the point of the pencil in between the two sets of concentric circles and focus on it, remaining at your normal reading distance.

3. Move the pencil slowly toward your eyes, leaving the illustration where it is. Keep focusing on the point of the pencil, but be aware of the circles beyond it as you do. You should begin to see three, rather than two, sets of concentric circles when the pencil is approximately six inches from your eyes. The set in the middle (the one that's not really there) should appear as a three-dimensional figure, farther away from you than the larger ones and resembling a cup or flower pot. Keep the pencil still, and keep looking at it. Your eyes should feel as if they're crossing (they're actually just pulling in toward each other).

4. Relax your focus and look away from the illustration for a second or two, then look back at the illustration and see if you can regain the image. This may take some practice.

5. Repeat step 4 until it is easy to maintain and hold the center image.

Do this technique for several minutes every day. Alternate it with convergence relaxation, the next technique. Convergence stimulation and convergence relaxation exercise the same set of eye muscles, but pull them in different directions. If one of the techniques is much easier for you than the other, concentrate on the one that's more difficult until you can do it as easily as the other one.

Convergence Relaxation

Convergence relaxation is the opposite of convergence. It's the ability of the eyes to relax—that is, to diverge from their converged position—as they focus on a distant object. Excessive near-point work can cause the eyes to have trouble relaxing, so practicing convergence relaxation is good for breaking up your day if you do a lot of reading or computer work. The technique helps with binocular coordination, depth perception, and attention maintenance. You'll once again need Figure 3.11, below, plus a blank wall. To practice convergence relaxation:

1. Stand at least ten feet away from the blank wall and focus your eyes on it.

2. Slowly bring the illustration into your line of sight at your normal reading distance, but keep your eyes focused on the wall. You can hold the illustration just above the point on the wall where your eyes are focused. You should see three sets of concentric circles, just as you did in the convergence-stimulation technique. But this time, while the center set of circles should still seem to be three-dimensional, it should also appear to be closer to you than the outside circles and resemble upside-down cups or flower pots. The other sets of circles, which will be in your peripheral vision, may appear this way, too.

3. Relax your focus and look away from the illustration for a second or two, then look back at the illustration and see if you can regain the image. This may take some practice.

4. Repeat step 3 until it is easy to maintain and hold the center image.

Do this technique for several minutes every day. Alternate it with convergence stimulation, the previous technique.

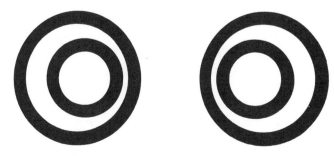

Figure 3.11. Convergence Stimulation and Convergence Relaxation.

Palming

Palming is a relaxation technique to use between other techniques and throughout the day. It allows you to relax your mind and your eyes because you don't focus on anything but blackness. It can also increase your visualization skills. Palming is adapted from the Bates method. To do palming:

1. Close your eyes and cover them with your hands. Keep your palms over, but not touching, your eyelids. Your fingers should overlap near your hairline, and you should have enough room to breathe easily. Rest your elbows on a table. All you should see is complete blackness. If you see flashes of light, just let them go, and allow the blackness to return. You can either continue to focus on the blackness, or you can now start to visualize a relaxing scene of your own choosing.

2. Take a deep breath and feel the muscles around your eyes completely relax. Breathe deeply and slowly eight times.

Do this technique as needed, at least eight times a day, preferably before you start an intense near-point task, such as reading or computer work.

Head Rolling

Head rolling is another relaxation technique based on the Bates method. It increases the blood flow, which increases the flow of life-maintaining oxygen, to the brain and eyes. It also feels good!

1. While seated, gently drop your head forward, reaching your chin toward your chest. Then, slowly roll your head around from one shoulder to the other, making a complete circle. Keep your shoulders level and maintain regular breathing. Make two or three complete revolutions with your head.

2. Repeat step 1, rolling your head in the other direction.

Do this technique first thing in the morning and again later in the afternoon for a relaxation break. It is also good to do this technique as a short break from computer work.

Appendix

Glossary

accommodation. The ability of the eye to adjust its focus for near or distance vision.

acquired immune deficiency syndrome (AIDS). A virus that impairs the body's immune system, and leaves the person highly susceptible to infections, malignancies, and neurologic disease.

acuity. *See* visual acuity.

acupressure. An ancient Chinese medical practice that involves the use of finger pressure to stimulate specific points in the body that assist in healing. *See also* acupuncture.

acupuncture. An ancient Chinese medical practice that involves the use of extremely fine needles to stimulate specific points in the body that assist in healing. *See also* acupressure.

aftercataract. *See* secondary cataract.

albinism. A genetic condition in which all the normal pigmentation in the body is absent.

amblyopia. *See* lazy eye.

amino acid. One of the chemical substances that are the building blocks of protein.

antihistamine. A type of medication used to suppress allergic reactions. Antihistamines can cause increased pressure in the eyes, and should not be used by people who have glaucoma.

antioxidant. A substance that blocks oxidation reactions in the body, some of which can lead to cellular dysfunction and destruction. The antioxidant nutrients include beta-carotene, vitamin C, vitamin E, and selenium. Other antioxidants are the amino acid glutathione, and the enzymes superoxide dismutase (SOD), peroxidase, and catalase.

anti-reflective lens coating. A coating that is applied to an eyeglass lens to allow the passage of more light through the lens, and to decrease the scattering of light from the surface of the lens.

aqueous fluid. *See* aqueous humor.

aqueous humor. A watery fluid that surrounds the iris and lens in the front part of the eye, and provides some nutrition to the adjoining parts of the eye. Also called the aqueous fluid.

artificial intraocular lens. An artificial lens that is often inserted following cataract surgery to take over the focusing that the eye's own lens can no longer do. Present artificial intraocular lenses cannot change focus the way the eye's lens can, but focus-changing lenses should soon be available. *See also* lens.

astigmatism. A condition in which the cornea is shaped more like a barrel than a ball, causing the light passing through it to be spread over a diffuse area of the retina rather than focused into a single point; a refractive error. *See also* emmetropia; farsightedness; nearsightedness; presbyopia; refractive error.

atherosclerosis. A condition in which fats are deposited in the body's arteries. It is associated with high blood pressure, high blood levels of cholesterol and triglycerides, obesity, smoking, diabetes, stress, family history of atherosclerosis, physical inactivity, and the male sex.

Bates method. A system of techniques devised by Dr. William Bates to improve eyesight. Dr. Bates theorized that stress is the cause of most vision problems, and that relaxation is the cure.

beta-carotene. A nutrient related to vitamin A that is used by the body to manufacture vitamin A.

bifocal contact lens. A contact lens that compensates for presbyopia by correcting both distance and near vision. *See also* contact lens.

bifocal lens. A lens that contains two segments—one

for distance viewing and one for near viewing. *See also* lens; trifocal lens.

binocular. Two-eyed.

binocular coordination. The ability to use both eyes in a smooth, efficient manner.

biofeedback. A technique for controlling autonomic (normally uncontrollable) body functions. It involves learning to respond to a signal, such as a tone, when changes occur in the pulse, blood pressure, or other autonomic body function.

bioflavonoids. A diverse group of compounds found in most plants, including fruits and vegetables. They can act as antioxidants, immune-system regulators, and anti-inflammatory agents.

blepharitis. A condition in which the eyelid is inflamed.

blink reflex. A reflex in which the eyes automatically close in response to the sudden movement of an object toward them.

blue light. Light with a wavelength of between 400 and 500 nanometers. It can cause damage to the retina.

blue-blocker sunglasses. Sunglasses with lenses that block out blue light.

board certification. In medicine, a designation indicating that a practitioner has met standards above and beyond those required for a license to practice, and has passed a specialty examination in a particular field, such as ophthalmology.

carotene. A yellow pigment present in some plants and animals. It is abundant in yellow vegetables such as carrots, squash, and corn, and is convertable to vitamin A in the human liver.

cataract. A condition in which the lens inside the eye loses its transparency and begins to become opaque, eventually preventing light from reaching the retina. *See also* congenital cataract; glass blower's cataract; secondary cataract; senile cataract.

central vision. The direct, line-of-sight vision. Also called the macular vison. *See also* peripheral vision; visual field.

chalazion. A condition in which the duct of one of the meibomian glands in the eyelid becomes plugged, resulting in inflammation. Also called a meibomian cyst. *See also* stye.

choroid. A layer between the retina and sclera, con-

sisting primarily of blood vessels that provide nourishment to the retina.

closed-angle glaucoma. *See* narrow-angle glaucoma.

collagen. A fibrous protein found in the connective tissues in the skin, bones, ligaments, and cartilage.

color deficiency. A condition in which a person either is missing a certain type of color cone in the retina or has cones that are deficient in the ability to process color signals. Most people who are labeled colorblind are actually color deficient. *See also* colorblindness.

color receptors. *See* cones.

colorblindness. Strictly speaking, a complete absence of color vision. The condition is extremely rare. *See also* color deficiency.

complete protein. Dietary protein that contains the full complement of amino acids, especially the eight that the body cannot produce on its own. *See also* protein.

complex carbohydrate. A carbohydrate that includes fiber, which slows the release of sugar from the carbohydrate into the bloodstream and provides dietary fiber as well. The sources of complex carbohydrates include whole grains, fruits, and vegetables. *See also* simple carbohydrate.

cones. The specialized cone-shaped cells in the retina of the eye. They are responsible for color vision. Also called color receptors. *See also* photoreceptors; rods.

congenital cataract. A cataract that is present at birth. *See also* cataract.

conjunctiva. The membrane that covers the sclera and the insides of the eyelids, and contains glands to moisten the front of the eyeball.

conjunctivitis. *See* pinkeye.

contact lens. An artificial lens that rests on the cornea of the eye, and corrects for refractive errors. *See also* bifocal contact lens; daily-wear contact lens; disposable contact lens; extended-wear contact lens; flexible-wear contact lens; gas-permeable contact lens; hard contact lens; lens; rigid gas-permeable contact lens.

convergence. The moving of the two eyes toward each other. This normally happens when the eyes change focus from distance to near.

cornea. The outermost, transparent part of the outer protective layer of the eye. Its bulging curvature is responsible for most of the refraction that occurs in the eye.

corneal abrasion. A small cut or scrape on the front

surface of the cornea.

corneal ulcer. A loss of tissue in the cornea due to a progressive erosion or loss of cells.

CR-39. A type of plastic material used to make eyeglass lenses.

cross-eyed. Having an eye that turns inward toward the nose while the other eye looks straight ahead. *See also* strabismus; wall-eyed.

cytomegalovirus. A common virus of the herpes family that can cause disease in infants and in persons with compromised immune systems.

daily-wear contact lens. A contact lens designed to be worn on a full-time basis, but not overnight. *See also* contact lens.

depth perception. The ability to perceive size and distance relationships among objects in space.

deuteranopia. A defect in the perception of the color green. *See also* protanopia.

developmental optometry. The specialty of optometry that pertains to the visual development of children through adulthood. Developmental optometrists commonly treat visual-perception difficulties, strabismus, and other vision-related disabilities.

diabetes mellitus. A disorder of carbohydrate metabolism in which the body is unable to use glucose (sugar) properly. It is usually caused by a lack of the hormone insulin or an inability to utilize insulin.

diabetic retinopathy. A disorder of the blood vessels in the retina stemming from diabetes. It is one of the leading causes of blindness in the United States.

diopter. A unit of measurement used to describe the focusing power of a lens.

diplopia. *See* double vison.

directionality. The ability to distinguish right from left on another person or object without reference to your own body.

disposable contact lens. A contact lens designed to be discarded after the prescribed wearing time, which is usually one to two weeks. *See also* contact lens.

distance vision. The vision used to see objects twenty or more feet away. *See also* intermediate vision; near vision.

doll's-eye reflex. A reflex in which a baby's eyes continue to look at a certain person as his or her head is slowly turned or nodded back and forth.

double vision. The condition of seeing double. Also called diplopia.

dyslexia. An inability to read and understand written language despite having normal intelligence.

edema. Swelling that results from an accumulation of fluid.

emmetropia. The condition of the optically normal eye. When light passes through the cornea, it comes to a focus directly on the retina. *See also* astigmatism; farsightedness; nearsightedness; presbyopia; refractive error.

enzyme. A type of protein that is capable of inducing chemical changes in other substances without being changed itself.

extended-wear contact lens. A contact lens designed to be kept in overnight for several days. *See also* contact lens.

extracapsular cataract extraction. A technique used in cataract surgery in which the cataract-covered lens is removed, but the capsule surrounding the lens is left intact. *See also* intracapsular cataract extraction.

extract. A concentrated essence, such as of an herb, made by leaching the active properties using either alcohol or water. *See also* infusion; tincture.

extraocular. Outside the eyeball. Used to describe the muscles that move the eyeball. *See also* intraocular.

eye pressure. *See* intraocular pressure.

farsightedness. A condition in which the eye is too short or the cornea too flat, causing the light passing through the cornea to come to a focus behind the retina when viewing a distant object; a refractive error. The farsighted person can see distant objects clearly, but sees near objects as blurry. Also called hyperopia. *See also* astigmatism; emmetropia; nearsightedness; presbyopia; refractive error.

figure-ground discrimination. The ability to distinguish an object from its background. Some optical illusions are interesting because it is not clear which part is the figure and which is the ground.

fine motor. Referring to the small muscles of the body, such as those of the fingers. *See also* gross motor.

flexible-wear contact lens. A contact lens designed to be either taken out each night or left in overnight according to the wearer's wishes. *See also* contact lens.

floaters. Small bits of protein or cells within the vitreous of the eye. They vary in size and shape, and are occasionally visible as specks before the eyes.

focusing flexibility. The ability of the eye to easily change its focusing power from distance to near to distance again.

form perception. The ability to perceive the shapes of objects, including those of words on a page.

gas-permeable contact lens. A contact lens made of a material that allows the passage of oxygen and carbon dioxide. *See also* contact lens.

glass blower's cataract. A cataract that results from constant exposure to infrared light. It is found in glass blowers who work without eye protection. *See also* cataract.

glaucoma. A condition in which the pressure within the eye is increased, causing compression of the retina and optic nerve, as well as a reduction in the blood flow to the eye. If untreated, it can lead to blindness. *See also* narrow-angle glaucoma; open-angle glaucoma.

glucose. A sugar that is formed in the body during digestion. It is essential to the chemistry of the body.

gross motor. Referring to the large muscles of the body, such as those of the legs, arms, trunk, and head. *See also* fine motor.

hand-eye coordination. The ability to use the eyes and hands together to accomplish a task.

hard contact lens. A rigid plastic contact lens that does not allow the passage of oxygen or carbon dioxide. *See also* contact lens.

hemoglobin. The iron-containing pigment in red blood cells. Its function is to carry oxygen from the lungs to the rest of the body.

hemorrhage. Profuse or abnormal bleeding.

herpes viruses. A group of viruses, including herpes simplex and herpes zoster, that can infect the eyes, mouth, genitals, and other parts of the body.

hydrophilic. Literally means "water-loving." It is used to describe a type of plastic utilized in making soft contact lenses.

hyperopia. *See* farsightedness.

hyphema. A condition in which blood has collected in the anterior chamber of the eye.

infection. A condition in which the body is invaded by an organism that multiplies and produces injurious effects.

inflammation. The response of the body to an injury. It usually involves swelling, redness, heat, pain, and impaired functioning of the affected area.

infrared light. Light with a wavelength of more than 700 nanometers, which puts it above the range of the human visual spectrum. Also called infrared radiation.

infrared radiation. *See* infrared light.

infusion. A preparation made by steeping herbs in hot water; tea. *See also* extract; tincture.

intermediate vision. The vision used to see objects at roughly arm's length away. *See also* distance vision; near vision.

international unit (IU). A unit of potency based on an accepted international standard. Vitamins A and E, among other supplements, are usually measured in international units.

intracapsular cataract extraction. A technique used in cataract surgery in which both the cataract-covered lens and the capsule surrounding it are removed. *See also* extracapsular cataract extraction.

intraocular. Inside the eyeball. Used to describe the eye muscles that control focusing, as well as the eye's lens and other structures. *See also* extraocular.

intraocular lens, artificial. *See* artificial intraocular lens.

intraocular pressure. The pressure within the eyeball. An increased level of intraocular pressure is known as glaucoma. Also called eye pressure.

iris. The colored portion of the eye that surrounds the pupil. Its expansion decreases the amount of light entering the eye through the pupil, and its contraction increases the amount of light.

iritis. A condition in which the iris is inflamed.

Irlen lenses. Colored lenses developed by Dr. Helen Irlen that help some people with a certain form of dyslexia to read with more ease and comprehension.

keratoconus. A condition in which the cornea has a conelike bulge.

keratomileusis. A surgical procedure in which an outer layer of the cornea is removed, reshaped, and then sewn back in a effort to reshape the cornea and correct for a refractive error.

lacrimal gland. A gland located just above the eyeball that produces tears to wet the eye.

laser. A device that emits intense heat and power at

close range. It is used in surgery and some diagnostic procedures. Its name is an acronym for "light amplification by stimulated emission of radiation."

laser-assisted intrastromal keratomileusis (LASIK). A surgical procedure in which a microkeratome is used to make a flap in the cornea and a laser is then used to remove a wedge from the cornea in an effort to reshape the cornea and correct for a refractive error.

laterality. The ability to distinguish right from left on another person or object with reference to your own body.

lazy eye. A condition in which a healthy eye cannot achieve 20/20 vision with any corrective device. It usually results from the brain suppressing the vision in that eye to avoid seeing two different images from the two eyes. Also called amblyopia.

legal blindness. See low vision.

lens. The resilient, transparent structure in the eye that focuses light on the retina by changing the curvature of its front surface. It is located near the front of the eye, directly behind the pupil. Also, a transparent device that corrects for refractive errors by causing light to be focused on the retina of the eye. It includes eyeglass lenses, contact lenses, and the artificial intraocular lenses that are implanted after cataract surgery. See also artificial intraocular lens; bifocal lens; contact lens; trifocal lens.

light sensitivity. A condition in which the eyes are extremely sensitive to light. Also called photophobia.

low vision. A condition is which the best visual acuity, with correction, is less than 20/200 or the visual field extends less than 20 degrees in each direction from the point where the attention is focused. Also called legal blindness.

macula. The central area of the retina that is used for direct, central vision. In humans, it has only cones, no rods.

macular degeneration. Irreversible and progressive damage to the macular portion of the retina, resulting in a gradual loss of fine, or reading, vision. It is a leading cause of blindness in the United States, and is usually associated with aging.

macular vision. See central vision.

meibomian cyst. See chalazion.

meibomian gland. A sebaceous gland within the structure of the eyelid that secretes an oily substance that lubricates the edge of the eyelid and helps to pre-vent tears from evaporating. Each eyelid has twenty to thirty meibomian glands.

metabolic rate. The rate at which the body carries out its metabolic functions.

metabolism. The entire complex of physical and chemical processes necessary to sustain life. It includes the breaking down of certain substances (such as foods) to release energy, and the synthesis of others (such as proteins) for the growth and repair of tissues.

migraine headache. A type of headache that is severe and frequently involves just one side of the head. It may last for several days, and may be associated with nausea, distorted vision, and the appearance of flashes of light.

milligram (mg). A unit of measurement equivalent to one one-thousandth of a gram. It is used to measure weight.

mineral. An inorganic substance that occurs in nature. Some minerals, such as iron and calcium, are essential to the proper functioning of the human body.

minus lens. A lens that decreases the focusing power of the light passing through it, causing the light to focus farther back, on the retina. It is used to correct for nearsightedness. See also lens; nearsightedness; plus lens.

monovision. A technique in which one contact lens is prescribed for distance vision and the other is prescribed for near vision. It is used an as alternative to bifocal contact lenses.

motor development. Pertaining to the development of the muscles and their coordination.

multiple sclerosis. An inflammatory disease of the central nervous system. It can cause visual disturbances because it often affects both the optic nerve and the nerves that control the muscles of the eyes.

myopia. See nearsightedness.

nanometer (nm). A unit of measurement equal to one one-billionth of a meter. It is used to measure the wavelength of light.

narrow-angle glaucoma. A form of glaucoma in which the drainage channel for the eye fluids is blocked. Also called closed-angle glaucoma. See also glaucoma; open-angle glaucoma.

nasal side. The side closest to the nose, as opposed to the ear. It is used to describe the location of structures in the eye and other parts of the face. *See also* temporal side.

near vision. The vision used to see objects sixteen inches away or closer. *See also* distance vision; intermediate vision.

nearsightedness. A condition in which the eye is too long, the cornea too steeply curved, or the lens unable to relax, causing the light passing through the cornea to come to a focus in front of the retina when viewing a distant object; a refractive error. The nearsighted person can see near objects clearly, but sees distant objects as blurry. Also called myopia. *See also* astigmatism; emmetropia; farsightedness; presbyopia; refractive error.

oculomotor. Referring to the movement of the eyeball.

open-angle glaucoma. A form of glaucoma in which there is sufficient space for the eye fluids to drain, yet the pressure in the eye is still increased. *See also* glaucoma; narrow-angle glaucoma.

ophthalmologist. A medical doctor who specializes in eye diseases and eye surgery. *See also* optician; optometrist.

ophthalmoscope. An instrument with a mirror and light system that is used to view the interior of the eye, especially the retina, optic nerve, and choroid.

optic disk. The portion of the optic nerve that is formed by the gathering of all the transparent nerve fibers from the retina. The optic disk itself is not light-sensitive.

optic nerve. The bundle of fibers that carries the visual impulses from the retina to the brain.

optician. A licensed technician who makes and dispenses eyeglasses according to prescriptions from optometrists and ophthalmologists. In some states, opticians can also fit contact lenses. *See also* ophthalmologist; optometrist.

optometric vision therapy. A therapy program designed to realign and alter the functioning of the visual system. It includes techniques and other activities to reduce the visual stress, guide the development of the visual system, improve the visual skills, and enhance visual performance. Also called vision therapy.

optometrist. A licensed eye-care practioner who examines and treats the eyes and visual system for refractive errors, eye-brain coordination problems,

and signs of injury and disease. *See also* ophthalmologist; optician.

orbit. The area of the skull in which the eyeball and its associated parts are situated.

orthokeratology. A program of progressive contact lens fitting that gradually reduces the amount of nearsightedness and / or astigmatism.

peripheral vision. The part of the visual field that is outside the direct line of vision; the side vision. *See also* central vision; visual field.

phacoemulsification. A technique used in cataract surgery in which the eye's lens is disintegrated and then evacuated through a vacuum tube.

photochromic. Capable of changing color when exposed to ultraviolet light.

photochromic lens. An eyeglass lens that is capable of changing color when exposed to ultraviolet light.

photophobia. *See* light sensitivity.

photoreceptors. Sensory cells that are stimulated by light. In humans, they are the rods and cones of the retina. *See also* cones; rods.

pinguecula. A small raised yellowish area on the sclera, usually on the nasal side. It is a benign growth, and does not grow onto the cornea.

pinkeye. An inflammation of the conjunctiva. It can be caused by an infection, allergy, or irritation. Also called conjunctivitis.

plus lens. A lens that increases the focusing power of the light passing through it, causing the light to focus farther forward, on the retina. It is used to correct for farsightedness and presbyopia. *See also* farsightedness; lens; minus lens; presbyopia.

polarizing lens. An eyeglass lens that reduces glare by decreasing the scattering of the incoming light rays.

polycarbonate. A type of plastic material used to make eyeglass lenses. It has a higher refractive index and more impact resistance than CR-39.

presbyopia. A condition in which the eye's lens has hardened and lost its focusing flexibility, causing difficulty with near vision; a refractive error. It usually occurs after the age of forty. *See also* astigmatism; emmetropia; farsightedness; nearsightedness; refractive error.

progressive addition lens (PAL). A type of multifocal lens in which the transition from the distance segment to the intermediate segment and then to the near segment of the lens is gradual and uninterrupted. *See also* lens; trifocal lens.

protanopia. A defect in the perception of the color red. *See also* deuteranopia.

protein. A naturally occurring combination of amino acids that forms the basis of living cells. *See also* complete protein.

pterygium. A wing-shaped growth on the front of the eye, normally starting on the sclera on the nasal side and slowly growing over the cornea.

pupil. The round hole in the center of the iris through which light passes. It ordinarily appears black because very little light comes from the dark chamber behind it.

pupil reflex. A reflex in which the pupils constrict in response to light. Both pupils should constrict when a light is shined into either eye.

radial keratotomy. A surgical procedure in which radial cuts are made into the cornea in an effort to flatten it and correct for a refractive error.

refraction. The bending of a light ray when it passes from one transparent medium into another of a different optical density. Also, the portion of a vision examination in which corrective lenses are used to sharpen the vision to within the normal limits.

refractive error. A condition in which the light passing through the cornea is refracted incorrectly and therefore does not come to a focus on the retina, causing blurred near and/or distance vision. *See also* astigmatism; emmetropia; farsightedness; nearsightedness; presbyopia.

refractor. An instrument used for diagnosing refractive errors.

resolving power. The ability to distinguish two points from each other at a given distance. It is a measure of visual acuity.

retina. The inner lining of most of the back chamber of the eye. It contains layers of nerve cells that are sensitive to light.

retinal detachment. A condition in which the inner layer of the retina detaches from the outer layer. If it is detected early and treated promptly with surgery, it can be corrected and the vision restored.

retinitis pigmentosa. A condition in which the retina begins to deteriorate at around the age of ten, leading to night blindness, then loss of the peripheral vision,

and finally blindness. It is a progressive congenital disease with no cure. Also called tunnel vision.

rhodopsin. A light-sensitive pigment present in the rod cells of the retina. It is responsible for the transformation of light energy into nerve energy. Also called visual purple.

riboflavin. *See* vitamin B_2.

rigid gas-permeable contact lens. The modern version of a hard contact lens. A rigid lens allows the passage of oxygen and carbon dioxide. *See also* contact lens.

rods. The straight, thin cells in the retina of the eye. They contain rhodopsin, and are responsible for night vision and vision in dim light. *See also* cones; photoreceptors.

sclera. The tough, white, fibrous outer protective layer of the eye.

scotopic sensitivity syndrome (SSS). A condition in which the night vision is used at all times, which can lead to visual distortions and difficulty reading. It was first described by researcher Helen Irlen in the 1980s.

seasonal affective disorder (SAD). A condition marked by mental depression during the winter months. It is thought to be related to the lack of sunlight.

secondary cataract. The development of an opacity of the eye's lens capsule after cateract removal. Also called aftercataract. *See also* cataract.

seeing. The process of receiving light through the eyes and transmitting visual impulses to the brain for interpretation.

senile cataract. A cataract that develops in the later years. *See also* cataract.

simple carbohydrate. A simple sugar, such as glucose or lactose (milk sugar), that is rapidly absorbed into the bloodstream. *See also* complex carbohydrate.

slit lamp. A specialized microscope using a narrow slit of light and high magnification. It is used to examine the exterior portions of the eye.

Snellen chart. A chart imprinted with rows of black letters, with the letters graduating in size from the smallest on the bottom row to the largest on the top row. It was developed by Dutch ophthalmologist Herman Snellen (1834–1908), and is used for testing visual acuity.

soft contact lens. A contact lens made of a comfortable soft plastic with a high water content. *See also* contact lens.

strabismus. A condition in which the two eyes do not align properly while looking at a single object. One eye turns away (out, in, up, or down) from the point of regard. *See also* cross-eyed; wall-eyed.

stroke. A sudden loss of consciousness caused by an interruption of the blood supply to the brain.

stye. A condition in which the hair follicle of an eyelash becomes infected, resulting in inflammation, redness, and soreness. *See also* chalazion.

subconjunctival hemorrhage. Bleeding from broken blood vessels under the conjunctiva. It appears as a red spot on the white sclera. Though it looks alarming, it usually resolves without treatment.

temporal lobes. Areas of the brain located on both sides of the head surrounding the ears. The temporal lobes process auditory and some visual information.

temporal side. The side closest to the ear, as opposed to the nose. It is used to describe the location of structures in the eye and other parts of the face. *See also* nasal side.

thiamine. *See* vitamin B$_1$.

thyroid gland. A gland located in the neck that produces thyroid hormone.

thyroid hormone. The substances produced by the thyroid gland that play a role in the regulation of the metabolism. An overabundance of thyroid hormone is associated with damage to the eyes.

tincture. A concentrated essence, such as of an herb, made by extracting and concentrating the active properties using alcohol. *See also* extract; infusion.

tonometer. An instrument used to measure the pressure in the eye. It is used to screen for glaucoma.

toric contact lens. A contact lens designed to treat astigmatism. *See also* contact lens.

tracking. The ability to follow a moving target.

trifocal lens. A lens that contains three segments—one for distance viewing, one for intermediate viewing, and one for near viewing. *See also* bifocal lens.

tunnel vision. *See* retinitis pigmentosa.

20/20 vision. The visual acuity in the optically normal human eye. The term comes from the ability to read a specific row of letters or other symbols on a chart such as the Snellen chart from a distance of twenty feet.

Deviations from the norm are expressed as, for example, 20/30, which indicates the ability to read at twenty feet what an optically normal person can read at thirty feet.

ultraviolet (UV) light. Light with a wavelength of less than 400 nanometers, which puts it below the range of the human visual spectrum.

vision. The entire visual process of receiving light through the eyes, the eyes transmitting visual impulses to the brain, and the brain interpreting the various aspects of the impulses and initiating the body's response to them.

vision therapy. *See* optometric vision therapy.

visual acuity. The acuteness or keenness of vision; the ability to discriminate the fine details of objects. The normal visual acuity is 20/20. Also called acuity.

visual field. The entire area that can be seen without shifting the position of the eyes. It includes the central and peripheral vision. *See also* central vision; peripheral vision.

visual impulse. The sensation caused by light striking a photoreceptor. The sensation is then transmitted to the brain by nerves.

visual memory. The ability to remember objects and other information based on having perceived them visually.

visual purple. *See* rhodopsin.

visualization. The ability to form a mental image of an object that is not actually present.

vitamin. An essential organic compound necessary for human metabolism, but not manufactured by the human body. Vitamins must be taken in wholly or partly from nutrient sources.

vitamin B$_1$. Among its functions, it helps to maintain the health of the retina. Also called thiamine.

vitamin B$_2$. Among its functions, it contributes to the metabolism of nutrients in the retina, and plays a role in maintaining the oxygen supply to the cornea. Also called riboflavin.

vitreous humor. A clear jellylike substance that fills the posterior (back) chamber of the eye, and serves as a support structure for the retina.

wall-eyed. Having an eye that turns outward toward the ear while the other eye looks straight ahead. *See also* cross-eyed; strabismus.

Recommended Suppliers

The following list of suppliers is included so that you can find and use the supplements and remedies recommended in this book. It is not intended to be an exhaustive list of all possible sources of these products. Rather, the author recommends them because he has found their products to be of good quality. Also, please be aware that the addresses and phone numbers are subject to change.

HERBAL PRODUCTS

Brion Herbs
9200 Jeronimo Road
Irvine, CA 92718
800–333–HERB

Products include Chinese herbal combinations.

DY-Medias, Inc.
4800 Whitesburg Drive
Suite 30-164
Huntsville, AL 35802
205–881–5670

Products include Visioplex Eye Concentrate With Eyebright.

Herbs, Etc.
1340 Rufina Circle
Santa Fe, NM 87501
800–634–3727

Herb-Pharm
P.O. Box 116
William, OR 97544
503–846–6262

McZand Herbal Inc.
P.O. Box 5312
Santa Monica, CA 90409
310–822–0500

Nature's Herbs
P.O. Box 336
Orem, UT 84059
800–HERBALS

Nature's Way Products, Inc.
10 Mountain Springs Parkway
Springville, UT 84663
801–489–1520

Super Salve
606 Lake Mary Road
Flagstaff, AZ 86001
602–774–8910

Wyoming Wildcrafters
Wilson, WY 80304
307–733–6731

HOMEOPATHIC REMEDIES

Boericke and Tafel, Inc.
1011 Arch Street
Philadelphia, PA 19107
215–922–2967

Boiron
6 Campus Boulevard
Building A
Newtown Square, PA 19073
800–BLU–TUBE

Products include Optique 1 and Thyroidium. Products available only through physicians.

Boiron-Borneman
1208 Amosland Road
Norwood, PA 19074
215–532–2035

Dolisos America, Inc.
3014 Rigel Avenue
Las Vegas, NV 89102
702–871–7153

Hahnemann Pharmacy
828 San Pablo Avenue
Albany, CA 94706
510–527–3003

Homeopathic Educational
Services
2124 Kittredge Street
Berkeley, CA 94704
510–649–8930

Luyties Pharmacal Company
4200 Laclede Avenue
St. Louis, MO 63108
800–325–8080

Millen Medical Products
15 Pecunit
Canton, MA 02021
800–649–4372

Products include Similisan No. 1.

Standard Homeopathic Company
P.O. Box 61604
436 West Eighth Street
Los Angeles, CA 90014
213–321–4284

LIGHTING EQUIPMENT AND INFORMATION

Duro-Test Corporation
9 Law Drive
Fairfield, NJ 07007
800–289–3876

General Electric Company
Lighting Information Center
Nela Park
Cleveland, OH 44112
216–266–3900

NUTRITIONAL SUPPLEMENTS

Advanced Medical Nutrition
2247 National Avenue
P.O. Box 5012
Hayward, CA 94540-5012

Products available only through physicians.

Alacer Corporation
14 Morgan Street
Irvine, CA 92718
714–951–9660

Betatene
71-77 Taunton Drive
Cheltenham, Victoria 3192
Australia
61–3–9584 4588

Products include Carotenoid Complex.

Ethical Nutrients
971 Calle Negocio
San Clemente, CA 92673
714–366–0818

Health Shoppe
41 Charles Street
Toronto, Ontario M4Y 2R4
Canada
800–387–2749

Products include OptiZinc zinc supplement.

Lane Labs-USA, Inc.
172 Broadway
Woodcliff Lake, NJ 07675
800–526–3001

Products include Benefin Shark Cartilage.

Miracle Exclusives Inc.
3 Elm Street
P.O. Box 349
Locust Valley, NY 11560
516–676–0220

Natren, Inc.
3105 Willow Lane
Westlake Village, CA 91361
805–371–4742

Pine Health Works
8813 North Cedarcrest Drive
Kickapoo, Illinois 61528-9616
888–278–0068

Products include Pycnogenol Pine Bark Extract.

Rainbow Light Nutritional Systems
207 McPherson Street
P.O. Box 3033
Santa Cruz, CA 95060
408–429–9089
800–635–1233

Vision Pharmaceuticals
1022 North Main
Mitchell, SD 57301
800–325–6789

Products include Viva-Drops vitamin-A drops.

Wakunaga of America Company Ltd.
23501 Madero
Mission Viejo, CA 92691
714–855–2776

Resource Organizations

The following organizations can answer questions, provide referrals, and tell you how to find more information. Some organizations sell literature or offer classes and workshops to help you broaden your understanding of their areas of specialty. Use them liberally in your investigation of the best ways to care for yourself and your family.

BLINDNESS AND LOW VISION

American Council of the Blind, Inc.
1211 Connecticut Avenue, NW
Suite 506
Washington, DC 20036
202–833–1251

American Foundation for the Blind
15 West 16th Street
New York, NY 10011
800–232–5463

Regional offices:
Chicago, IL   312–269–0095
Atlanta, GA   404–525–2303
Dallas, TX   214–352–7222
San Francisco, CA   415–392–4848
Washington, DC   202–492–0358

Association for the Education and Rehabilitation
  of the Blind and Visually Impaired
206 North Washington
Suite 320
Alexandria, VA 22314
703–548–1884

National Association for the Visually Handicapped
305 East 24th Street
New York, NY 10010
212–889–3141

National Federation of the Blind
1800 Johnson Street
Baltimore, MD 21230
301–659–9314

Prevent Blindness America
500 East Remington Road
Schaumburg, IL 60173
312–843–2020
800–331–2020

Research to Prevent Blindness, Inc.
598 Madison Avenue
New York, NY 10022
212–752–4333

Trace Research and Development Center
S-151 Waisman Center
1500 Highland Avenue
Madison, WI 53705
608–262–6966
608–263–5408 (TDD)
608–262–8848 (Fax)

A multidisciplinary research and resource center on technology and human disability.

DYSLEXIA AND LEARNING DISABILITIES

American Speech-Language-Hearing Association
10801 Rockville Pike
Rockville, MD 20852
301–897–5700

Association for Children and Adults With
  Learning Disabilities
4156 Library Road
Pittsburgh, PA 15234
412–341–1515

Irlen Institute for Perceptual and Learning
  Disabilities
4425 Atlantic Avenue
Suite A-14
Long Beach, CA 90807
213–422–2723

The Orton Dyslexia Society
724 York Road
Baltimore, MD 21204
301–296–0232

HERBAL THERAPY

Institute for Traditional Medicine and Preventive
  Health Care
2442 SE Sherman Avenue
Portland, OR 97214
503–233–4907

Oriental Healing Arts Institute
1945 Palo Verde Avenue
Suite 208
Long Beach, CA 90815
562–431–3544

OPTOMETRIC VISION THERAPY

College of Optometrists in Vision Development
243 North Lindbergh Boulevard
Suite 310
St. Louis, MO 63141
888–268–3770

Optometric Extension Program Foundation, Inc.
1921 East Carnegie
Suite 3L
Santa Ana, CA 92705
714–250–8070

ORTHOKERATOLOGY

National Eye Research Foundation
International Orthokeratology Section
910 Skokie Boulevard
Suite 207A
Northbrook, IL 60062
800–621–2258

SPECIFIC CONDITIONS

American Diabetes Association
P.O Box 25757
Alexandria, VA 22313
703–549–1500
800–232–3472

Benign Essential Research Foundation
P.O. Box 12468
Beaumont, TX 77726-2468
409–832–0788
409–832–0890 (Fax)

Blepharospasm information and support groups.

Foundation for Glaucoma Research
490 Post Street
Suite 1042
San Francisco, CA 94102
415–986–3162

The International Albinism Center
Box 485 UMHC
The University of Minnesota Hospital and Clinic
420 Delaware Street SE
Minneapolis, MN 55455
612–624–0144

*A center for research about albinism and health care
for albinism.*

National Multiple Sclerosis Society
205 East 42nd Street
New York, NY 10017
212–986–3240

The National Organization for Albinism and
  Hypopigmentation (NOAH)
1530 Locust Street #29
Philadelphia, PA 19102-4415

*NOAH provides information and support for persons
with albinism, their families, and health professionals.
NOAH publishes a newsletter, answers individual
questions, and conducts conferences.*

Retinitis Pigmentosa Foundation
1401 Mt. Royal Avenue
Baltimore, MD 21217
301–225–9400
800–638–2300
301–225–9409 (TDD)

SPORTS VISION

National Academy of Sports Vision
200 South Progress Avenue
Harrisburg, PA 17109
717–652–8080
MISCELLANEOUS

American Academy of Ophthalmology
655 Beach Street
P.O. Box 7424
San Francisco, CA 94120-7424
415–561–8500

American Academy of Optometry
4330 East West Highway
Suite 1117
Bethesda, MD 20814-4408
301–718–6500

American Optometric Association
243 North Lindbergh Boulevard
St. Louis, MO 63141
314–991–4100

American Society of Cataract and Refractive Surgery
4000 Legato Road
Suite 850
Fairfax, VA 22033
703–591–2220

College of Syntonic Optometry
21 East 5th Street
Bloomsburg, PA 17815
717–784–2131

*Professional organization and referral source
for color therapy.*

Corporate Vision Consulting
842 Arden Drive
Encinitas, CA 92024
760–944–1200
800–383–1202 (Voicemail/fax)
E-mail: eyedoc@adnc.com
Web site: http://www.cvconsulting.com

Offers the Eye-CEE System for VDT Users.

Eye Bank Association of America, Inc.
1511 K Street, NW
Suite 830
Washington, DC 20005-1401
202–628–4280

National Academy of Opticianry
10111 Martin Luther King, Jr. Highway
Suite 112
Bowie, MD 20720
301–577–4828

Bibliography for Further Reading

DIET AND NUTRITION

Cheraskin, E.W., M. Ringsdorf, and J.W. Clark. *Diet and Disease.* New Canaan, CT: Keats Health Science, 1977.

Davidson, S., J.E. Passmore, and A.S. Trusswell. *Human Nutrition and Dietetics*, 7th edition. New York: Churchill Livingstone, 1979.

Kirschmann, John D. *Nutrition Almanac.* New York: McGraw-Hill Book Company, 1979.

Lieberman, Shari, and Nancy Bruning. *The Real Vitamin and Mineral Book*, 2nd edition. Garden City Park, NY: Avery Publishing Group, 1997.

Messinger, Lisa. *Why Should I Eat Better?* Garden City Park, NY: Avery Publishing Group, 1993.

Shute, Wilfred. *The Vitamin E Book.* New Canaan, CT: Keats Publishing Company, 1975.

Simone, Charles. *Cancer and Nutrition.* Garden City Park, NY: Avery Publishing Group, 1992.

Wright, J.V. *Dr. Wright's Guide to Healing With Nutrition.* Emmaus, PA: Rodale Press, 1984.

HERBAL MEDICINE

Castleman, M. *The Healing Herbs.* Emmaus, PA: Rodale Press, 1991.

Griggs, B. *Green Pharmacy: A History of Herbal Medicine.* London, England: Robert Hale, 1981.

Hallowell, Michael. *Herbal Healing.* Garden City Park, NY: Avery Publishing Group, 1994, 1985.

Lust, John. *The Herb Book.* New York: Bantam Books, 1982.

Tenney, Louise. *Health Handbook.* Pleasant Grove, UT: Woodland Books, 1994.

HOMEOPATHY

Boericke, William. *Materia Medica With Repertory.* Philadelphia: Boericke & Tafel, 1988.

Cummings, S., and D. Ullman. *Everybody's Guide to Homeopathic Medicines.* Los Angeles: J.P. Tarcher, 1984.

Kent, J.T. *Lectures on Homeopathic Materia Medica.* New Delhi, India: Homeopathic Publications, 1905.

Kruzel, T. *The Homeopathic Emergency Guide.* Berkeley, CA: North Atlantic Books, 1992.

Murphy, R. *Homeopathic Medical Repertory.* Pagosa Springs, CO: Hahneman Academy of North America, 1993.

Panos, Maisemond B., and J. Heimlich. *Homeopathic Medicine at Home.* Los Angeles: J.P. Tarcher, 1982.

Phatak, S.R. *Phatak's Materia Medica of Homeopathic Medicines.* London, England: Foxlee-Vaughan, 1988.

Stevenson, J.H. *Helping Yourself With Homeopathic Remedies.* San Francisco: Thorsons, 1976.

NATURAL MEDICINE

Balch, James F., and Phyllis A. Balch. *Prescription for Nutritional Healing*, 2nd edition. Garden City Park, NY: Avery Publishing Group, 1997.

Lininger, Skye, Jonathan Wright, Steve Austin, Donald Brown, and Alan Gaby. *The Natural Pharmacy.* Rocklin, CA: Prima Publishing, 1998.

Trattler, R. *Better Health Through Natural Healing.* New York: McGraw-Hill, 1985.

TRADITIONAL CHINESE MEDICINE

A Barefoot Doctor's Manual: The American Translation of the Official Chinese Paramedical Manual. Philadelphia: Running Press, 1977.

Connelly, D.M. *Traditional Acupuncture: The Law of the Five Elements.* Columbia, MD: The Centre for Traditional Acupuncture, 1979.

MISCELLANEOUS

Irlen, Helen. *Reading by the Colors: Overcoming Dyslexia and Other Reading Disabilities Through the Irlen Method.* Garden City Park, NY: Avery Publishing Group, 1991.

Rosenthal, Odeda, and Robert H. Phillips, PhD. *Coping With Colorblindness.* Garden City Park, NY: Avery Publishing Group, 1997.

NEWSLETTERS

Health Facts. Published monthly by the Center for Medical Consumers, 237 Thompson Street, New York, NY 10012; 212–674–7105.

Herbal Gram: The Journal of the American Botanical Council and the Herb Research Foundation. Write P.O. Box 201660, Austin, TX 78720; 512–331–8868.

Nutrition Action. Published by the Center for Science in the Public Interest, 1875 Connecticut Avenue, NW, Suite 300, Washington, DC 20009-5728; 202–667–7438.

Index